Cytopathology of Infectious Diseases

ESSENTIALS IN CYTOPATHOLOGY

Dorothy L. Rosenthal, MD, FIAC, Series Editor

Editorial Board

Syed Z. Ali, MD
Douglas P. Clark, MD
Yener S. Erozan, MD

For further volumes:
http://www.springer.com/series/6996

Liron Pantanowitz, MD, MIAC

Pam Michelow, MBBCh, MSc (Med Sci)

Walid E. Khalbuss, MD, PhD, FIAC

Cytopathology of Infectious Diseases

Including Chapters 2 & 14 Co-authored by:
Tanvier Omar, MB BCH, FC Path (S.A.)
Chapters 3, 9, 10 & 13 Co-authored by:
Sara E. Monaco, MD
Chapter 4 Co-authored by:
Gladwyn Leiman, MBBCh, FIAC, FRCPath
Lynne S. Garcia, MS, CLS, FAAM
Chapter 5 Co-authored by:
R. Marshall Austin, MD, PhD
Chapter 6 Co-authored by:
Rodolfo Laucirica, MD
Chapter 7 Co-authored by:
Robert M. Najarian, MD
Helen H. Wang, MD, PhD
Chapter 8 Co-authored by:
Anil V. Parwani, MD, PhD
and Chapter 15 Co-authored by:
Robert A. Goulart, MD
Rafael Martínez-Girón, MD, PhD

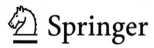 Springer

Liron Pantanowitz, MD, MIAC
Department of Pathology
University of Pittsburgh
Medical Center
Pittsburgh, PA 15232, USA
pantanowitzl@upmc.edu

Walid E. Khalbuss, MD, PhD, FIAC
Department of Pathology
University of Pittsburgh
Medical Center
Pittsburgh, PA 15232, USA
khalbussw2@upmc.edu

Pam Michelow, MBBCh,
MSc (Med Sci)
Department of Anatomical
Pathology, University of the
Witwatersrand & National Health
Laboratory Service
Johannesburg 2000, South Africa
pamela.michelow@nhls.ac.za

ISSN 1574-9053   e-ISSN 1574-9061
ISBN 978-1-4614-0241-1   e-ISBN 978-1-4614-0242-8
DOI 10.1007/978-1-4614-0242-8
Springer New York Dordrecht Heidelberg London

Library of Congress Control Number: 2011932800

Printed on acid-free paper

Springer is part of Springer Science+Business Media (www.springer.com)

This book is dedicated to my wife Heidi and children
Joshua and Maya.

Liron Pantanowitz, MD, MIAC

To my husband Alan and children Gina, Matt, and Aaron.

Pam Michelow, MBBCh, MSc (Med Sci)

To my family, mentors, trainees, and friends
for their encouragement and support.

Walid E. Khalbuss, MD, PhD, FIAC

Foreword

Although it is long overdue, finally there is a textbook developed entirely to the cytology diagnosis of infectious diseases, despite the fact that since the early twentieth century there were a number of reports documenting the utility of cytology examination. Greig and Gray were the first to describe fine needle aspiration (FNA) cytology for the diagnosis of infectious disease in their 1904 report of biopsies of lymph nodes from fifteen patients with sleeping sickness. Proscher used FNA cytology of lymph nodes for the diagnosis of spirochetal infections in 1907, along with other investigators reporting the use of FNA cytology for the diagnosis of filariasis, bubonic plague, and spirochetes in secondary syphilis. In 1921, Guthrie reported FNA biopsy of lymph nodes using air-dried, Romanowsky-stained smears in cases of syphilis, tuberculosis, simple adenitis, and trypanosomiasis. Guthrie also reported the use of special stains for organisms including Ziehl-Neelsen stain for acid fast bacilli, along with dark field examination for spirochetes and reported bacteria such as streptococci and staphylococci in lymph node aspirates.

Despite these early successes in the use of cytology for the diagnosis of infectious disease, beginning in 1925 at Memorial Hospital in New York, FNA began to be used mainly to diagnose neoplastic conditions, although infectious diseases such as tuberculosis, syphilis, and actinomyces were occasionally encountered. However, the dynamic explosion of FNA cytology for the diagnosis of neoplastic disease initially took place in Scandinavia by clinician/cytopathologists. Following their seminal contributions,

FNA cytology had a rebirth in the USA due to the contributions of a number of outstanding cytopathologists.

It has been over 20 years since I have had the opportunity to publish a text on FNA of infectious and inflammatory diseases and other nonneoplastic disorders. Since that time, there has been a renewed interest in the cytologic diagnosis of infectious disease coinciding with increased incidence of common and unusual infections due to the AIDS epidemic, expansion of organ transplantation, and aggressive treatment of neoplastic diseases resulting in an increasing population of immunocompromised patients.

Now stepping forward to fill the void are Pantanowitz, Michelow and Khalbuss with their associates, who have written the first text devoted entirely to the cytopathology of infectious diseases. The authors' format is user friendly, presenting in a very concise format the clinical, cytomorphologic features, differential diagnosis, pitfalls, and ancillary studies of a wide range of infectious diseases that can be appreciated in cytology specimens. I believe the reader, whether in training or a practicing pathologist, will benefit from the authors' extensive experience in the cytologic diagnosis of infectious agents that can be encountered both in developing and industrial nations. It is with great pleasure to have this opportunity to recognize the outstanding cytopathologists who share their extensive experience in this much-needed cytology monograph.

Jan F. Silverman, MD
Pittsburgh, PA, USA

Series Preface

The subspeciality of cytopathology is over 60 years old and has become an established and reliable discipline in medicine. As expected, cytopathology literature has expanded in a remarkably short period of time, from a few textbooks prior to the 1980s to a currently substantial library of texts and journals devoted exclusively to cytomorphology. The *Essentials in Cytopathology* Series does not presume to replace any of the distinguished textbooks in cytopathology. Instead, the Series has published generously illustrated and user-friendly guides for both pathologists and clinicians. The Series has met with gratifying success, and we now present volume 10, with more than five volumes scheduled to come.

Built on the amazing success of The Bethesda System for Reporting Cervical Cytology, now in its second edition, the Series has utilized a similar format, including minimal text, tabular criteria, and superb illustrations based on real-life specimens. *Essentials in Cytopathology* has, at times, deviated from the classic organization of pathology texts. The logic of decision trees, elimination of unlikely choices, and narrowing of differential diagnosis via a pragmatic approach based on morphologic criteria are some of the strategies used to illustrate principles and practice in cytopathology.

Most of the authors for *Essentials in Cytopathology* are faculty members in The Johns Hopkins University School of Medicine, Department of Pathology, Division of Cytopathology. They bring to each volume the legacy of John K. Frost and the collective experience of a preeminent cytopathology service. The archives at Hopkins are meticulously catalogued and form the framework for text and illustrations. Authors from other institutions have been selected on the basis of their national reputations, experience, and enthusiasm for cytopathology. They bring to the series, complementary viewpoints and enlarge the scope of materials contained in the photographs.

The editor and the authors are indebted to our students, past and future, who challenge and motivate us to become the best that we possibly can be. We share that experience with you through these pages, and hope that you will learn from them as we have from those who have come before us. We would be remiss if we did not pay tribute to our professional colleagues, the cytotechnologists, and preparatory technicians, who lovingly care for the specimens that our clinical colleagues send to us. We are also grateful to Springer and its production staff for their enthusiasm, responsiveness, and patience.

And finally, we cannot emphasize enough throughout these volumes the importance of collaboration with the patient care team. Every specimen comes to us with questions begging answers. Without input from the clinicians, complete patient history, results of imaging studies, and other ancillary tests, we cannot perform optimally. It is our responsibility to educate our clinicians about their role in our interpretation, and for us to integrate as much information as we can gather into our final diagnosis, even if the answer at first seems obvious.

We hope you will find this Series useful and welcome your feedback as you place these handbooks by your microscopes and into your book bags.

Dorothy L. Rosenthal
Baltimore, MD, USA
drosenthal@jhmi.edu

Contents

Contributors

R. Marshall Austin, MD, PhD
Professor of Pathology, Department of Pathology,
Magee-Women's Hospital of University of Pittsburgh
Medical Center, Pittsburgh, PA, USA

Lynne S. Garcia, MS, CLS, FAAM
Director, LSG and Associates, Santa Monica, CA, USA

Robert A. Goulart, MD
Director of Surgical Pathology and Hospital Pathology Services,
Associate Director of Cytopathology Services, New England
Pathology Associates, Mercy Medical Center of Sisters
of Providence Health System/Catholic Health East,
Springfield, MA, USA

Walid E. Khalbuss, MD, PhD, FIAC
Associate Professor of Pathology, Director of Cytology
and Cytopathology Fellowship Program,
Department of Pathology, University of Pittsburgh Medical
Center, Pittsburgh, PA, USA

Rodolfo Laucirica, MD
Associate Professor of Pathology and Immunology,
Director of the Cytopathology Fellowship Program,
Director of Cytology, Department of Pathology
and Immunology, Baylor College of Medicine,
Ben Taub General Hospital, Houston, TX, USA

Gladwyn Leiman, MBBCh, FIAC, FRCPath
Director of Cytopathology, Fletcher Allen Health Care,
Professor of Pathology, University of Vermont,
Burlington, VT, USA

Rafael Martínez-Girón, MD, PhD
Professor of Cytopathology, CF Anatomía Patológica y Citología,
Instituto de Piedras Blancas, Piedras Blancas, Asturias, Spain

Pam Michelow, MBBCh, MSc (Med Sci), MIAC
Chief Medical Officer, Faculty of Health Sciences,
Cytology Unit, Department of Anatomical Pathology,
University of the Witwatersrand and National Health
Laboratory Service, Johannesburg, Gauteng, South Africa

Sara E. Monaco, MD
Assistant Professor, Associate Director of Cytopathology
Fellowship, Department of Pathology, University of Pittsburgh
Medical Center, Pittsburgh, PA, USA

Robert M. Najarian, MD
Staff Pathologist and Consultant in Gastrointestinal
and Hepatobiliary Pathology, Department of Pathology,
Beth Israel Deaconess Medical Center/Harvard Medical School,
Boston, MA, USA

Tanvier Omar, MB BCH, FC Path (S.A.)
Principal Pathologist, Division of Cytopathology, Department
of Anatomical Pathology, National Health Laboratory Service
and University of Witwatersrand, Johannesburg, Gauteng,
South Africa

Liron Pantanowitz, MD, MIAC
Associate Professor of Pathology and Biomedical Informatics,
Department of Pathology, University of Pittsburgh Medical
Center, Pittsburgh, PA, USA

Anil V. Parwani, MD, PhD
Associate Professor of Pathology and Biomedical Informatics,
Department of Pathology, University of Pittsburgh Medical
Center, Pittsburgh, PA, USA

Helen H. Wang, MD, PhD
Director of Cytopathology, Associate Professor of Pathology,
Department of Pathology, Beth Israel Deaconess Medical Center/
Harvard Medical Center, Boston, MA, USA

1
Introduction

Liron Pantanowitz[1] and Pam Michelow[2]
[1]Department of Pathology, University of Pittsburgh Medical Center, 5150 Centre Avenue, Suite 201, Pittsburgh, PA 15232, USA

[2]Cytology Unit, Department of Anatomical Pathology, University of the Witwatersrand and National Health Laboratory Service, Johannesburg, Gauteng, South Africa

> *We believe that the examination of fluid removed from lymphatic glands will prove to be a much more rapid and satisfactory method of diagnosing early cases of sleeping sickness than the examination of blood. At first the glands were excised, but this was soon found to be unnecessary, as it is easy to puncture a superficial gland with a hypodermic syringe (Grieg 1904).*

Cytopatholgy provides a rapid, inexpensive, simple, and effective mechanism to diagnose and manage a wide range of infectious diseases. A variety of ancillary techniques such as special stains, immunocytochemistry, and molecular studies can be applied to cytology samples, thereby increasing the specificity and sensitivity of this procedure. As a result, cytology specimens can reliably provide timely and specific diagnoses as well as classify many microorganisms including viruses, bacteria, fungi, and parasites. While it may be impossible to detect individual viruses by light microscopy, the cytopathic changes they induce on infected cells are often readily visible, even in routine preparations. The advantages of cytology in the work-up of patients with infectious diseases include:

- *Specimen procurement*: Rapid, minimally invasive, and cost-effective procedure with minimal contamination. Specimens submitted for cytologic evaluation may be obtained via exfoliation, abrasion, aspiration, or touch preparation.

L. Pantanowitz et al., *Cytopathology of Infectious Diseases*,
Essentials in Cytopathology 17, DOI 10.1007/978-1-4614-0242-8_1,
© Springer Science+Business Media, LLC 2011

- *Specimen triage*: Rapid assessment with submission of additional material for cell block preparation, cultures, special stains, flow cytometry, and molecular tests.
- *Specimen diagnosis*: Rapid diagnostic procedure to guide early patient management, including timely implementation of infection control procedures if required. In many cases a diagnosis can be obtained sooner than microbiology testing or tissue biopsy. Mycobacterial and fungal cultures, for example, often take several weeks to yield an answer.

Cytology specimens can be obtained from clinics and outpatient settings, hospitalized, and even critically ill or intraoperative patients. The emergence of opportunistic infections in transplant recipients and AIDS patients has increased the need for minimally invasive rapid diagnostic methods. The resurgence of previously rare infections is also largely due to the increasing incidence of immunocompromised patients. Fine needle aspiration (FNA) biopsy permits the evaluation of superficial and deep masses. Cytologists can play a key role in the immediate interpretation of material, rapidly identifying infectious cases at the patient's bedside that may benefit from additional material and/or ancillary studies. Consequently, cytology as an accepted modality to reliably diagnose infectious disease has come a long way from one of the first recorded instances in 1904 when FNA was employed to diagnose trypanosomiasis.

Microorganisms are frequently encountered in cytology specimens. The identification of these microorganisms based upon cytomorphologic appearance can on occasion be challenging and hence require ancillary studies. For example, numerous collapsed pneumocystis cysts may appear to be "budding," while capsule deficient cryptococcus may be mistaken for other microorganisms such as histoplasmosis. Evaluation of the host response to organisms provides important clues to the diagnosis of infections. The potential to render a false positive diagnosis of malignancy exists when inflammatory atypia and/or repair accompanies an infection. Conversely, there is increased risk for a false negative diagnosis when neoplasms have a prominent inflammatory component or concomitant infection. Endogenous structures and contaminants may also mimic pathogens. There have been numerous texts describing the microbiology and pathology of microorganisms seen in tissue specimens.

However, very few books deal with the cytomorphologic features of these infectious diseases. Major changes in the screening, treatment, and prevention (e.g., vaccination) of certain infections such as human papillomavirus (HPV) have recently impacted the field of cytopathology.

This book deals entirely with the cytopathology of infectious diseases. This textbook covers the cytomorphology, differential diagnoses, and pitfalls of common and uncommon infectious diseases, and provides a practical approach to their diagnosis. Many color images are included along with tables and simple diagrams that serve as quick reference guides. The content also provides advice on specimen procurement and handling, processing of material in the cytology laboratory, and incorporates recent advances in the field. With the advent of immunocytochemistry, in situ hybridization and advanced molecular studies, no longer are cytologists limited to identifying pathogens using only morphological and limited special stain characteristics.

Suggested Reading

Atkins KA, Powers CN. The cytopathology of infectious diseases. Adv Anat Pathol. 2002;9:52–64.

Grieg EDW, Gray ACH. Note on the lymphatic glands in sleeping sickness. Br Med J. 1904;1:1252.

Jannes G, De Vos D. A review of current and future molecular diagnostic tests for use in the microbiology laboratory. Methods Mol Biol. 2006;345:1–21.

Kradin RL, editor. Diagnostic pathology of infectious disease. Philadelphia: Saunders Elsevier; 2010.

Lal A, Warren J, Bedrossian CW, Nayar R. The role of fine needle aspiration in diagnosis of infectious disease. Lab Med. 2002;11:866–72.

Powers CN. Diagnosis of infectious diseases: a cytopathologist's perspective. Clin Microbiol Rev. 1998;11:341–65.

Silverman JF, Gay RM. Fine-needle aspiration and surgical pathology of infectious lesions. morphologic features and the role of the clinical microbiology laboratory for rapid diagnosis. Clin Lab Med. 1995;15:251–78.

2
Specimen Collection and Handling

Pam Michelow[1], Tanvier Omar[2], and Liron Pantanowitz[3]
[1]Cytology Unit, Department of Anatomical Pathology,
University of the Witwatersrand and National Health
Laboratory Service, Johannesburg, Gauteng, South Africa

[2]Division of Cytopathology, Department of Anatomical Pathology,
National Health Laboratory Service and University of Witwatersrand,
Johannesburg, Gauteng, South Africa

[3]Department of Pathology, University of Pittsburgh Medical Center,
5150 Centre Avenue, Suite 201, Pittsburgh, PA 15232, USA

Cytology is often performed in the investigation of patients with suspected infection. This is because cytology provides a safe, rapid, and cost-effective means to diagnose many infections, allowing correct management to be instituted. Moreover, cytology permits appropriate ancillary investigations to be undertaken either at the time of specimen procurement (e.g., triage of material for microbiology culture) (Fig. 2.1) or after material is processed (e.g., special stains for microorganisms using cell block sections). The use of ancillary investigations (e.g., cell block preparation, special stains, immunocytochemistry, molecular studies) in cytopathology is covered in Chap. 14. Appropriate specimen collection and handling are essential to the diagnosis of infectious diseases. Sample collection for pathogens needs to be coordinated. This requires effective communication with clinicians, radiologists, and microbiologists, particularly if an uncommon infectious process is suspected. Universal precautions must be followed when handling specimens.

L. Pantanowitz et al., *Cytopathology of Infectious Diseases*,
Essentials in Cytopathology 17, DOI 10.1007/978-1-4614-0242-8_2,
© Springer Science+Business Media, LLC 2011

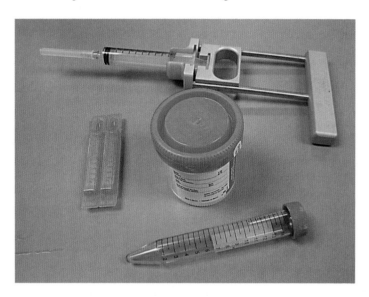

Fig. 2.1. Aspirated material obtained by FNA can be submitted by the cytologist for microbiology studies such as culture using suitable sterile containers or tubes (*orange* capped examples shown), along with some sterile saline (two *pink* sterile saline solution packs shown) or placed on moistened filter paper. Bacteriostatic saline or formalin should not be used. Drying of specimens during transport may compromise the recovery of viable organisms. Alternatively, sterile culture media can be used at the time of specimen collection to directly transfer specimens obtained by FNA.

- *Virology.* Methods used to diagnose viral infections include antigen detection, virus isolation, serology, and molecular techniques. While antigen detection is rapid, there may be many false positives and negatives. The primary method to diagnose many viruses (except EBV, for example) is with viral isolation in cell culture, but this can take weeks. Specimens submitted to culture viral agents may require special transport medium, although media designed for transporting bacteria are often acceptable. Viral detection in culture is carried out by visual examination of culture cells for viral cytopathic effect (CPE)

TABLE 2.1. Characteristic viral inclusions observed in culture.

Virus	Nuclear inclusions	Cytoplasmic inclusions	Syncytia
Herpes simplex virus	Yes	No	Yes
Cytomegalovirus	Yes	Yes	No
Influenza	No	No	No
Respiratory syncytial virus	No	No	Yes
Adenovirus	Yes	No	No
Measles	Yes	Yes	Yes

(Table 2.1). Serology (detection of circulating antibodies) relies on demonstrating a rise in antibody titers in sequential samples.

- *Bacteriology.* Bacteria are diagnosed by direct examination (Gram and acid-fast staining) and culture (aerobic and anerobic) using specific culture media (Fig. 2.2). Specimens for anerobic culture should ideally be submitted in anerobic containers and immediately transported to the laboratory. A specimen submitted in an anerobic container can also be used for aerobic, mycobacterial, and fungal cultures. Mycobacteria are cultured on both solid (e.g., Lowenstein-Jensen and Middlebrook agars) and broth (e.g., BACTEC system, Mycobacterium Growth Indicator Tube or MGIT) media.
- *Mycology.* Fungi can be identified using direct examination (e.g., calcofluor white fluorescent stain, India ink), antigen detection (e.g., cryptococcal antigen), and fungal culture (e.g., Sabouraud agar). Yeasts (unicellular with budding) form small bacterial-like creamy colonies in culture, whereas molds (multicellular with hyphae) make large fuzzy colonies.
- *Parasitology.* Parasites are usually not cultured. They are usually diagnosed on direct examination using both wet mounts and stained slides (e.g., modified acid-fast stains for *Cryptosporidium*, *Cyclospora*, and *Isospora*). Wet mounts are useful to identify motile trophozoites and cysts (often with iodide added). Serology is of limited use in parasitology.

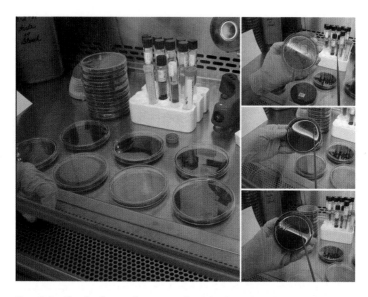

FIG. 2.2. Cytologic specimens received in the microbiology laboratory get plated under a culture hood (*left*) onto various media such as (*top right*) MacConkey agar, (*middle right*) chocolate agar, and (*bottom right*) blood agar. Most pathogens are able to grow on blood agar, which is used to initially culture most specimens. Other culture media like MacConkey agar provide a selective and differential medium for specific bacteria (e.g., Gram-negative bacilli).

Specimen Type

- *Pap test* (*smear*) involves scraping of the cervix with a cervical brush, broom, or wooden/plastic spatula. For anal Pap tests a small brush or cotton-tipped rod is inserted into the anus. Rinsing the collection device or detaching and placing it in a vial containing proprietary preservative fluid (liquid-based cytology) permits material to be processed for ancillary studies (e.g., DNA testing for HPV, gonorrhea, and Chlamydia) and for infections that cannot be reliably identified morphologically. Conventional smears can also be used for ancillary studies (e.g., HPV tests), by scraping material off slides.

- *Wet prep* can be performed at the patient bedside to provide immediate microscopic examination of vaginal specimens (swab or secretions) for the presence of *Trichomonas vaginalis*, clue cells, and yeast in a saline suspension (e.g., 2 mL 0.9% NaCl) with/without potassium hydroxide (20% KOH with dimethyl-sulfoxide).

- *Tzanck test* is a scraping of an ulcer base to look for infected cells with herpetic changes due to herpes simplex virus (HSV) or varicella-zoster virus (VSV). As these are often prepared by clinicians and received on prepared slides, they are subject to air-drying artifact without residual material to perform immunocytochemistry. Due largely to sampling issues, there is a high rate of false-negative results even when the virus is present.

- *Scrapings, swabs, or impressions* may be performed to diagnose oropharyngeal (e.g., *Candida*) as well as conjunctival and corneal (e.g., Herpes simplex keratitis and trachoma) infections. The technique for performing impression cytology of the ocular surface is described in Chap. 12.

- *Washings, brushings, and lavage* typically involve an invasive procedure (e.g., bronchoscopy) with infusion and reaspiration of sterile saline solution. Samples can be submitted for cytological evaluation and culture.

- *Fluids* from effusions and other anatomic sites (e.g., CSF, urine, joints) can be shared for cytological evaluation and a variety of microbiology tests (e.g., serology, culture. PCR). Cytologic preparation techniques include cytocentrifuge (larger volumes), cytospins (smaller volumes <5 mL), membrane filtration, liquid-based preparations, and cell blocks. The sensitivity of microscopy can be improved by increasing the concentration of the specimen. Specimens should be prepared soon after collection to prevent degeneration. If this is not possible, refrigeration and/or addition of equal volume of 50% alcohol can be used. At least 2–5 mL is required for bacterial culture and >10 mL for fungi and/or mycobacteria because these latter organisms are generally present in low numbers.

- *Fine needle aspiration* (*FNA*) permits procured material to be immediately evaluated on site for appropriate triage. Aspirated material can be used to make smears and liquid based preparations and cell blocks, or sent for culture, flow cytometry and molecular studies. Material submitted for culture requires the use of sterile containers into which patient's material is added along with minimal sterile saline. Isolation of pathogens in fine needle aspirates is almost always considered significant and not due to contamination.

Specimen Sites

- *Genital tract.* Collection of genital specimens includes Pap smears, swabs, Tzanck preparations of ulcers, and infrequently FNA. Typically, specimens in female patients to detect pathogens are acquired at the time of performing a Pap test. Many common and uncommon pathogens can be identified on a Pap smear (see Chap. 5). A wet preparation can be used to make a rapid diagnosis of vaginitis. A definitive diagnosis of certain pathogens may require culture, especially in cases of suspected sexual abuse.
- *Urinary tract.* The normal urinary tract is usually devoid of bacteria, except for microflora of the urethral mucosa. Nevertheless, urine can become contaminated with bacteria of the vaginal canal or perineum. For urinary tract infections, a midstream "clean-catch" urine specimen is preferable. A 24-h urine sample is recommended for suspected schistosomiasis. Catheterized urine can be collected, but not urine from catheter bags. Other specimens from the urinary tract that may be required to diagnose infection include suprapubic aspirates (used mainly in neonates and small children), upper tract brushings and washings, urinary diversions (e.g., ileal conduit), and kidney FNA.
- *Respiratory tract.* Sputum is often submitted for the diagnosis of infection. Multiple, early morning specimens improve sensitivity because they harbor pooled overnight secretions, and hence they are more likely to contain concentrated bacteria. All cytopreparatory techniques (pick and smear, Saccomanno, cytocentrifugation, liquid based) are suitable. Sputa should be processed as soon as possible, because after 20 h of refrigeration there is a significant decrease in recoverable organisms. For pneumocystis, the yield from sputum is generally low. Various grading schemes (e.g., Bartlett grading system, Murray and Washington

grading system) have been used to assess the quality of sputum samples for Gram staining. These schemes use the number of squamous epithelial cells and leukocytes as well as the presence of mucus in sputum samples. For example, greater numbers of epithelial cells indicates oropharyngeal contamination. These grading schemes do not apply for all infections (e.g., Legionella spp., mycobacteria, fungi, and viruses). Bronchial washings, brushings, and bronchoalveolar lavage specimens are recommended for the optimal recovery of microorganisms. Organisms seen in sputum and specimens collected via bronchoscopy may be present due to contamination from the oral cavity rather than true infection of lungs. Transbronchial and percutaneous FNA may be required in some patients.

- *Central nervous system.* Specimens that can be submitted for microbiology studies include CSF obtained by lumbar puncture or other means (subdural tap, ventricular aspiration, or collected from a shunt), stereotactic FNA (e.g., abscess), and tissue biopsy. Specimens should be prepared as soon as possible after collection. If this is not possible, addition of an equal amount of 50% alcohol may help preserve the specimen. Refrigeration may adversely affect the recovery of certain microorganisms. Rapid diagnostic tests are available including India ink preparation for *Cryptococcus neoformans* and wet preparation for free-living amebae. FNA may identify toxoplasmosis, mycobacteria, cryptococcus, ameba, and cysticercosis.

- *Gastrointestinal system.* A variety of cytologic specimens can be obtained from the gastrointestinal tract including stool samples, ano-rectal swabs, secretions, and FNA. The development of fiber-optic endoscopy has greatly expanded the ability to obtain specimens for cytological evaluation (e.g., esophageal and gastric brushings and washings), including endoscopic ultrasound FNA of the liver and pancreas, as well as bile duct brushings.

- *Musculoskeletal system.* Usually such specimens are obtained by FNA, which includes aspiration of joint fluid. Joint fluid clots quickly, and if not submitted into appropriate containers that contain anticoagulant cell counts cannot be performed.

- *Skin.* Cytologic specimens include superficial scrapings, swabs and for vesicles, bullae, pustules, and deep palpable subcutaneous lesions FNA.

- *Fluids.* Effusions due to bacterial infection (e.g., *Staphylococcus* spp., *Streptococcal* spp.) appear turbid and purulent macroscopically while mycobacterial-infected effusions often have a shiny green appearance. Fungi (e.g., *Candida*, *Cryptococcus*) and parasites (e.g., *Echinococcus*, *ameba*, *Strongyloides*) may produce a purulent or serous effusion, whereas viral infected-fluids (e.g., coxsackie, herpes) are usually serous.

Suggested Reading

Murray PR, Witebsky FG. The clinician and the microbiology laboratory. In: Mandell GL, Bennett JE, Dolin R, editors. Principles and practice of infectious diseases. 7th ed. Philadelphia: Churchill Livingstone Elsevier; 2010. p. 233–65.

Winn W, Allen S, Janada W, Koneman E, Procop G, Schreckenberger P, et al. Koneman's color atlas and textbook of diagnostic microbiology. 6th ed. Philadelphia: Lippincott Williams & Wilkins; 2006. p. 67–110.

Woods GL, Gutierrez Y. Diagnostic pathology of infectious diseases. Philadelphia: Lea & Febiger; 1993. p. 539–637.

3
Host Reactions to Infection

**Sara E. Monaco[1], Walid E. Khalbuss[2],
and Liron Pantanowitz[3]**
[1-3]Department of Pathology, University of Pittsburgh Medical Center,
Pittsburgh, PA 15232, USA

The reaction of a human host to infectious stimuli can differ and manifest in various ways (Table 3.1). These reaction patterns depend on the target (i.e., organism or antigen) and immune status of the patient. Knowledge of these reactions and their cytomorphologic features can help identify potential infectious agents. Characteristic host reaction patterns are the focus of this chapter.

Acute (Purulent) Inflammatory Response

- An acute inflammatory exudate composed predominantly of neutrophils.
- An abscess is a localized area of liquefactive necrosis packed with neutrophils associated with cell debris and often organisms.
- This is a common response to bacterial or fungal organisms (Fig. 3.1).

Cytomorphologic Features

- Abundant neutrophils with degenerated cells and acellular debris.
- Examination at high power may reveal intracellular or extracellular organisms, such as the negative image of mycobacteria seen on Diff-Quik (DQ) stained smears within macrophages or background material.

L. Pantanowitz et al., *Cytopathology of Infectious Diseases*,
Essentials in Cytopathology 17, DOI 10.1007/978-1-4614-0242-8_3,
© Springer Science+Business Media, LLC 2011

TABLE 3.1.   Different host reactions to infection.

Usual reactions and inflammatory patterns
  Acute purulent inflammation
  Eosinophilia and allergic mucin
  Granulomatous inflammation
  Necrosis
  Viral cytopathic effect
  Reactive epithelial atypia and mesenchymal repair

Unusual reactions and inflammatory patterns
  Immune reconstitution inflammatory syndrome (IRIS)
  Hemophagocytosis and emperipolesis
  Ciliocytophthoria
  Xanthogranulomatous inflammation
  Malakoplakia
  Pseudotumor/inflammatory pseudotumor reaction
  Crystal formation
  Inclusions in granulomatous inflammation
  Splendore-Hoeppli phenomenon

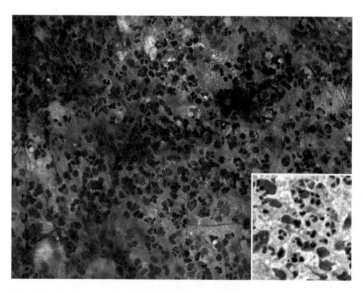

FIG. 3.1. Acute suppurative lymphadenitis (Diff-Quik stain, high magnification; *inset*: Pap stain, high magnification). The smears are cellular and show numerous neutrophils in a background of acute inflammatory debris.

Differential Diagnosis

- Cat scratch disease
- Mycobacterial infection in children or immunocompromised patients, when the body cannot mount a granulomatous response
- Mimics include cellular degeneration, apoptosis (karyorrhectic debris that mimics neutrophils), Kikuchi lymphadenitis, eosinophilia (eosinophils mimic neutrophils, especially on Papanicolaou stained smears)

Ancillary Studies

- Special stains and/or immunostains for organisms
- Microbial cultures

Eosinophilia and Allergic Mucin

- This is a type I immediate hypersensitivity response that may occur with allergies, parasites, and certain fungal infections.
- It is typically seen in the nasal sinuses (rhinosinusitis) or lower respiratory tract (asthma, pulmonary infiltrates, and bronchiectasis) (Fig. 3.2).

Cytomorphologic Features

- Viscous allergic mucin is seen with numerous eosinophils and possibly Charcot Leyden crystals, which are needle or rhomboid-shaped eosinophilic crystals.
- Material should be carefully examined for fungus, particularly *Aspergillus* spp.

Differential Diagnosis

- Noninfectious inspissated mucin
- Fungi other than *Aspergillus* such as mucormycosis and dematiaceous fungi like *Bipolaris spicifera* or *Curvularia lunata*

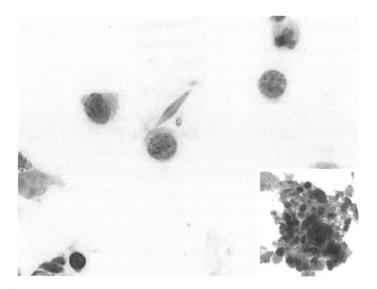

FIG. 3.2.   Charcot-Leyden crystals (Pap stain, high magnification). Needle-shaped eosinophilic crystals are seen in association with numerous eosinophils (*inset*), which have weakly orangeophilic cytoplasmic granules and bilobed nuclei.

Ancillary Studies

- Special stains (PAS, GMS) and/or immunostains for fungal organisms
- Fungal cultures

Granulomatous Inflammation

- A chronic inflammatory response comprised of aggregates of epithelioid macrophages (histiocytes) with or without other inflammatory cells.
- Granulomas can be subclassified into necrotizing (caseating with central necrosis) and non-necrotizing (without central necrosis) granulomatous inflammation.

- Granulomas may form cohesive clusters of macrophages (e.g., tuberculoid leprosy, syphilitic gumma) or present as a diffuse population of macrophages (e.g., lepromatous leprosy). Diffuse macrophage infiltration is often seen in patients with impaired cell-mediated immunity.
- Granulomas with a polymorphous exudate that includes neutrophils may be seen with tuberculosis, actinomycosis, cysticercosis, filariasis, rhinosporidiosis and other fungal infections.
- Foreign body-type granulomas occur in response to parasitic eggs or cuticular fragments or certain parasitic worms.

Cytomorphologic Features

- Epithelioid macrophages have kidney bean or boomerang-shaped nuclei, prominent nucleoli, and abundant ill-defined cytoplasm.
- Multinucleated giant cells may be seen including Langhans giant cells (with nuclei arranged around the periphery of the cell in a horseshoe pattern) or foreign body-type giant cells (with scattered nuclei).
- There may be evidence of phagocytosis of microorganisms or other debris within macrophages.
- Intermixed inflammatory cells are usually lymphocytes and plasma cells, but neutrophils may also be seen.
- Aspirates may have suboptimal cellularity if procured from long-standing hyalinized granulomas.

Differential Diagnosis

- Necrotizing granulomatous inflammation: *Mycobacterium tuberculosis* infection, fungal infection, cat-scratch disease.
- Non-necrotizing granulomatous inflammation: Atypical mycobacterial infection (nontuberculous mycobacteria), fungal infection (Cryptococcus), sarcoidosis, foreign body.
- Granulomatous inflammation with neutrophils: *M. tuberculosis*, cat scratch disease, fat necrosis.

- Granulomas associated with malignancy: Lymphoma, seminoma, squamous cell carcinoma.
- Xanthogranulomas (see uncommon host reactions).
- Malakoplakia (see uncommon host reactions).
- Mimics: low-grade neoplasia (e.g., renal cell carcinoma), spindle cell neoplasms (e.g., spindle cell melanoma).
- Pitfall: False positive diagnoses due to overcalling granulomas as malignancy, particularly in cases of necrotizing granulomas.

Ancillary Studies

- Special stains, immunostains, and/or PCR for organisms
- Microbial cultures (Figs. 3.3–3.5 and Table 3.2)

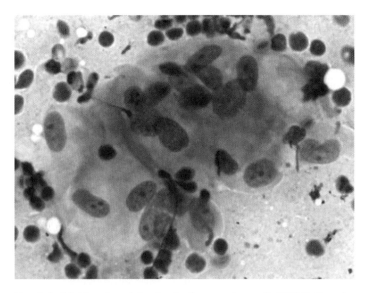

Fig. 3.3. Multinucleated foreign body-type giant cell (Diff-Quik stain, high magnification). A large cell with multiple scattered vesicular nuclei within abundant ill-defined cytoplasm.

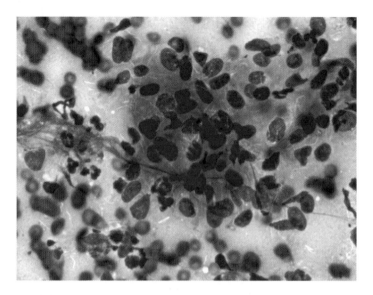

FIG. 3.4. Non-necrotizing granulomatous inflammation (Diff-Quik stain, high magnification). Cohesive cluster of macrophages seen in an atypical mycobacterial infection. Note the negative image (clear rods) of mycobacteria seen within the histiocytes and in the background.

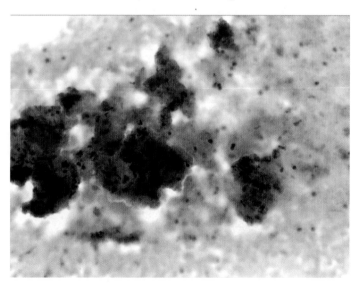

FIG. 3.5. Necrotizing granulomatous inflammation (Pap stain, medium magnification). Cohesive granulomas (*left*) are present in a background of necrotic inflammatory material (*right*).

TABLE 3.2. Cytomorphology of granulomatous and reactive host reactions compared to neoplasia.

Cytomorphologic features	Granulomatous inflammation	Reactive atypia	Neoplasia
Cellularity	Mild–moderate	Low–moderate	Usually high
Range of cell types	Continuum (benign to reactive)	Continuum (benign to reactive)	Two populations (normal and tumor)
Multinucleated giant cells	Frequent	Uncommon	Uncommon
Nuclei	Boomerang to oval with smooth contours	Smooth nuclear membrane	Large with irregular nuclear membrane
Nucleoli	Present in epithelioid macrophages	Uniform and small	Prominent and irregular
Cytoplasm	Vacuolated and ill-defined	Depends on cell type, often dense squamoid with scalloped edges	Scant cytoplasm
Background	Necrotic or non-necrotizing	Clean or inflammatory	Necrotic

Necrosis

- Necrosis is the end result of cell death and an irreversible form of cell injury that occurs with benign conditions (infection, inflammation, infarction) and neoplasms (Fig. 3.6).

Cytomorphologic Features

- The gross appearance of aspirated necrosis is thick yellow-tan, pus-like material. It is often easy to make smears with necrotic material. More peripheral sampling of a lesion may be required to see viable material.
- Necrotic material forms amorphous, somewhat granular, thick acellular debris, which can form linear rolls or lines on the slides in some cases. Necrotic material may exhibit variable staining with different stains.

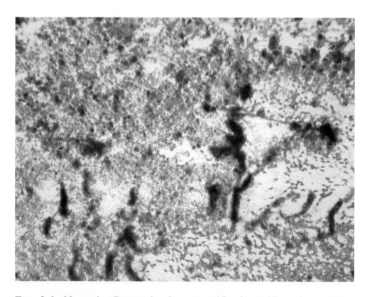

FIG. 3.6. Necrosis (Pap stain, low magnification). Necrotic acellular debris with a granular appearance can clump in a linear arrangement when smeared on slides.

- Coagulative necrosis contains ghost cells that have loss of nuclei but preserved cell shape.
- A careful search for microorganisms, atypical or tumor cells is important.

Differential Diagnosis

- Necrotizing granulomatous inflammation
- Fat necrosis
- Tumor necrosis
- Inspissated cyst contents
- Postprocedural necrosis (after previous FNA biopsy). Be cautious not to over-interpret reactive atypia in a necrotic background

Ancillary Studies

- Special stains and/or immunostains for organisms
- Microbial cultures

Viral Cytopathic Effect

- Viruses can induce cellular changes associated with infection that may result in nuclear and/or cytoplasmic structural changes or inclusions. These are degenerative changes often associated with viral replication or cell lysis.

Cytomorphologic Features

- Nuclear changes may include nuclear enlargement (e.g., cytomegalovirus), smudgy chromatin (e.g., adenovirus in bronchial epithelial cells), glassy chromatin (e.g., human polyoma virus in urine), multinucleation (e.g., herpes simplex virus), large prominent macronucleolus (e.g., owl eye appearance of cytomegalovirus), intranuclear inclusions (margination of chromatin or eosinophilic Cowdry bodies seen with Herpes simplex virus), or koilocytic change (human papillomavirus in cervical Pap tests).

- Cytoplasmic changes may include giant cell formation and intracytoplasmic inclusions (e.g., respiratory syncytial virus and measles in respiratory samples).
- Nuclear changes may be more easily appreciated on alcohol-fixed Pap stained slides than air-dried Diff-Quik or Romanowsky stained slides.

Differential Diagnosis

- Treatment (radiation, chemotherapy) related change
- Degenerative change, which usually lacks multinucleation and inclusions
- Malignancy

Ancillary Studies

- Immunocytochemical stains for viral infections
- Serology for viral infections

Reactive Epithelial and Mesenchymal Repair

- Reactive atypia or repair includes squamous metaplastic or other epithelial atypia (e.g., of bronchial epithelium), mesenchymal spindle cells with atypia, and granulation tissue.
- These changes can occur in response to certain infections (e.g., cavitary fungal lesions, chronic abscess, or in response to ulceration), but may also be seen after treatment (radiation, chemotherapy) or infarction (Fig. 3.7 and Table 3.2).

Cytomorphologic Features

- Specimens display a continuum of changes from benign cells to cells with reactive or repair features. Unlike neoplasms there is a lack of two distinct populations (i.e., normal and tumor cells).
- Atypical cells have uniform nuclear membranes, occasional small nucleoli, and collectively exhibit uniform repair-type atypia ("school of fish" appearance) often with cohesive cell

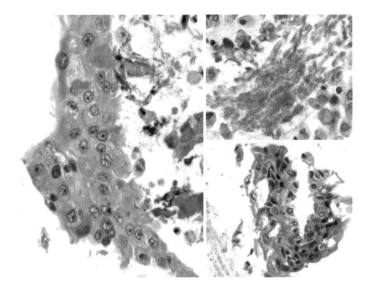

FIG. 3.7. Reactive epithelial atypia (H&E stain, high magnification). In this bronchoalveolar (BAL) specimen, all of the squamous cells show similar cytologic atypia in association with an *Aspergillus* infection (*upper right*).

groups and maintenance of polarity. High cellularity, loss of cohesion, three-dimensional cell groups, irregular nuclear contours, increased nuclear-to-cytoplasmic ratios, and many mitoses are concern for malignancy.
- The background can be inflammatory and necrotic, particularly with cavitary infections.

Differential Diagnosis

- Reactive cellular atypia unrelated to infection (e.g., infarction)
- Chemotherapy or radiation effect
- Malignancy

Ancillary Studies

- Special stains and/or immunostains for organisms

Reactions with Impaired Cell-Mediated Immunity

- In patients with impaired cell-mediated immunity (e.g., AIDS), their immune system cannot effectively kill microbes or form granulomas. As a result, the host reaction to infection in these patients is often atypical.
- Host response to infection in these cases may result in (a) no or scant inflammation (e.g., *Cryptococcus* and *Pneumocystis jirovecii* infection), or (b) a diffuse infiltration of macrophages that are packed with numerous intracellular organisms (e.g., *Mycobacterium avium-intracellulare*, leishmaniasis, histoplasmosis).

Cytomorphologic Features

- Microorganisms like yeast may be seen without associated inflammatory cells.
- Samples may contain diffuse sheets of macrophages with abundant foamy cytoplasm and numerous organisms.

Differential Diagnosis

- Granulomatous inflammation
- Conditions with numerous foamy histiocytes such as fat necrosis, lipoid pneumonia, and Gaucher disease
- Malignant histiocytosis

Ancillary Studies

- Special stains and/or immunostains for organisms
- Microbial cultures

Immune Reconstitution Inflammatory Syndrome

- The immune reconstitution inflammatory syndrome (IRIS) is a florid inflammatory response that may occur in HIV infected patients shortly after starting highly active antiretroviral therapy (HAART).
- IRIS is usually triggered in HIV-positive individuals who have an underlying coinfection (e.g., tuberculosis, CMV, Cryptococcus) or disease (e.g., Kaposi sarcoma).

- Clinically it presents as a paradoxical worsening of disease or pre-existing infection in HIV patients, shortly after starting antiretroviral treatment. This may be a life-threatening condition.

Cytomorphologic Features

- Marked florid granulomatous inflammation or other inflammatory response.
- Microorganisms may not be identified at the site of inflammation.

Differential Diagnosis

- Newly acquired infection

Ancillary Studies

- Concomitant drop in HIV levels with improvement in CD4 cell count
- Special stains and/or immunostains for organisms
- Microbial cultures

Hemophagocytosis and Emperipolesis

- Hemophagocytosis is the ingestion and often destruction of blood cells by macrophages. Emperipolesis is the penetration of an intact cell into and through a larger phagocytic cell.
- Hemophagocytic syndrome is due to activated macrophages in different organs that phagocytose other cells such as red blood cells (RBCs) and lymphocytes.
- This host reaction can be seen with a viral-associated (secondary) hemophagocytic syndrome (EBV, HIV, CMV, Parvovirus B19), as well as a variety of other noninfectious primary (familial) clinical disorders like hemophagocytic lymphohistiocytosis (HLH). Some gene mutations have been implicated (e.g., such as perforin, IL-2, and purine nucleoside phosphorylase).
- Hemophagocytosis is not specific and can be seen in up to 50% of patients with bone marrow examination as part of a workup for fever (Fig. 3.8).

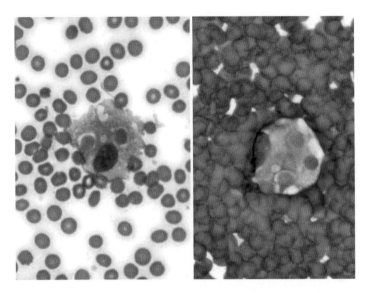

FIG. 3.8. Hemophagocytosis (Diff-Quik stain, high magnification). Macrophages are shown with engulfed intracytoplasmic red blood cells and a surrounding clear halo.

Cytomorphologic Features

- The hallmark finding is macrophages with abundant cytoplasm and peripherally located ingested RBCs or leukocytes.
- Phagocytosed cells may be intact or fragmented, and with emperipolesis may be surrounded by a thin cytoplasmic membrane or halo.
- Histiocytes are immunoreactive with CD68 and S100, but are negative for CD1a.

Differential Diagnosis

- Sinus histiocytosis with massive lymphadenopathy (Rosai-Dorfman disease)
- Noninfectious primary hemophagocytic lymphohistiocytsosis (HLH)
- Associated T-cell lymphoma
- Malignant histiocytosis with atypical histiocytes

Ancillary Studies

- Immunostains to characterize macrophages (S100 and CD68 positive)
- Immunostains, serology and/or further microbiology studies to detect an underlying viral infection

Ciliocytophthoria

- Ciliocytophthoria refers to the finding of anucleate apical portions of ciliated epithelial cells (also referred to as detached ciliary tufts). This may be seen in respiratory, gynecologic and peritoneal cytology specimens.
- Ciliocytophthoria can occur as a result of certain viral infections (e.g., adenovirus infection in the lung), but may also be traumatic in nature (Fig. 3.9).

Cytomorphologic Features

- Single or multiple detached tufts of cilia without nuclei.

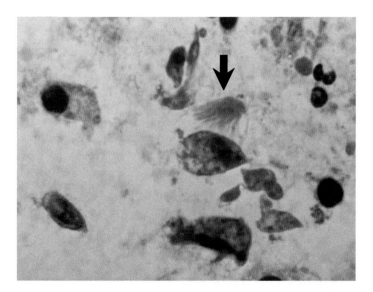

FIG. 3.9. Ciliocytophthoria (Pap stain, high magnification). A detached ciliary tuft is seen (*arrow*) in this sputum specimen.

Differential Diagnosis

- Noninfectious cause such as idiopathic or traumatic etiology.
- Mimics: Ciliated microorganisms (e.g., *Balantidium coli*), parasites, foreign material.

Ancillary Studies

- Immunostain for viral infections (e.g., Adenovirus)

Xanthogranulomatous Inflammation

- This is an uncommon form of granulomatous inflammation characterized by many lipid-laden foamy macrophages.
- Such inflammation mainly involves the kidney (xanthogranulomatous pyelonephritis) or biliary system (xanthogranulomatous cholecystitis). It is often observed in patients with diabetes and/or some other form of immunocompromise.
- The condition is most commonly associated with *Proteus*, *Escherichia coli*, or Pseudomonas spp. infection (Fig. 3.10).

Cytomorphologic Features

- There are numerous histiocytes with vacuolated or lipid-laden cytoplasm (foam cells), as well as chronic inflammatory cells.
- Occasionally multinucleated giant cells may be seen, including Touton giant cells with nuclei placed around the periphery of the cell.

Differential Diagnosis

- Other granulomatous or histiocytic processes
- Malignancy such as renal cell carcinoma or adenocarcinoma

Ancillary Studies

- Gram stain for associated bacteria
- Immunostains to characterize macrophages (S100 and CD68 positive)

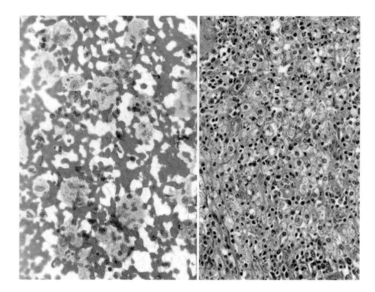

Fig. 3.10. Xanthogranulomatous inflammation. FNA showing (*left*) a predominance of foamy macrophages with ill-defined cytoplasmic borders (Pap stain, high magnification) that (*right*) form sheets in cell block material (H&E stain, high magnification).

Malakoplakia

- This is an uncommon chronic granulomatous inflammatory reaction of unknown etiology, thought to be due to the inability of macrophages to eliminate Gram-negative coliforms (e.g., *E. coli* or *Proteus*).
- It commonly affects the genitourinary tract (bladder), but has also been described in a variety of different tissues.
- In the urinary tract, malakoplakia is associated mainly with *E. coli*. Pulmonary malakoplakia is a known complication of *Rhodococcus equi* pneumonia in AIDS patients.
- Macrophages contain Michaelis-Guttman bodies, which are thought to represent mineralized bacterial fragments (Fig. 3.11).

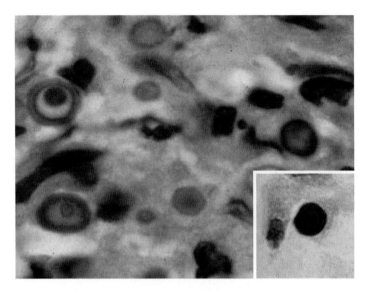

FIG. 3.11. Malakoplakia (H&E stain, high magnification; *inset*: Pap stain, high magnification). Macrophages are shown with characteristic eosinophilic cytoplasm and targetoid, round intracytoplasmic inclusions known as Michaelis-Guttman bodies.

Cytomorphologic Features

- Specimens contain numerous macrophages (von Hansemann cells) that have eosinophilic granular cytoplasm containing cytoplasmic Michaelis-Guttman bodies.
- Michaelis-Guttman bodies are round-to-oval, laminated inclusions surrounded by a membrane or halo, that typically have a calcified or clear core. These inclusions are usually PAS positive, Grocott (GMS) positive, and von Kossa positive due to their calcium composition.
- Numerous bacteria may be seen among acute or chronic inflammation.

Differential Diagnosis

- Other infectious granulomatous disease (e.g., tuberculosis)
- Intracellular yeast forms or other organisms
- Foreign body-type granulomas with foreign material engulfed
- Noninfectious granulomatous disease, particularly sarcoidosis which may have similar Schaumann bodies (round, concentrically laminated calcium inclusions). The other inclusions described with sarcoidosis are stellate-shaped asteroid bodies and clear calcium oxalate Hamazaki-Wesenberg bodies
- Psammomatous calcification

Ancillary Studies

- Special stains for Michaelis-Guttman bodies (PAS positive, GMS positive, von Kossa positive)
- Gram stain to identify associated bacteria
- Immunostains to characterize macrophages (S100 and CD68 positive)
- Microbial culture (e.g., urine culture)

Inflammatory Pseudotumor Reaction

- This rare mass lesion (pseudotumor) can be seen in any organ tissue, commonly described in patients with HIV infection. The clinical and imaging impression is often concern for malignancy.
- Such a localized inflammatory mass may develop in response to a viral infection (e.g., CMV, EBV), mycobacteria, or parasite.

Cytomorphologic Features

- Cytology specimens contain a reactive spindle cell and/or myofibroblastic proliferation with intermixed histiocytes and inflammatory cells.
- The inciting microorganism (e.g., parasitic worm) may be present.

Differential Diagnosis

- Granulation tissue
- Granulomatous inflammation
- Spindle cell neoplasms: Renal cell carcinoma, melanoma, mesenchymal neoplasms including Kaposi sarcoma (LNA-1 immunoreactive for HHV8) and EBV-associated smooth muscle tumors

Ancillary Studies

- Special stains for organisms (e.g., acid fast stains for mycobacterial spindle cell pseudotumor)
- EBV in situ hybridization (EBER) positivity may be seen in EBV-associated smooth muscle tumors
- PCR for mycobacteria
- Immunostains to characterize lesional cells (macrophages are S100 and CD68 positive, ALK negative, and myofibroblastic cells may express smooth muscle actin)

Crystal Formation

- Charcot-Leyden crystals are seen in association with eosinophilia. They consist of lysophospholipase, which is produced by eosinophils, and results from the breakdown of eosinophils.
- Birefringent calcium oxalate crystals may be seen in association with *Aspergillus* infection, particularly with *Aspergillus niger.* Crystals are believed to form when oxalic acid precipitates and undergoes crystallization when produced via a fermentation process by *Aspergillus.*

Cytomorphologic Features

- Calcium oxalate crystals form rosettes or wheat sheaf-like clusters and polarize under polarized microscopy (Fig. 3.12).
- Charcot-Leyden crystals are needle- or rhomboid-shaped eosinophilic crystals seen in association with eosinophilic inflammation (Fig. 3.2).
- The background may be inflammatory or necrotic.

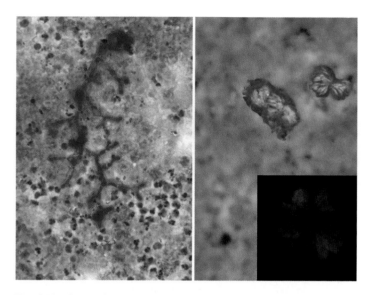

Fig. 3.12. Crystal formation in *Aspergillus* infection (Diff-Quik stain, high magnification; *Inset*: polarization microscopy, high magnification). Acute inflammatory cells and necrotic debris with fungal hyphal elements showing narrow-angle branching (*left*) associated with calcium oxalate crystals (*right*).

Differential Diagnosis

- Calcium oxalate crystals: *Aspergillus* spp.
- Charcot-Leyden crystals: Eosinophilic inflammation (allergy, asthma, parasites)
- Other crystals or foreign material

Ancillary Studies

- Special stains (PAS, GMS) for fungal elements
- Fungal culture for *Aspergillus* spp.

Splendore-Hoeppli Phenomenon

- The Splendore-Hoeppli phenomenon (also called asteroid bodies) describes the formation of eosinophilic crystalline material around microorganisms (fungi, bacteria, and parasites) or biologically inert substances.

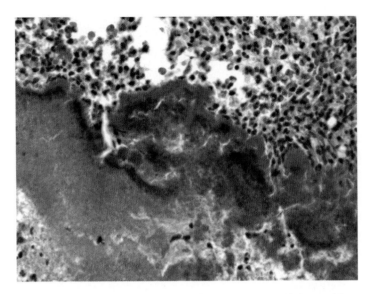

Fɪɢ. 3.13. Splendore-Hoeppli phenomenon (H&E stain, high magnification). A case of *Actinomyces* infection in the bone in which an eosinophilic stellate band can be seen at the edge of the filamentous organisms (sulfur granule) and surrounding acute inflammatory cells.

- These eosinophilic structures may be seen in association with filamentous bacilli (actinomycoses, nocardiosis), other bacterial infections (*Staphylococcus aureus*, *Pseudomonas aeruginosa*), botryomycosis, schistisoma, and microfilaria.
- The formation of this material is thought to be a localized host reaction made up of glycoprotein or antigen-antibody complexes, in addition to tissue debris and fibrin. This reaction probably prevents phagocytosis and intracellular killing of the insulting organism (Fig. 3.13).

Cytomorphologic Features

- The characteristic finding is a stellate or club-shaped acellular band-like structure surrounding microorganisms or sulfur granules (in the case of actinomycosis), which separates them from the background inflammatory cells and debris.

Differential Diagnosis

- Foreign, crystalline, or necrotic material
- Fibrin deposition
- Tophaceous lesions of gout
- Granulomatous inflammation with keratin debris

Ancillary Studies

- Special stains for microorganisms

Suggested Reading

Brummer E. Human defenses against *Cryptococcus neoformans*: an update. Mycopathologia. 1999;143:121–5.

Gupta M, Venkatesh SK, Kumar A, Pandey R. Fine-needle aspiration cytology of bilateral renal malakoplakia. Diagn Cytopathol. 2004;31:116–7.

Hadziyannis E, Yen-Lieberman B, Hall G, Procop GW. Ciliocytophthoria in clinical virology. Arch Pathol Lab Med. 2000;124:1220–3.

Kradin RL, Mark EJ. The pathology of pulmonary disorders due to Aspergillus spp. Arch Pathol Lab Med. 2008;132:606–14.

Kumar N, Jain S, Murthy NS. Utility of repeat fine needle aspiration in acute suppurative lesions: follow-up of 263 cases. Acta Cytol. 2004;48:337–40.

Pantanowitz L, Balogh K. Charcot-Leyden crystals: pathology and diagnostic utility. Ear Nose Throat J. 2004;83:489–90.

Pantanowitz L, Omar T, Sonnendecker H, Karstaedt AS. Bone marrow cryptococcal infection in the acquired immunodeficiency syndrome. J Infect. 2000;41:92–4.

Rodig SJ, Dorfman DM. Splendore-Hoeppli phenomenon. Arch Pathol Lab Med. 2001;125:1515–6.

Sereti I, Rodger AJ, French MA. Biomarkers in immune reconstitution inflammatory syndrome: signals from pathogenesis. Curr Opin HIV AIDS. 2010;5:504–10.

Zeppa P, Vetrani A, Ciancia G, Cuccuru A, Palombini L. Hemophagocytic histiocytosis diagnosed by fine needle aspiration cytology of the spleen: a case report. Acta Cytol. 2004;48:415–9.

4
Microbiology

Liron Pantanowitz[1], Gladwyn Leiman[2], and Lynne S. Garcia[3]

[1] Department of Pathology, University of Pittsburgh Medical Center,
5150 Centre Avenue, Suite 201, Pittsburgh, PA 15232, USA

[2] Fletcher Allen Health Care, Professor of Pathology,
University of Vermont, Burlington, VT, USA

[3] LSG & Associates, 512-12th Street, Santa Monica, CA 90402, USA

Cytologists are likely to encounter infectious diseases either because a cytology sample was obtained for diagnostic purposes or incidentally when an infectious process or microorganism is discovered in the material they are reviewing. In order to render an accurate diagnosis, and correctly identify clinically important species or microorganisms, a good understanding and knowledge of microbiology is essential. This chapter provides a broad overview of microbiology that is relevant to the practicing cytologist, but is not intended to replace standard microbiology texts.

Viruses

- Viruses replicate only inside host cells. Their particles (called virions) consist of DNA or RNA and a capsid (coat) that may be surrounded by a lipid envelope. Once they attach to and penetrate cells, they uncoat and replicate so that their progeny may be released following host cell lysis.
- Viral infection may cause cell death, proliferation, or neoplastic transformation (oncogenesis) (Table 4.1). Tumor viruses may promote cancer by expression of viral oncoproteins (or oncogenes) and/or inactivation of tumor suppressor genes.

L. Pantanowitz et al., *Cytopathology of Infectious Diseases*,
Essentials in Cytopathology 17, DOI 10.1007/978-1-4614-0242-8_4,
© Springer Science+Business Media, LLC 2011

TABLE 4.1.   Viral induced tumors.

Virus	Tumor
Epstein-Barr virus (EBV)	Non-Hodgkin lymphoma (e.g., Burkitt lymphoma, post-transplant lymphoproliferative disorder, plasmablastic lymphoma)
	Hodgkin lymphoma
	Carcinoma (e.g., nasopharyngeal carcinoma, gastric carcinoma)
	Smooth muscle tumor
	Follicular dendritic cell sarcoma
Kaposi sarcoma herpesvirus/ human herpesvirus-8 (KSHV/HHV8)	Kaposi sarcoma
	Non-Hodgkin lymphoma (e.g., primary effusion lymphoma)
	Castleman disease
Human papillomavirus (HPV)	Anogenital dysplasia and carcinoma
	Oropharyngeal dysplasia and carcinoma
Hepatitis viruses (HBV, HCV)	Hepatocellular carcinoma
Human T-cell lymphotropic virus type 1 (HTLV-1)	Adult T-cell leukemia/lymphoma
Merkel cell polyomavirus (MCPyV)	Merkel cell carcinoma

- In general, viruses are too small to be identified directly by light microscopy. Viruses that remain latent often do not cause apparent changes to infected cells. However, several viruses may cause cytopathic changes (Fig. 4.1) that affect the nucleus (e.g., inclusions, margination, multinucleation), cytoplasm (e.g., koilocytosis, syncytial giant cell formation), and/or entire cell (e.g., cytomegaly, ciliacytopthoria). Recognition of these changes can be life-saving as this would initiate confirmatory studies and/or therapy (Fig. 4.2).
- Superinfection by pyogenic bacteria is a complication of many viral infections that may mask subtle viral changes.

Papillomaviruses

- Papillomaviruses (genus) are nonenveloped viruses that contain double-stranded circular DNA molecules that replicate exclusively in skin and/or mucosal keratinocytes. They belong to the *Papillomaviridae* family.

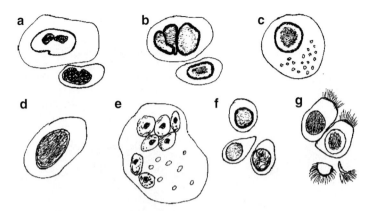

Fig. 4.1. Viral cytopathic changes. (**a**) HPV showing a large binucleate koilocyte and adjacent smaller high grade squamous intraepithelial lesion (HSIL) cell. (**b**) Herpes simplex virus showing a large multinucleated epithelial cell with cowdry A inclusions and a smaller cell with an intranuclear cowdry B inclusion. (**c**) CMV infected cell showing enlargement (cytomegaly), an intranuclear inclusion ("owl's-eye" appearance), and intracytoplasmic inclusions. (**d**) *Molluscum contagiosum* infection showing a keratinocyte with an intranuclear inclusion (molluscum body). (**e**) Measles (or RSV) infected syncytial giant cell with intranuclear inclusions. (**f**) BK polyomavirus infected epithelial cells (decoy cells) showing early (ground glass) and late ("fish-net stocking") intranuclear inclusions, as well as a comet cell in the middle with eccentric cytoplasm. (**g**) Adenovirus infected pneumocytes showing "smudge cells" with inclusions filling the nucleus and decapitated ciliated cells (ciliocytophthoria).

- Their genome is divided into an early (E) region that encodes genes E1–E7, and a late region (L) that encodes the capsid genes L1 and L2. In oncogenic human papillomavirus (HPV) types, the genes E6 (binds to p53) and E7 (binds to retinoblastoma [Rb] protein) are key players in transforming cells.
- HPV infection causes various diseases including warts (verruca), anogenital lesions (condylomata acuminata, intraepithelial neoplasia) and cancer, epidermodysplasia verruciformis (genodermatosis), oral and laryngeal papillomas, as well as orpharyngeal and conjunctival cancer. Genital HPV infection is covered in greater detail in Chap. 5.

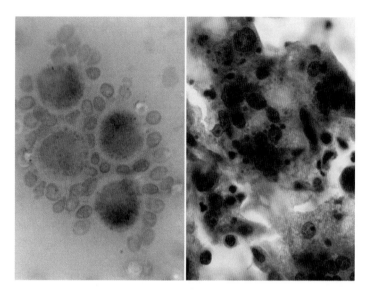

Fig. 4.2. Viral cytoplasmic inclusions. (*Left*) Cytomegalovirus infected cells (MGG stain, high magnification). (*Right*) Measles infected cells (Phloxine tartrazine stain, high magnification) (image courtesy of Dr. Pawel Schubert, University of Stellenbosch, Cape Town).

Herpesviruses

- Herpesvirues (family Herpesviridae) are DNA viruses that may cause latent or lytic infections. Reactivation of latent viruses has been implicated in a number of diseases.
- A major hallmark of herpes infection is the ability to infect mainly epithelial mucosal cells and/or lymphocytes. Cytomegalovirus (CMV) can infect many cells types including epithelial cells, endothelial cells, neuronal cells, smooth muscle cells, and monocytes.
- There are eight types of herpesvirus that may infect humans (Table 4.2). They include the Alphaherpesviruses (HSV and Varicella-Zoster virus [VZV]), Betaherpesviruses (CMV, HHV6, HHV7), and Gammaherpesviruses (Epstein-Barr virus [EBV] and KSHV). EBV and KSHV are oncogenic.
- *Herpes simplex virus types 1 and 2 (HSV-1 and HSV-2)* have similar characteristics. Viral infection typically results in the

TABLE 4.2. Human herpesviruses (HHV).

HHV type	Virus name	Target cells	Disease
HHV1	Herpes simplex virus type 1 (HSV-1)	Mucoepithelium	Oral and/or genital herpes
HHV2	Herpes simplex virus type 2 (HSV-2)	Mucoepithelium	Oral and/or genital herpes
HHV3	Varicella-Zoster virus (VZV)	Mucoepithelium	Chickenpox
			Shingles
HHV4	Epstein-Barr virus (EBV)	Lymphocytes and epithelium	Infectious mononucleosis
			Non-Hodgkin lymphoma
			Hodgkin lymphoma
			Nasopharyngeal carcinoma
			Lymphomatoid granulomatosis
			Gastric carcinoma
			Oral hairy leukoplakia
HHV5	Cytomegalovirus (CMV)	Epithelium, monocytes, lymphocytes	Acute (mono-like) illness
			Systemic illness (e.g., pneumonia, hepatitis)
			Retinitis
HHH6	Roseolovirus	T lymphocytes and others	Sixth disease (roseola infantum or exanthem subitum)
HHV7	Human herpes virus-7 (HHV-7)	T lymphocytes and others	Sixth disease (roseola infantum or exanthem subitum)
HHV8	Kaposi's sarcoma-associated herpes virus (KSHV)	Lymphocytes and endothelium	Kaposi sarcoma
			Non-Hodgkin lymphoma
			Multicentric Castleman disease

formation of Cowdry type A and B inclusions. Both types of HSV can infect oral (e.g., cold sores) or genital mucosa. HSV-2 is normally spread sexually, which is why genital herpes is usually the result of HSV-2 infection. Infection may also cause herpes keratitis, gladiatorum (skin lesions), visceral and CNS infection, and neonatal herpes.

- *VZV* typically causes chickenpox (Varicella) in childhood and shingles (Zoster) in adults, which is usually severe in patients with acquired immunodeficiency syndrome (AIDS). Approximately 15% of patients may develop pneumonia. Infection in utero can cause congenital varicella syndrome. The cytopathic effect of VZV infection is similar to that seen with HSV.

- *EBV* has a tropism for epithelial cells (e.g., oral and nasopharynx) and B lymphocytes, binding to its receptor (CD21). Primary infection may cause infectious mononucleosis. Infected B-cells activate T-cells, the cause of atypical lymphocytosis in infectious mononucleosis. Latent infection in cells is characterized by the expression of latent membrane proteins (LMP) 1 and 2, EBV nuclear antigens (EBNAs), and EBV-encoded RNAs [EBERs]. EBV-associated malignancies are associated with latent gene expression (Table 4.3).

- *CMV* is the largest virus to infect humans. It produces cytomegalic cells with characteristic "owl's eye" nuclear inclusions. Most infections are asymptomatic. However, in immunosuppressed persons CMV can be a major problem. CMV pneumonia is the most common life-threatening complication after transplantation.

- *Human herpes virus 6 and 7 (HHV6 and HHV7)* both infect T cells. They cause sixth disease typically in children, where a transient skin rash on the trunk and neck follows an episode of fever.

- *Kaposi's sarcoma-associated herpes virus/Human herpesvirus-8 (KSHV/HHV8)* was the eighth herpes virus to be discovered. Most viral genes are expressed in lytic infection. The five genes expressed in latent infection are key to oncogenesis, which includes the latency-associated nuclear antigen (LANA). The immunohistochemical stain LNA-1 targets LANA within the nuclei of KSHV infected cells. KSHV has an etiologic role in Kaposi sarcoma, certain lymphomas like primary effusion lymphoma (PEL), and multicentric Castleman disease.

TABLE 4.3. Patterns of latent gene expression in EBV.

| EBV gene | Acute infection | Latency I | Latency II | | Latency III | |
		Burkitt lymphoma	Hodgkin lymphoma	Nasopharyngeal carcinoma	PCNSL	PTLD
EBNA1	+	+	+	+	+	+
EBNA2	+	–	–	–	+	+
EBNA3	+	–	–	–	+	+
LMP1	+	–	+	+	+	+
LMP2	+	–	+	+	+	+
EBER	+	+	+	+	+	+

PCNSL primary central nervous system lymphoma; *PTLD* post-transplant lymphoproliferative disorder

Respiratory Viruses

- *Influenza* and *Parainfluenza viruses* can cause severe respiratory tract disease (e.g., pneumonia, bronchitis, and bronchiolitis). As infection usually does not cause characteristic cytologic findings, the diagnosis requires isolation and identification of the virus in the laboratory or a rise in serum antibodies.
- *Coronavirus* causes illness ranging from the common cold to severe acute respiratory syndrome (SARS). Respiratory samples may show atypical reactive pneumocytes with or without background inflammation and marked fibrin exudate in cases with diffuse alveolar damage (DAD).
- *Respiratory syncytial virus* (*RSV*) causes lower respiratory tract infections mainly in childhood. RSV belongs to the same Paramyxoviridae family as measles (Rubeola) and mumps viruses. Both RSV and measles pneumonia can cause multinucleated syncytial giant cells containing intranuclear and inconspicuous usually paranuclear cytoplasmic inclusions. Multinucleated giant cells are usually rare, but when identified may contain up to 35 nuclei.
- *Adenoviruses.* They were named after being first isolated from adenoid samples. There are 55 described serotypes in humans that cause respiratory tract infections (e.g., pharyngitis, pneumonia). Infection may also cause gastroenteritis, conjunctivitis, hemorrhagic cystitis, meningoencephalitis, hepatitis, and disseminated disease. Early infected cells may display small eosinophilic inclusions. With late infection, basophilic intranuclear inclusions eventually obscure the nucleus producing a characteristic "smudge cell."

Polyomaviruses

- Most people are infected with these viruses and hence are seropositive for polyomaviruses. These double-stranded DNA viruses tend to only cause infection in immunosuppressed individuals, and are all potentially oncogenic. They fall under the SV40 (Simian vacuolating virus 40) clade seen in monkeys, except for Merkel cell polyomavirus.
- *BK virus* (BKV) has a tropism for cells of the genitourinary tract. BKV may cause nephropathy in 1–10% of renal transplant

patients resulting in the loss of their renal allograft. Reactivation in the kidneys and urinary tract results in shedding of infected cells, virions, and/or viral proteins in the urine. Infection can thus be diagnosed using urine cytology looking for cells with polyomavirus inclusions of the nucleus, as well as PCR. BKV may also cause ureteral stenosis in renal transplant patients and asymptomatic hemorrhagic cystitis, usually after bone marrow transplantation.

- *JC virus (JCV)* may infect the respiratory tract, kidneys, or brain. CNS infection can cause fatal progressive multifocal leukoencephalopathy (PML) in AIDS patients.
- *Merkel cell polyomavirus (MCV or MCPyV)*. This recently discovered virus (in 2008) causes around 80% of Merkel cell carcinomas. Although lymphocytes may serve as a tissue reservoir for MCV infection, only rare (approximately 2%) of hematolymphoid malignancies show evidence for MCPyV infection by DNA PCR.

Poxviruses

- *Molluscum contagiosum virus.* Infection involves the skin and occasionally the mucous membranes. There are four types of MCV (MCV-1–4). Skin lesions are self-limited and pearly in appearance with an umbilicated (dimpled) center. Infected cells are characterized by molluscum bodies (also called Henderson-Paterson bodies). Unlike herpes, this virus does not remain latent. As patients do not develop permanent immunity, repeated infections can occur.

Retroviruses

- Retroviruses are enveloped viruses that belong to the viral family *Retroviridae*. They are RNA viruses that replicate in host cells using the enzyme reverse transcriptase to produce DNA from its RNA genome. DNA is then incorporated into the host genome.
- *Human immunodeficiency virus (HIV), types 1 and 2.* HIV belongs to the retrovirus family. Infection causes AIDS. Details are covered in greater detail in Chap. 13.
- *Human T-cell lymphotrophic virus (HTLV), types 1 and 2.* HTLV-1 is the first recognized retrovirus that causes adult T-cell

leukemia/lymphoma (ATLL). Infection may also be involved in certain demyelinating diseases. Infected lymphocytes in the peripheral blood produce characteristic "flower cells."

Miscellaneous Viruses

- *Hepatitis viruses*. Several viruses may cause hepatitis including Hepatitis A (RNA picornavirus), Hepatitis B (DNA hepadnavirus), Hepatitis C (RNA flavivirus), Hepatitis E (RNA calicivirus), and Hepatitis D (Delta agent). They usually do not cause viral cytopathic changes seen in cytology samples. However, in liver tissue chronic hepatitis B virus (HBV) can cause a ground-glass appearance of hepatocytes due to the accumulation of HBsAg within the endoplasmic reticulum. Chronic infection with HBV and hepatitis C (HCV) may lead to cirrhosis, liver dysplasia, and ultimately hepatocellular carcinoma.
- *Parvoviruses.* These are among the smallest known DNA viruses. Parvovirus B19 (B19V) causes fifth disease (erythema infectiosum) and arthropathy. Infection of erythroid precursors in the bone marrow may cause severe anemia characterized by giant normoblasts and intranuclear inclusions with a ground glass appearance that tend to compress the chromatin against the nuclear membrane. Cells with parvovirus B19 inclusions have been reported in cytology fluid specimens from fetal cases with hydrops fetalis.

Bacteria

- Bacteria (singular: bacterium) are single-celled microorganisms that measure 0.5–5.0 μm in length. Mycoplasma spp. are among the smallest bacteria. Bacteria have a wide range of shapes. Most are spherical (cocci) or rod-shaped (bacilli), but they may also be curved or spiral-shaped (e.g., spirochaetes, *Helicobacter pylori*). Some bacteria are described as being coccobacilli because they have the ability to exist as a coccus, bacillus, or intermediate form (e.g., *Haemophilus influenzae*, *Rhodococcus equi*, *Bartonella* spp.). Bacteria may also form pairs (e.g., diploids), chains (e.g., Streptococcus), or clusters (e.g., Staphylococcus). Some bacteria may also have flagella.

- Anerobic bacteria do not need oxygen for growth. Some anerobes die when oxygen is present (obligate anerobes), whereas others will utilize oxygen if it is present (facultative anaerobes). They are found in normal flora (e.g., *Fusobacterium* in the mouth, *Bacteroides fragilis* in the large bowel, *Lactobacillis* in the vagina). These bacteria can usually be isolated from abscesses, aspiration pneumonia, empyema, and wounds. Material being collected from sites that do not harbor indigenous flora (e.g., body fluids other than urine and fine needle aspirates) should always be cultured for anaerobic bacteria.

- Bacteria, along with some fungi (mainly *Candida* spp.) and archaea (single-celled microorganisms), make up the normal human flora of the skin, mouth, gastrointestinal tract, conjunctiva, and vagina (lactobacilli). Loss of normal flora may permit the unfavorable growth of harmful pathogens that can lead to infection.

- Some bacteria form biofilms, which are bacterial aggregates embedded within a self-produced matrix (slime). These bacterial clusters, seen associated with amorphous mucoid material, may be encountered in cytology specimens related to catheter infections, *Pseudomonas aeruginosa* pulmonary infections in cystic fibrosis, middle ear infections, joint prostheses, and dental (gingival) disease.

Gram-Positive and Gram-Negative Bacteria

- Bacteria can generally be divided into Gram-positive and Gram-negative bacteria on the basis of their reaction to the Gram stain. Most bacteria can be classified into one of the following four groups: Gram-positive cocci, Gram-positive bacilli, Gram-negative cocci, and Gram-negative bacilli.

- *Gram-positive bacteria* stain dark blue (violet) by Gram staining because they retain the crystal violet stain as a result of the abundant peptidoglycan in their cell wall. Gram-positive cell walls typically lack the outer membrane found in Gram-negative bacteria.

- *Gram-negative bacteria* cannot retain the crystal violet stain. Hence, they take up the counterstain (safranin or basic fuchsin) instead and with Gram staining appear red or pink (Figs. 4.3 and 4.4).

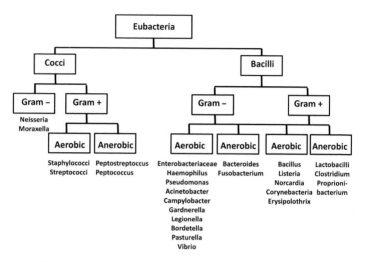

Fig. 4.3. Bacteria divided according to their shape (cocci or bacilli), Gram staining properties, and dependence upon oxygen for growth.

Mycobacteria

- Mycobacteria are aerobic Gram-positive rod-shaped bacilli that are acid–alcohol fast (so-called AFB) with acid fast stains (Fite, Ziehl-Neelsen, Kinyoun, and auramine rhodamine stains). *Mycobacterium tuberculosis* are strongly acid fast positive (stain deep red), thin, and slightly curved bacilli that measure 0.3–0.6 × 1–4 nm (Fig. 4.5). The bacteria of MAI are typically short and cocobacillary like. Beading may be seen in some mycobacteria, which represents nonuniform staining of the bacillus. For example, *M. kansasii* are characteristically long and broad and exhibit a cross-banded or barred appearance.

- Acid-fast staining of morphologically similar bacteria such as *Nocardia* and *Legionella* is a possible pitfall in the cytologic diagnosis of mycobacterial infection. Other organisms known to be acid-fast positive include micrococcus species, the oocysts of cryptosporidium species, *Isospora belli*, and sarcocystis.

- Mycobacteria are grouped on the basis of their appearance and rate of growth in culture (slow, intermediate, and rapidly growing). According to the Runyon classification there are three

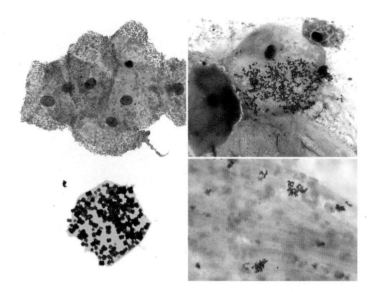

FIG. 4.4. Commonly encountered bacteria. (*Top left*) Lactobacilli are shown in a Pap test associated with normal squamous cells. These were discovered by the German gynecologist Albert Döderlein in 1892. (*Bottom left*) Sarcina forms seen attached to an oral squamous cell in a BAL specimen, showing its characteristic appearance in tetrads (buckets of eight elements). This type of bacteria is frequently observed as a commensal flora to the mouth (GMS stain, high magnification). (*Top right*) Sputum showing Gram positive diplococci of *Streptococcus pneumoniae* (Gram stain, high magnification). (*Bottom right*) Lung abscess FNA showing clusters of Gram positive *Staphyloccus aureus* (Gram stain, high magnification).

slow growing groups (photochromogens that develop pigments with light exposure such as *M. kansasii* and *M. marinum*, scotochromogens which become pigmented in darkness such as *M. scrofulaceum*, and nonchromogens such as *M. avium complex* [MAC]). Rapid growers include *M. chelonae* and *M. fortuitum*.

- For diagnostic and treatment purposes they can be classified into three main groups:
  ○ *M. tuberculosis complex*. This includes *M. tuberculosis*, *M. bovis*, *M. africanum*, *M. microti*, *BCG* and *M. canetti*. Infection causes tuberculosis. The response to Bacillus Calmette-Guerin (BCG)

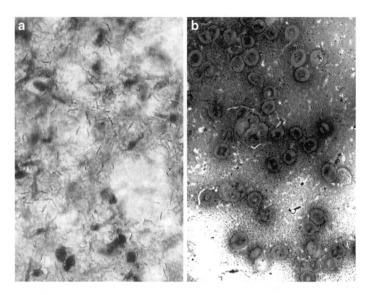

FIG. 4.5. *Mycobacterium tuberculosis* can be identified (**a**) with an acid stain (Ziehl-Neelsen stain, high magnification) or (**b**) negative staining of bacterial rods (Diff-Quik stain, high magnification).

vaccine in some infants and immunocomprised patients may cause postvaccinial disseminated infection presenting with lymphadenitis, osteomyelitis, and hepatic granulomas. BCG vaccine contains attenuated live bacilli of *M. bovis*.

○ *Mycobacterium leprae* which causes leprosy (Hansen's disease).

○ *Nontuberculous mycobacteria* (NTM), which include all of the other mycobacteria. These are also known as atypical mycobacteria, mycobacteria other than tuberculosis (MOTT), or environmental mycobacteria. Infections with these mycobacteria are increasingly being seen in immunosuppressed patients. Infection causes lung disease but may also disseminate to involve the hematopoietic system, gastrointestinal tract, as well as skin and soft tissue. While most NTM can be detected microscopically with an acid-fast stain, culture and/or molecular studies may be required to identify these species.

Filamentous Bacteria

- Bacteria can be elongated to form filaments (e.g., *Actinobacteria*, *Nocardia*, *Rhodococcus*, *Streptomyces*, *Actinomadura*). They can sometimes form complex, branched filaments that morphologically resemble fungal mycelia (mass of branching hyphae).
- These bacteria are usually part of the normal oral flora. Most infections are acquired by inhalation of the bacteria or via trauma.
- *Actinomyces* (genus) belong to the *Actinobacteria* (class of bacteria). Infection (actinomycosis) with these Gram-positive bacteria forms multiple abscesses and sinus tracts that may discharge sulfur granules. Actinomycosis is most frequently caused by *Actinomyces israelii*.
- *Nocardia* (genus) are weakly-staining Gram-positive bacteria that form partially acid-fast beaded branching filaments. There are a total of 85 species, although *Nocardia asteroides* is the species that most frequently causes infection (nocardiosis). Nocardial disease (norcardiosis) includes pneumonia, endocarditis, encephalitis, and/or brain abscess, as well cutaneous infections such as actinomycotic mycetoma (Figs. 4.6 and 4.7).

Chlamydia

- *Chlamydiae* are obligate intracellular Gram negative bacteria. They are classified taxonomically into a separate order (*Chlamydia*) because of their unique life cycle.
- Organisms occur in two forms: an elementary body (0.3 μm) that exists outside the host and infects host cells where it transforms into a reticulate body (0.6 μm). Following replication, new elementary bodies are released from the infected host cell when it ruptures.
- *Chlamydia* inclusion bodies may be identified within infected cells. However, the cytologic findings (e.g., in a Pap test) are not considered reliable. When stained with iodine, reticulate bodies can be visualized as intracytoplasmic inclusions. They can also

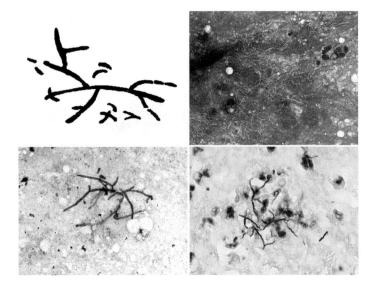

Fig. 4.6. *Nocardia.* (*Top left*) Diagrammatic illustration of branched filamentous bacteria. (*Top right*) Negative image of *Nocardia* in a direct smear from a brain abscess (Diff-Quik stain, high magnification). (*Bottom left*) *Nocardia* bacteria are shown highlighted with a GMS stain (high magnification). (*Bottom right*) Weakly Gram positive *Nocardia* (high magnification).

be stained with Giemsa or Gimenez methods as well as immunocytochemistry.

- Organisms are better detected by culture (gold standard) or other laboratory tests (e.g., enzyme immunoassay, leukocyte esterase test in urine, rapid *Chlamydia* test, and nucleic acid tests).
- Three species of *Chlamydia* are known to produce human disease:
  ○ *Chlamydia pneumonia* (also *Chlamydophila pneumoniae* and previously known as the TWAR agent). Infection causes pharyngitis, bronchitis, and atypical pneumonia. Less common infections include meningoencephalitis, arthritis, and myocarditis. An association with atherosclerosis and possibly lung cancer has been reported.

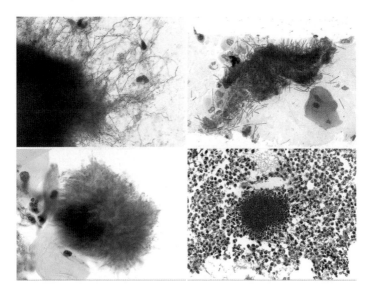

FIG. 4.7. *Actinomyces.* (*Top left*) Clump of long filamentous bacteria are shown (May-Grünwald-Giemsa stain, high magnification). (*Top right*) *Actinomyces* from the mouth contaminating a bronchoalveolar lavage ThinPrep specimen (Pap stain, high magnification). (*Bottom left*) Typical "dust bunny" seen on a cervical Pap test (Pap stain; high magnification). (*Bottom right*) Sulfur granule is shown in the center of the cell block preparation aspirated from an actinomycotic liver abscess (H&E stain, intermediate magnification).

- ○ *Chlamydia trachomatis* (previously called TRIC agent). This includes three human biovars: trachoma (serovars A, B, Ba or C), urethritis (serovars D-K), and lymphogranuloma venereum (LGV, serovars L1, 2 and 3). Infection causes inclusion conjunctivitis (trachoma), pneumonia in neonates, and sexually transmitted disease in adults (e.g., cervicitis, urethritis, salpingitis, proctitis, epididymitis).
- ○ *Chlamydia psittaci* (also called *Chlamydophila psittaci*) causes respiratory psittacosis and is acquired from birds (Fig. 4.8).

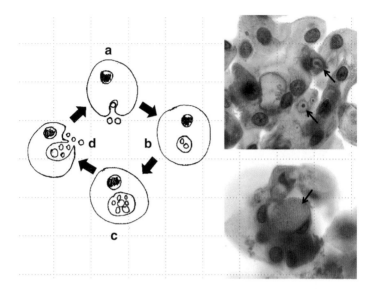

Fig. 4.8. Chlamydia. (*Left*) Chlamydia developmental cycle. Infectious elementary bodies that infect a host cell (**a**) transform into noninfectious reticulate bodies (**b**) which then multiply (**c**). Elementary bodies are then released following cell lysis that can infect new cells (**d**). *Chlamydia* inclusions containing (*top right*) elementary bodies (*arrows*) and (*bottom right*) reticulate bodies (*arrow*) are shown in squamous cells of a Pap test (Pap stain, high magnification).

Fungi

- On the basis of morphologic forms fungi can be divided into yeasts and hyphae.
- *Yeasts* are unicellular fungi. They reproduce by budding (forming *blastoconidia*) or fission. The term "yeast" is used only to describe a morphological form of a fungus and is of no taxonomic significance.
- *Hyphae* (single hypha) are multicellular fungi. Morphologically they are branching, thread-like tubular structures. Hyphae may lack cross walls (coenocytic or aseptate) or have cross walls (septate). A *mold* is a mass of hyphal elements (also called *mycelium*).

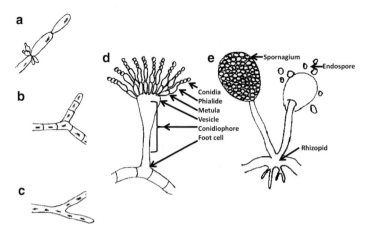

Fig. 4.9. Fungal morphology. Hyphae may be characterized as (**a**) pseudohyphae (e.g., *Candida* spp.), (**b**) septate (e.g., *Aspergillus*) or (**c**) coenocytic (aseptate) hyphae (e.g., Zygomycetes). Conidia (spores) develop from asexual fruiting structures such as (**d**) a conidiophore or (**e**) enclosed in a sac called a sporangium, in which case they are then called endospores.

- Hyphae can produce *conidia* (synonymous with *spores*). Large complex conidia are called macroconidia. Smaller more simple conidia are termed microconidia. When these conidia are enclosed in a sac (the *sporangium*) they are called *endospores*. A sporangium-bearing hypha is referred to as a sporangiophore.
- Dimorphism (*dimorphic fungi*) is the condition whereby a fungus can exhibit either the yeast form or the hyphal form, depending on growth conditions (Fig. 4.9).

Candida

- *Candida* is a polymorphic fungus that undergoes a yeast-to-mycelial transition. In clinical specimens, they produce pseudohyphae (hyphae that show distinct points of constriction resembling sausage links), rarely true septate hyphae, and budding yeast forms (blastoconidia).
- The yeast-like forms (blastoconidia) are oval and measure 3–5 μm in diameter

- Although typically seen extracellularly, intracellular *Candida* can mimic other small fungi such as *Histoplasma*. *Candida* usually exhibit variably sized yeast cells, lack a pseudocapsule, and elicit more of a suppurative reaction than a granulomatous response.
- *Candida* yeasts form part of the normal flora on the skin and mucous membranes of the respiratory, gastrointestinal, and female genital tracts. They often contaminate cytology samples from these sites. They may also colonize tissue (e.g., after prolonged antibiotic use, prolonged skin moisture, and in patients with diabetes).
- Infection may result from overgrowth or when introduced into the body (e.g., intravenously). Superficial infections include oropharyngeal and vulvovaginal candidiasis (thrush). Candidiasis may also become a systemic illness causing widespread abscesses, endocarditis, thrombophlebitis, endocarditis, eye infections, or involve other organs.
- *Candida albicans* is clinically the most significant member of this genus. *Candida glabrata* (previously known as *Torulopsis glabrata*) is a nondimorphic species (only has a yeast form) (Fig. 4.10).

Cryptococcus

- Cryptococci are small (5–15 μm) pleomorphic (ovoid to spheroid) yeasts that are characterized by often having a thick gelatin-like capsule and demonstrating narrow-based (teardrop-shaped) budding. They have thin walls and are occasionally refractile. Their capsules may have a diameter of up to five times that of the fungal cell, and form a halo on Diff-Quik, Pap, and India ink stains.
- Smaller (2–5 μm) capsule-deficient cryptococci can resemble other organisms with similar microforms (e.g., *Histoplasma*, *Candida*, and immature spherules of *Coccidioides immitis*). In such cases, with careful examination some weakly encapsulated yeasts can still be detected. Loss of capsular material usually elicits an intense inflammatory reaction characterized by suppuration and granulomas.
- Yeasts usually produce single buds, but multiple buds and even chains of budding cells may rarely be present.

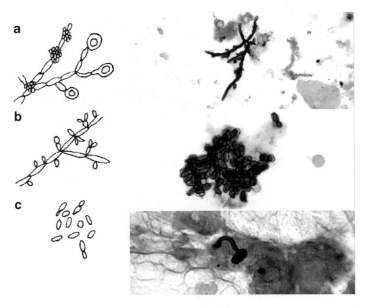

Fig. 4.10. *Candida* morphology. Pseudohyphae and yeast are shown of (**a**) *Candida albicans* and (**b**) *C. tropicalis*. (**c**) *C. glabrata* (*torulopsis*) only has a yeast form. The images of *Candida* on the *right* show classic examples of (*top*) pseudohyphae with distinct points of constriction along the fungal filaments, (*middle*) oval yeasts with a separate budding form present in the top right field of the image, and (*bottom*) a germ tube (germinating outgrowth) (GMS stains, high magnification).

- The presence of pseudohyphae-like elements and germ tube-like structures may be detected in some cases, mimicking *Candida*. However, this is rare and reported to be observed in older lesions of cryptococcosis where aberrant forms are frequently seen.
- Infection (cryptococcosis) arises mainly in immunosuppressed patients and may cause very little inflammation.
- *Cryptococcus neoformans* causes most infections, such as meningitis and meningoencephalitis in HIV positive patients.
- *Cryptococcus gattii* (formerly *Cryptococcus neoformans var gattii*), endemic in tropical areas of Africa and Australia, may cause cryptococcosis in immunocompetent individuals (Fig. 4.11).

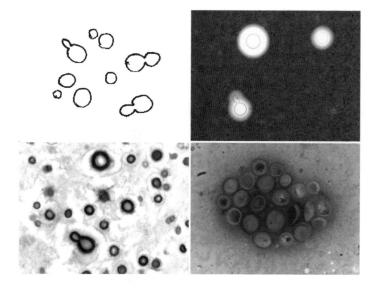

FIG. 4.11.   *Cryptococcus.* (*Top left*) Diagram showing the pleomorphic yeast-like cells of *C. neoformans*, which have thin walls and exhibit narrow based budding forming teardrop structures. (*Top right*) India ink preparation of a CSF specimen from a patient with AIDS associated cryptococcal meningitis demonstrates unstained halos around the microorganisms due to their thick capsules (high magnification). (*Bottom left*) A mucicarmine stain demonstrates the mucinous capsules surrounding cryptococci (high magnification). (*Bottom right*) Cryptococci are shown with ovoid and cup-shaped forms that may resemble *Pneumocystis* organisms (Diff-Quik stain, high magnification).

Aspergillus

- *Aspergillus* genus consists of many mold species. Pathogenic species include *Aspergillus fumigatus* and *Aspergillus flavus*.
- These fungi consist of septate hyphae that branch at 45° angles. Other dichotomous hyphae that may mimic *Aspergillus* include the hyalinohyphomyces (e.g., *Fusarium*, *Penicillium*) and dermatophytes.
- Species specific conidiophores called fruiting bodies have swollen vesicles lined by phialides that give rise to many conidia. The presence of fruiting bodies in cytology samples are usually only seen in samples obtained from cavities or other well oxygenated areas.

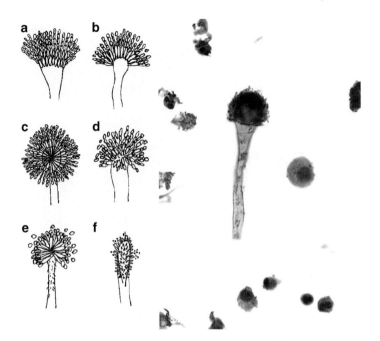

FIG. 4.12. Fruiting bodies of *Aspergillus* spp. (*Left*). Illustrations of the varied microscopic morphology of common *Aspergillus* spp. including (**a**) *A. nidulans* and *A. terreus*, (**b**) *A. fumigatus*, (**c**) *A. niger*, (**d**) *A. glaucus* group, (**e**) *A. flavus*, and (**f**) *A. clavatus*. (*Right*) Fruiting body of *A. fumigatus* is shown in a ThinPrep BAL specimen from a patient with a cavitary lung lesion (Pap stain, high magnification).

- Diseases caused by *Aspergillus* spp. (aspergillosis) include sinusitis, allergic bronchopulmonary aspergillosis, aspergilloma ("fungus ball") within lung cavities, and invasive disseminated aspergillosis (Figs. 4.12 and 4.13).

Zygomycetes

- The zygomycetes belong to the phylum Zygomycota (Table 4.4). The two orders that contain fungi causing human disease are the Mucorales and Entomophthorales. Most illness is linked to Rhizopus spp. of the Mucorales.

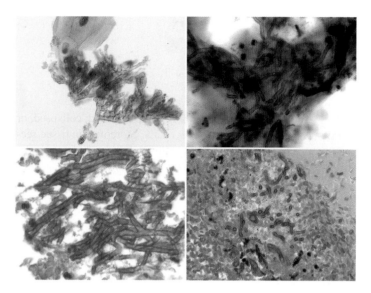

FIG. 4.13. *Aspergillus* hyphae with branching at 45° angles are shown (*top left*) in a ThinPrep specimen (Pap stain, high magnification), (*top right*) direct smear (Pap stain, high magnification), (*bottom left*) with a PAS stain (high magnification), and (*bottom right*) in a cell block (H&E stain, high magnification).

TABLE 4.4. Zygomycetes taxonomy.

Phylum	Zygomycota		
Class	Zygomycetes		
Order	Mucorales		Entomophthorales
Family	Mucoraceae	Cunninghamellaceae	
Genus	Absidia Apophysomyces Mucor Rhizomucor Rhizopus	Mortierellaceae Saksenaceae Syncephalastraceae Thamnidaceae	Ancylistaceae Basidioboaceae

- Zygomycetes are fungi characterized by the formation of spores (zygospores) and a vegetative mycelium. They have broad, ribbon-like, aseptate hyaline hyphae (coenocytic hyphae) with wide-angle branching. These morphological features are helpful in differentiating the zygomycetes from other fungal agents of infection that may be seen in cytologic specimens (Table 4.5).
- In cytology samples hyphal forms may be twisted, collapsed, or wrinkled making them hard to evaluate. Moreover, in tissue sections from biopsies or cell block material, folds and creases in the section may cause the hyphae to appear as if they have septae.
- In respiratory samples, the zygomycetes can be distinguished from dimorphic fungi and yeasts as they do not produce a yeast phase in this anatomic site.
- Samples are often associated with extensive necrosis and inflammation.
- Their isolation in the clinical laboratory reflects either environmental contamination or clinical disease (zygomycosis). Human zygomycosis is usually an opportunistic infection in immunocompromised hosts such as patients with diabetes mellitus, neutropenia, or using immunosuppressive therapy.
- Infection is associated with angioinvasive disease causing thrombosis, tissue infarction, and subsequent dissemination.
- Disease manifestations include rhinocerebral and pulmonary disease, and infrequently cutaneous, gastrointestinal, and allergic diseases (Fig. 4.14).

Dimorphic Fungi

- Dimorphic fungi can exist both as a mold form that consists of hyphae (when grown at room temperature outside the host) and as yeast (when grown at body temperature in the host). Therefore, in clinical samples obtained from patients the cytologist will encounter yeasts from these organisms (Table 4.6). Several such fungal species are potential pathogens.
- *Blastomyces*. The yeasts are 8–15 μm in size, have a double-contour refractile wall, and demonstrate broad-based budding. The most well-known species of this genus is *Blastomyces dermatitidis*, endemic to the United States (especially the southeastern, south central, and midwestern states) and Canada.

TABLE 4.5. Comparison between zygomycetes, *Aspergillus* spp., and *Candida* spp.

Morphologic feature	*Aspergillus*	Zygomycetes	*Candida*
Pap stain appearance			
Hyphal type	Septate	Aseptate	Pseudohyphae
Hyphal width	Consistently thin (2–3 μm wide)	Variable and wide (6–16 μm wide)	Consistently thin (2–3 μm wide)
Branching	45° angles	90° angles	Variable angles
Blastoconidia	Absent	Absent	Present
Sporulation	Present with air exposure	Absent	Absent

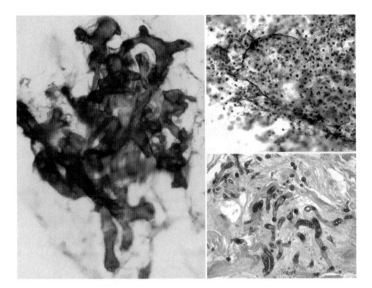

FIG. 4.14. Zygomycetes. (*Left and top right*) Zygomycete hyphae are shown characterized by broad, aseptate (coenocytic) hyphae that display wide-angle branching (Pap stain, *left* high magnification, *top right* intermediate magnification). (*Bottom right*) Fungal hyphae are shown immunoreactive with a specific immunostain for zygomycetes (high magnification).

Infection (blastomycosis) occurs by inhalation of the fungus from its natural soil habitat. Infection may involve virtually any organ including the lungs, skin, bones, and brain (Fig. 4.15).

- *Coccidioides.* This fungus presents with endospores contained within thick-walled spherules that vary in size (20–150 μm). Endospores measuring 3–5 μm may be seen scattered singly if the spherule ruptures. When free endospores occur within macrophages, they can imitate other intracellular yeasts. The causative agents of infection (coccidioidomycosis) are *C. immitis* and *C. posadasii.* These fungi are endemic in American deserts. Infection causes granulomatous and miliary disease affecting largely the lungs. In endemic regions, fungus balls may develop within lung cavities.

TABLE 4.6. Morphology of commonly encountered yeasts and yeast-like cells.

Fungi	Yeast appearance	Yeast shape	Yeast size (μm)	Associated elements	Budding	Location
Candida		Oval	3–5	Pseudohyphae Rare hyphae	Narrow based	Mainly extracellular
Histoplasma		Oval to round	2–4	No hyphae	Narrow based	Mainly intracellular
Cryptococcus		Oval to round	5–15	Very rare pseudohyphae	Narrow based	Extracellular and intracellular
Blastomyces		Spherical	8–15	No hyphae	Broad based	Mainly intracellular

		Shape	Size	Hyphae	Budding	Location
Coccidioides		Oval	3–5	Within spherules	None	Mainly extracellular
Sporothrix		Round to elongated	3–5	Rare hyphae	Narrow based	Mainly extracellular
Pneumocystis		Round to crescent	5–8	No hyphae	None	Mainly extracellular
Penicilliosis		Round to elongated	2–3	Rare hyphae	None	Mainly intracellular

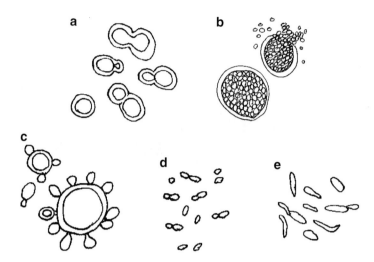

FIG. 4.15. Dimorphic fungi including (**a**) *Blastomyces dermatitidis*, (**b**) *Coccidioides immitis*, (**c**) *Paracoccidiodes brasiliensis*, (**d**) *Histoplasma capsulatum*, and (**e**) *Sporothrix schenckii.*

- *Paracoccidioides.* These yeasts measure 5–30 μm in size and are round to oval. Budding is characterized by a central yeast with multiple surrounding daughter buds, that morphologically resembles a "ship's wheel." Infection (paracoccidioidomycosis) is caused by *Paracoccidioides brasiliensis*, typically found in Brazil and elsewhere in South America. Primary infection (Valley Fever) is usually mild and self-limiting, but may progress into a systemic mycosis producing oral lesions, generalized lymphadenopathy, and miliary pulmonary lesions. Infection can also spread to bones, meninges, and the spleen.
- *Histoplasma.* This budding yeast is round to oval, on average 1–5 μm in size and observed mainly within macrophages (Fig. 4.16), but sometimes also within neutrophils. Narrow based round to oval budding may be noted, but because of their small size buds are often not seen. Intracellular yeasts are usually surrounded by a clear zone (halo). However, with cell disruption organisms may be spilled extracellularly. This fungus is usually found in bird and bat (guano) fecal material. There are a few

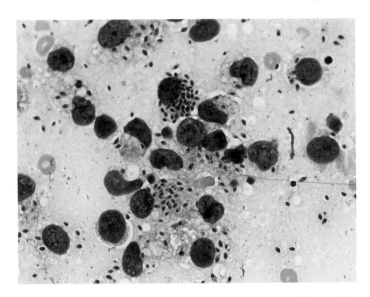

FIG. 4.16.   Histoplasmosis. Numerous small intracellular and extracellular yeasts of *H. capsulatum* are shown (GMS stain, high magnification).

species including *H. capsulatum*. *H. capsulatum var. capsulatum* are smaller (1–5 μm) than *H. capsulatum var. duboisii* which have larger sized budding yeast cells (5–12 μm). Although this fungus occurs worldwide, it is prevalent in certain regions (Ohio and Mississippi river valleys) of North America and in caves of southern and East Africa. Infection causes histoplasmosis which primarily affects the lungs and mediastinum, but may become disseminated presenting with hepatosplenomegaly, lymphadenopathy, ocular and skin disease, as well as enlarged adrenal glands.

- *Sporothrix*. Yeasts measure 3–5 μm in diameter, are round to cigar-shaped, and can show single or multiple buds. Rarely aseptate hyphae may be observed. The only active species is *Sporothrix schenckii*, which is the causative agent of sporotrichosis (rose-handler's disease). Initial cutaneous infections may spread via lymphatics and disseminate to joints, bones, and the central nervous system. Inhaled fungi can cause pulmonary sporotrichosis with lung nodules, cavities, fibrosis, and hilar lymphadenopathy.

- *Penicillium.* These fungi produce penicillin. *Penicillium marneffei* is the only known thermally dimorphic species. In cytology specimens, Penicillium present in the mold phase with septate and branched hyphae represent a contaminant. However, in immunosuppressed patients *P. marneffei* is an opportunistic infection that causes penicilliosis. There is a particularly high incidence of penicilliosis in AIDS patients from tropical Southeast Asia. Infection after inhalation spreads from the lungs to involve the hematopoietic system and skin. Yeast-like cells are present within macrophages and extracellularly. They are not true yeast cells, but rather arthroconidia. Intracellular "yeasts" measure 2–3 μm in diameter and are round to oval. Because they divide by binary fission, budding is not observed. The extracellular organisms tend to be more elongated, sometimes up to 13 μm, and can have "septae" (crosswalls from binary fission).

Pneumocystis

- *Pneumocystis jirovecii* (previously called *Pneumocystis carinii*) is a yeast-like fungus of the genus *Pneumocystis*, which is the causative organism of *Pneumocystis pneumonia* (or pneumocystosis, formerly referred to as PCP).
- The cysts often collapse forming crescent-shaped bodies.
- All stages of the life cycle are found within the lung alveoli. Once inhaled, unicellular trophozoites (1–4 μm, Giemsa positive) undergo binary fission to form a precyst (difficult to distinguish by light microscopy) and ultimately develop thick walled cysts (5–8 μm, GMS positive). Spores (eight) form within these cysts, which are eventually released on rupture of the cyst wall.
- This organism is often seen in the lungs of healthy individuals, but is an opportunistic pathogen in immunosuppressed people, especially those with AIDS.
- Extrapulmonary disease may be seen with advanced HIV infection presenting with involvement of the lymph nodes, spleen, liver, bone marrow, gastrointestinal tract, eyes, thyroid, adrenal glands, kidneys, and within macrophages in pleural effusions (Fig. 4.17).

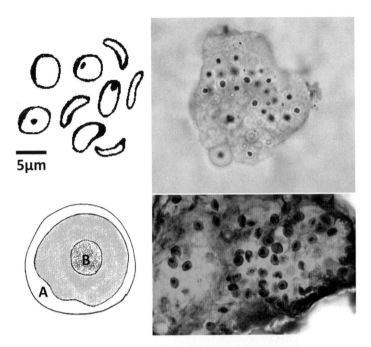

Fig. 4.17. *Pneumocystis.* (*Top left*) Diagram illustrating *P. jirovecii* thick walled cysts with a diameter (5 μm) approximately equal to that of a red-blood cell. When collapsed, some cysts assume a cup or crescent shape (crushed ping-pong ball appearance). (*Bottom left*) Schematic showing the ultrastructure of a cyst: The cyst wall is composed of an outer and inner layer that is focally thickened (**a**). The center of the cyst contains a tro-phozoite (**b**) with an ill-defined nucleus. (*Top right*) Bronchial washing from a patient showing a foamy alveolar cast containing *Pneumocystis* cysts (Pap stain, high magnification). (*Bottom right*) Localized areas of cyst wall thickening are best seen with a GMS stain also highlighting their central trophozoites (high magnification).

Dematiaceous Fungi

- The dematiaceous (naturally pigmented) group of fungi pro-duce melanin in their cell walls. As a result, fungal colonies are brown when cultured and in tissue samples fungal forms are characteristically pigmented. A Fontana-Masson stain can be used to confirm the presence of fungal melanin pigment.

- They cause several human infections including chromoblasto-mycosis (also called chromomycosis) and phaeohyphomycosis (or phaeomycotic cyst).

Dermatophytes

- Dermatophytes cause infections of the skin and hair (ringworm or tinea) as well as the nails (onychomycosis). The three genera that cause these diseases include *Microsporum*, *Epidermophyton*, and *Trichophyton*.
- A rapid scraping of the nail, skin, or scalp can be used to identify characteristic hyphae and sometimes spores associated with squamous cells or within broken hairshafts.

Hyalohyphomycoses

- Hyalohyphomycosis is the term used to group together invasive mycotic infections caused by hyaline septate hyphae. This includes species of *Aspergillus*, *Penicillium*, *Paecilomyces*, *Acremonium*, *Beauveria*, *Fusarium*, and *Scopulariopsis*. They may represent contamination or cause invasive disease in the immunosuppressed host.
- *Fusarium* hyphae are similar to those of *Aspergillus*, with septate hyphae that branch at acute and right angles. Sporulation may also occur in tissue with infection (fusariosis). Their macroconidia are crescent-shaped, orangeophilic, and septate structures that measure $80–120 \times 3–6$ μm in size.

Parasites

Protozoa

- Protozoa are unicellular motile organisms. They are traditionally divided according to their means of locomotion such as amebae, flagellates, and ciliates.
- Their life cycle often alternates between trophozoites (feeding–dividing stage) and cysts (dormant stage able to survive outside the host). Their characteristics (particularly the nuclei and cytoplasmic inclusions) help in species identification. Ingested cysts cause infection by excysting (releasing trophozoites) in the alimentary tract.

- *Amebae* (Sarcodina) pathogenic to humans include intestinal and free-living amebae.
  - *Intestinal amebae. Entamoeba histolytica* causes amebiasis that may manifest with dysentery, flask-shaped colon ulcers, a colonic ameboma, and possible extraintestinal abscesses that contain anchovy paste-like material within the liver, and infrequently spleen or brain. Several of the amebae such as *Entamoeba dispar* are harmless and some may be relatively common, such as *Entamoeba gingivalis* that is usually found in the mouth. Unlike other amebae, the cytoplasm of pathogenic *E. histolytica* contains ingested red blood cells.
  - *Free-living amebae.* These include *Acanthamoeba* spp., *Balamuthia mandrillaris*, and *Naegleria fowleri. Acanthamoeba* cause granulomatous amebic encephalitis (GAE), contact lens-associated *Acanthamoeba* keratitis, and skin lesions. *Balamuthia* also causes GAE. *N. fowleri* ("brain-eating" ameba) is associated with rapidly fatal primary amebic meningoencephalitis (PAM), most often seen in children swimming in fresh water ponds and rivers during which amebae enter the nasal passages and migrate to the brain via the olfactory nerve. These trophozoites can be seen in CSF specimens, but culture on nonnutrient agar plates seeded with *Escherichia coli* and/or a flagellation test is required for confirmation.
- *Flagellates* (Mastigophora) are organisms that have one or more flagella.
  - *Giardia.* There are approximately 40 species described, but the species that infects humans is *Giardia lamblia* (also called *G. intestinalis* or *G. duodenalis*). This parasite is the most common cause of protozoal gastroenteritis (giardiasis). Trophozoites (9–21 μm long and 5–15 μm wide) are kite (or pear)-shaped and have two nuclei, four pairs of flagella, and two central axonemes running down their middle. Their cysts (8–14×7–10 μm) seen in stool specimens are oval, thick walled, and contain four nuclei and multiple curved median bodies.
  - *Trichomonas.* There are several trichomonad species such as the intestinal *Pentatrichomonas hominis* which is a nonpathogenic organism. *Trichomonas vaginalis* is the anaerobic, flagellated protozoan that causes trichomoniasis (Fig. 4.18). Details of this sexually transmitted infection are covered in Chap. 5. Apart from urogenital infections, *T. vaginalis* has

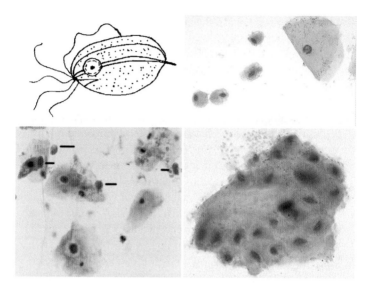

Fig. 4.18. *Trichomonas vaginalis*. (*Top left*) Illustration showing an oval organism (5–30 μm wide) that possess four anterior flagella, an undulating membrane, single large nucleus, and a central axostyle that projects from the posterior end. (*Bottom left*) *Trichomonas* organisms are shown in a sputum smear (indicated by *black bars*) with an oval shape and visible nuclei. Note that some of the squamous epithelial cells have typical perinuclear "trich halos" (Pap stain, high magnification) (image courtesy of Rafael Martinez Girón, Instituto de Piedras Blancas-Asturias, Spain). (*Right*) Several trichomonads are shown (*top right*) free in the background and (*bottom right*) attached to a squamous epithelial cell in a ThinPrep cervicovaginal Pap test (Pap stain, high magnification).

also been reported to cause pneumonia, bronchitis, and oral lesions. Pulmonary trichomoniasis is usually caused by aspirated *Trichomonas tenax* (mouth commensal) and less often *T. vaginalis* infection. An association between flagellated protozoa and asthma has been reported.

○ *Leishmania*. These parasites are acquired from the sandfly. Depending on the species, they may cause cutaneous (e.g., oriental sore), mucocutaneous (espundia or uta), or visceral (kala-azar) leishmaniasis (Table 4.7). There are two morphological forms: promastigote (with a flagellum) found in

TABLE 4.7. Comparison of skin, mucocutaneous, and visceral leishmaniasis.

| Type of infection | Pathogenic species | | Geographic location |
	Old world	New world	
Cutaneous	*L. major*	*L. mexicana*	South America, Middle
	L. tropica		East; North America
	L. aethiopica		(Southwestern USA)
Mucocutaneous	None	*L. braziliensis*	South America, China
Visceral	*L. donovani*	None	All continents except
	complex		Australia

the insect host and an amastigote (without flagella) present in the human host (Fig. 4.19). Diagnostic samples may be procured from skin lesions (cutaneous or mucocutaneous) or bone marrow aspirates (visceral). The morphologic hallmark is the presence of multiple small (2–5 µm) intracellular amastigotes within macrophages (Leishman-Donovan bodies). Amastigotes are spherical to ovoid in shape and have both a nucleus and ovoid or rod-shaped kinetoplast. The differential diagnosis for multiple small organisms within histiocytes includes *H. capsulatum* (with budding and only intracellular) and toxoplasmosis (more curved and mostly extracellular).

○ *Trypanosoma*. The major human diseases caused by trypanosomatids are African trypanosomiasis (sleeping sickness) caused by *Trypanosoma brucei* and American trypanosomiasis (Chagas disease) caused by *T. cruzi*. Trypomastigotes (30 µm in length) are usually found in peripheral blood. They have an undulating membrane, central nucleus, and kinetoplast at the anterior end.

• *Ciliates* (Ciliophora) include the parasitic species *Balantidium coli*, the only member of this phylum known to be pathogenic to humans. The trophozoite is relatively large (50–70 µm), has a ciliated surface, and contains a kidney bean-shaped macronucleolus. The cyst form may occasionally also have cilia. Cilicytophthoria may be sometimes mistaken for these ciliated organisms.

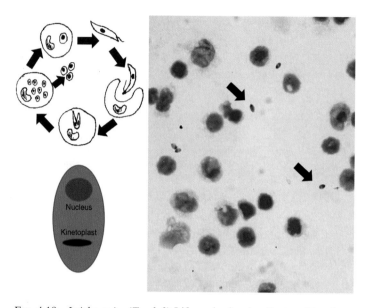

FIG. 4.19. *Leishmania.* (*Top left*) Life cycle showing the transition from a flagellated promastigote that occurs in the sandfly to small amastigotes without flagella in the human host: Promastigotes phagocytosed by macrophages multiply within these cells and disseminate when released. (*Bottom left*) Illustration of an ovoid amastigote shows a large nucleus and prominent rod-shaped kinetoplast. (*Right*) This FNA sample obtained from a Saudi Arabian child presenting with hepatosplenomegaly and lymphadenopathy from kala-azar shows few scattered amastigotes (*arrows*) among chronic inflammatory cells (Giemsa stain, high magnification).

Apicomplexans

- The Apicomplexa are a diverse group of protists that includes organisms such as coccidia (Sporozoa), *Plasmodium* spp. (cause malaria), and *Babesia* (cause babesiosis). Malaria and babesiosis are not discussed further because the diagnosis and speciation of these organisms primarily requires examination of peripheral blood smears and monoclonal antibody tests.
- Coccidian diseases include cryptosporidiosis (*Cryptosporidium* spp.), isosporiasis (*I. belli*), cyclosporiasis (*Cyclospora cayetanensis*), sarcocystis, and toxoplasmosis (*Toxoplasma gondii*).

The microsporidia, at one time a separate group (not coccidian), are now classified with the fungi.

- *Cryptosporidium* spp. *C. parvum* is the causative agent of cryptosporidiosis in humans and animals, a major cause of protracted diarrhea in patients with AIDS. Other species that cause human disease include *C. hominis*. These small (8–15 μm) oval parasites are identified within the brush border of the intestinal epithelium, and are discussed in the chapter on gastrointestinal infections. Ultrastructural studies have shown them to be intracellular but with an extracytoplasmic localization in enterocytes. Modified acid-fast thick-walled oocysts (4–6 μm) may be detected in stool samples. *Cryptosporidium* can disseminate beyond the intestine, especially in patients with AIDS, to involve the biliary tract, stomach, lungs, middle ear, and pancreas.

- *Microsporidia* include *Enterocytozoon bieneusi* and *Encephalitozoon intestinalis* (previously *Septata intestinalis*). Although these organisms are now considered fungi, parasitologists still maintain them in most books. In cytology specimens obtained from the small intestine, microsporidia appear as numerous small intracellular organisms within the apical portion of enterocytes. They stain well with Gram and silver stains (e.g., Warthin-Starry). Their spores (1–1.5 μm) may be found with a modified trichrome stain in stool samples as well as urine.

- *I. belli* and *Sarcocystis* infections very rarely have trophozoites that are detected. Their oocysts, however, may be seen when excreted in feces.

- *T. gondii* belongs to the genus *Toxoplasma*. Although infection can be acquired from the accidental ingestion of infective oocysts from cat feces (definitive host), most infections are acquired from eating infected rare or raw meats. Disease ranges from mild flu-like illness to fatal fetal infections. Latent infection may reactivate in immunosuppressed patients. Organisms may be found in samples from the brain, heart, eye, hematopoietic system, and lungs. Specimens may contain free (extracellular) tachyzoites which are small (3–5 μm), curved (banana-shaped) forms (Fig. 4.20). When parasites accumulate within macrophages (so-called "bag of parasites") they form a pseudocyst (parasitophorous vacuole) containing bradyzoites.

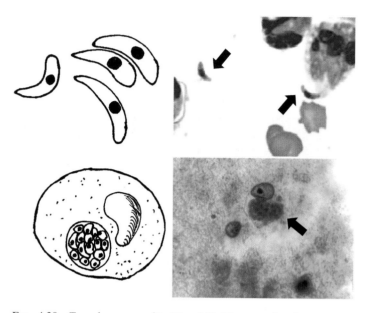

FIG. 4.20. *Toxoplasma gondii.* (*Top left*) Diagram showing crescent shaped tachyzoites (sometimes called endozoites) with a prominent nucleus: These trophozoites usually have a tapered anterior end and more blunt posterior end. (*Top right*) Free tachyzoites (*arrows*) can be seen in this BAL specimen (Giemsa stain, high magnification). (*Bottom left*) Diagram showing a macrophage with a pseudocyst containing multiple bradyzoites: Note that some of these microorganisms are still crescent shaped. The cysts are usually round in brain tissue, more elongated in muscle, and often very small and hard to identify in lung tissue. (*Bottom right*) An infected macrophage contains a cluster of bradyzoites (Pap stain, high magnification).

Helminths

- Helminths (parasitic worms) are categorized into three groups: cestodes (tapeworms), nematodes (roundworms), and trematodes (flukes) (Table 4.8). Flukes and tapeworms belong to the phylum platyhelminthes (flatworms).
- Clinical infection may be caused by adult worms, larvae, and/or eggs (Fig. 4.21). Infections are usually diagnosed by the characteristics of these different developmental stages.

TABLE 4.8. Common parasitic worms (helminthiases).

Helminth	Worm	Egg
Cestodes (tapeworms)		
Taenia saginata (beef tapeworm)	Scolex with four suckers and proglottids	Radially striated wall (30–40 μm)
Taenia solium (pork tapeworm)	Scolex with four suckers, hooklets and proglottids	Radially striated wall (30–40 μm)
Diphyllobothrium latum (fish tapeworm)	Scolex with wide proglottids	Oval with operculum and knob at either end (up to 60 μm)
Hymenolepis nana (dwarf tapeworm)	Very small (2–4 cm)	Wide inner and outer shells (30–47 μm), contain polar filaments
Echinococcus spp.	Protoscolices in hydatid cyst	Identical to *Taenia* (30–45 μm)
Nematodes (round worms)		
Trichuris trichiura (whipworm)	Whip-like anterior end	Barrel shaped with polar plugs at both ends (20–50 μm)
Ascaris lumbricoides	Large (up to 35 cm)	Rough mammillated shell (up to 75 μm)
Necator americanus (hookworm)	Mouthpart with cutting plates (adult worm)	Thin wall with internal morula (35–75 μm)
Ancyclostoma duodenale (hookworm)	Mouthpart with teeth (adult worm)	Thin wall with internal morula (35–75 μm)
Strongyloides stercoralis	Shorter buccal groove (mouth) than hookworm (rhabditiform larvae)	Identical to hookworm (35–75 μm), rarely seen
Enterobius vermicularis (pinworm)	Pointed pin-like tail	One side flattened (20–60 μm)
Trematodes (flukes)		
Fasciola hepatica (liver fluke)	Flat with cephalic cone	Very large (up to 150 μm), operculated (cannot distinguish from *Fasciolopsis buski*)
Fasciolopis buskii (intestinal fluke)	Flat with pointed head	Very large (up to 150 μm)
Clonorchis sinensis (liver fluke)	Flat with snout-like head	Small with shouldered operculum (12–20 μm)
Paragonimus westermani (lung fluke)	Flat ovoid worm	Oval with shouldered operculum (45–120 μm)

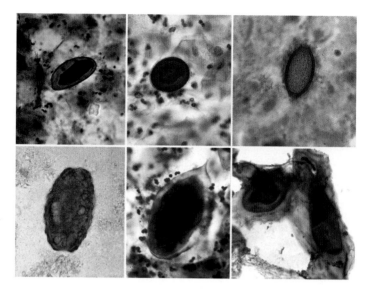

FIG. 4.21. Parasitic eggs are shown in cytologic preparations. (*Top left*) *Enterobius vermicularis.* (*Top middle*) *Taenia* (tapeworm). (*Top right*) *Trichuris trichiura.* (*Bottom left*) *Ascaris lumbricoides.* (*Bottom middle*) *Schistosoma haematobium.* (*Bottom right*) Pollen grain (belonging to the *Caryophyllaceae* family) that may be mistaken for *Toxocara* eggs (images courtesy of Dr. Pam Michelow, South Africa and Dr. Rafael Martinez Girón, Spain).

- The host response to these parasites includes eosinophilia, acute inflammation, and sometimes granulomas.
- *Cestodes.* These tapeworms usually parasitize humans after eating underprepared meat such as pork (*Taenia solium*), beef (*Taenia saginata*), or fish (*Diphyllobothrium* spp.), or food that is prepared in conditions of poor hygiene (e.g., *Echinococcus* spp.).
  - *Taenia.* Infection with the adult tapeworms occurs following ingestion of cysticerci in rare or poorly cooked beef or pork. *T. saginata* (beef) infection results in small intestinal infestation of adult worms (taeniasis). *T. solium* (pork) infection can also cause cysticercosis, as a result of the accidental ingestion of food or drink contaminated with tapeworm eggs from the feces. Cysticercosis is characterized by cysts

containing larvae located in several sites such as the brain (neurocysticercosis causes seizures), eye, as well as muscles and subcutaneous tissue (causes painful nodules). These cysts may cause eosinophilia, an inflammatory reaction and eventually they may calcify.

- ○ *Echinococcus*. Infection from the accidental ingestion of food or drink contaminated with tapeworm eggs results in hydatid disease, also known as echinococcosis. The larval cysts that develop can be found in virtually any site, grow slowly, and persist for many years until they cause symptoms or are discovered incidentally. Disruption of a cyst containing highly antigenic fluid may result in anaphylactic shock, and for this reason it has been recommended that they should not be biopsied. However, on the basis of published data adverse reactions are rare. Use of a fine gauge needle by a skilled operator is important to prevent fluid leakage during aspiration. There are three different forms of echinococcosis: cystic (unilocular) echinococcosis (caused by *Echinococcus granulosus*), alveolar (multilocular) echinococcosis (caused by *Echinococcus multilocularis*), and polycystic echinococcosis (caused by *Echinococcus vogeli* and rarely *Echinococcus oligarthus*). A hydatid cyst contains a thick outer (acellular) wall and thin inner germinal epithelium. Alveolar and polycystic echinococcosis cysts usually have multiple compartments. Hydatid cysts may contain several liters of fluid, daughter cysts, and hydatid sand (Fig. 4.22). Aspirated hydatid sand contains protoscolices (future scolices) and free hooklets. Viable protoscolices typically show a row of parallel hooklets whereas dead ones contain haphazardly attached hooklets.
- *Nematodes.* There are several roundworms (Table 4.7), but those likely to be seen in cytology specimens are *Enterobius vermicularis*, *Strongyloides stercoralis*, and the microfilariae.
  - ○ *E. vermicularis* (pinworm, also known as the threadworm in the United Kingdom) causes intestinal infestation (enterobiasis). The adult female worm migrates out onto the perianal area at night, and once exposed to oxygen she lays her eggs. This causes perianal pruritis and possibly vaginitis. Occasionally subcutaneous perineal nodules may develop. In such cases, Pap tests may contain an adult worm and/or eggs. The worm has a

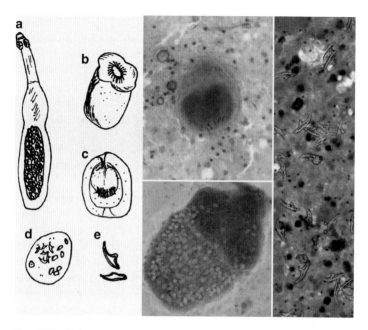

FIG. 4.22. *Echinococcus granulosus.* (*Left*) (**a**) Diagram showing an adult tapeworm that consists of a scolex (head) and three proglottids. The scolex has suckers and a crown of hooklets (adult worm not found in humans). Components of hydatid sand are illustrated including (**b**) evaginated protoscolex (usually occurs when placed into saline), (**c**) invaginated protoscolex with hooklets, (**d**) degenerated scolex with calcareous corpuscles, and (**e**) individual rostellar hooklets. (*Top middle*) Invaginated protoscolex (Pap stain, high magnification). (*Bottom middle*) Evaginated protoscolex (Pap stain, high magnification). (*Far right*) Free sickle shaped hooklets (MGG stain, high magnification) (cytology images courtesy of Pam Michelow and Dr. Pawel Schubert, South Africa).

characteristic pointed tail (Fig. 4.23). Their eggs are colorless, oval, thin walled, and flattened on one side,

○ *S. stercoralis.* This worm causes strongyloidiasis. After penetrating the skin, infective larvae pass through the lung (Loeffler syndrome). They are then coughed or swallowed and infest the duodenum. Here new autoinfective larvae may develop (autoinfection) leading to chronic infection. In immunocompromised patients, larvae may penetrate the intestinal wall

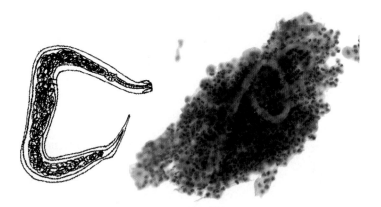

FIG. 4.23. *E. vermicularis* (pinworm). (*Left*) Diagram showing an adult female worm (8–33 mm long × 0.3–0.5 mm wide) that has a cephalic inflation and characteristic long, pointed tail. (*Right*) Pinworm shown among neutrophils in a Pap test. If the morphology of the worm is not definitive, then a diagnosis reporting a worm-like structure suggestive of pinworm is appropriate (Pap stain, intermediate magnification).

and disseminate via the bloodstream (called hyperinfection). Disseminated strongyloidiasis has a very high mortality rate. Cytology specimens including gastrointestinal and pulmonary (e.g., sputum) samples may contain larvae, either rhabditiform (noninfective) or filariform (infective) types.

○ *Filariae.* These roundworms cause filariasis. Microfilariae that may be periodically found in the peripheral blood include *Wuchereria bancrofti*, *Brugia malayi*, and *Loa loa*. *W. bancrofti* and *B. malayi* infest lymphatics leading to lymphadentitis and chronic lymphedema (elephantiasis). *L. loa* resides in subcutaneous tissue and the conjunctiva. Certain microfilariae such as *Mansonella perstans*, *Onchocerca volvulus*, *Dracunculus medinensis*, and *Dirofilaria immitis* are not readily found in blood smears. *M. perstans* inhabits body cavities such as the peritoneum and pleura (serous cavity filariasis). *O. volvulus* infects subcutaneous tissue forming nodules and the conjunctivae causing blindness (onchocerciasis or river blindness). *D. immitis* (dog heartworm) causes granulomatous nodules in the lung. Microfilariae are the diagnostic forms of infection. The presence or absence of a sheath and the pattern of nuclei in their tail are the main features used to distinguish the various species. Occult filariasis has been diagnosed by many bloody FNA procedures containing microfilariae, worms, or even eggs. Filarial morphology is best appreciated with a Giemsa stain. The background tissue response in cytology aspirates may include eosinophils, neutrophils, chronic inflammation, and even granulomas.

- *Trematodes.* The flukes are oval or worm-like helminthes that are parasites of molluscs and vertebrates. The liver flukes include *Fasciola hepatica* and *Clonorchis sinensis* that result in infestation of the bile ducts and subsequent biliary fibrosis. Infection with *C. sinensis* is a risk factor for cholangiocarcinoma. *Fasciolopis buskii* is an intestinal fluke that infests both the bile ducts and duodenum. *Paragonimus westermani*, the lung fluke, causes lung infestation with pulmonitis. Also included are the schistosomes (blood flukes).

  ○ *Schistosomes.* Infection by these trematodes causes schistosomiasis (bilharzia). There are three human schistosome pathogens: *Schistosoma mansoni* from Africa (Nile delta) which causes intestinal schistosomiasis, *S. haematobium* from Africa and the Middle East that infests the urinary bladder, and *S. japonicum* from China and Southeast Asia that primarily involves the liver. *S. haematobium* infection can lead to squamous cell carcinoma of the bladder. Microscopic identification of eggs in stool or urine specimens, as well as tissue biopsies, can provide a rapid diagnosis. The spines present on schistosome eggs help distinguish these different species. The egg of *S. haematobium* (oval) has a terminal spine, *S. mansoni* (oval) has a lateral spine, and *S. japonicum* (round) has a small knob-like lateral spine.

Algae

- Algae are ubiquitous and include a diverse group of simple organisms that range from unicellular to multicellular forms. The main algal groups include the cyanobacteria, green algae, and red algae (e.g., dinoflagellates).
- Most algae present in cytology samples are from contamination, discussed in greater detail in Chap. 15.

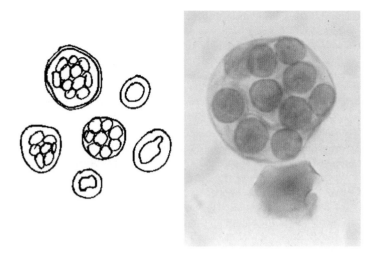

FIG. 4.24. *Prototheca.* (*Left*) Diagram of protothecae demonstrating variable morula formation: (*Right*) A sporangium of *P. wickerhamii* is shown in which endospores have a moruloid (daisy-like) pattern (Pap stain, high magnification) (image courtesy of Rafael Martinez Girón, Instituto de Piedras Blancas-Asturias, Spain).

- *Prototheca* is a genus of algae that lacks chlorophyll that causes the disease protothecosis. Most human cases are caused by *P. wickerhamii.* Infection may cause skin lesions or disseminated and systemic disease. Organisms may be seen within macrophages or extracellularly. They form spherical sporangia that range in size from 3 to 10 μm, have thick walls, and show no budding. These morular forms often contain endospores arranged symmetrically, typically in a daisy-like pattern (Fig. 4.24). They stain with most stains including H&E, PAS, and GMS stains.

Suggested Reading

Ash LR, Orihel TC. Ash & Orihel's atlas of human parasitology. 5th ed. Chicago: American Society for Clinical Pathology Press; 2007.

Bayón MN, Drut R. Cytologic diagnosis of adenovirus bronchopneumonia. Acta Cytol. 1991;35:181–2.

Bhambhani S, Kashyap V. Amoebiasis: diagnosis by aspiration and exfoliative cytology. Cytopathology. 2001;12:329–33.

Garcia LS. Diagnostic medical parasitology. 5th ed. Washington: ASM Press; 2007.

Gupta N, Arora SK, Rajwanshi A, Nijhawan R, Srinivasan R. Histoplasmosis: cytodiagnosis and review of literature with special emphasis on differential diagnosis on cytomorphology. Cytopathology. 2010;21:240–4.

Kumar B, Karki S, Yadava SK. Role of fine needle aspiration cytology in diagnosis of filarial infestation. Diagn Cytopathol. 2011;39:8–12.

Kumar PV, Omrani GH, Saberfirouzi M, Arshadi C, Arjmand F, Parhizgar A. Kala-azar: liver fine needle aspiration findings in 23 cases presenting with a fever of unknown origin. Acta Cytol. 1996;40:263–8.

Larone DH. Medically important fungi. A guide to identification. 3rd ed. Washington: ASM Press; 1995.

Onuma K, Crespo MM, Dauber JH, Rubin JT, Sudilovsky D. Disseminated nocardiosis diagnosed by fine needle aspiration biopsy: quick and accurate diagnostic approach. Diagn Cytopathol. 2006;34:768–71.

Sangoi AR, Rogers WM, Longacre TA, Montoya JG, Baron EJ, Banaei N. Challenges and pitfalls of morphologic identification of fungal infections in histologic and cytologic specimens: a ten-year retrospective review at a single institution. Am J Clin Pathol. 2009;131:364–75.

Takeuchi T, Fujii A, Okumiya T, Watabe S, Ishikawa T, Umeda A, et al. The study of cytopathological aspects induced by human cytomegalovirus infection. Diagn Cytopathol. 2004;31:289–93.

Williamson JD, Silverman JF, Mallak CT, Christie JD. Atypial cytomorphologic appearance of *Cryptococcus neoformans*: a report of five cases. Acta Cytol. 1996;40:363–70.

5
Gynecological Infections

**Liron Pantanowitz[1], R. Marshall Austin[2],
and Pam Michelow[3]**

[1]Department of Pathology, University of Pittsburgh Medical Center,
5150 Centre Avenue, Suite 201, Pittsburgh, PA 15232, USA

[2]Department of Pathology, Magee-Women's Hospital of University of
Pittsburgh Medical Center, 300 Halket Street, Pittsburgh, PA 15213, USA

[3]Cytology Unit, Department of Anatomical Pathology, University of the
Witwatersrand and National Health Laboratory Service, Johannesburg,
Gauteng, South Africa

Infections of the female genital tract, some of which are sexually
transmitted diseases (STDs), are common and hence an important cause of morbidity and mortality for women worldwide
(Table 5.1). Women with infections of the lower genital tract may
be asymptomatic or present with vaginal discharge, bleeding,
dysuria, dyspareunia, abdominal pain, fever, malaise or manifest
with more severe systemic illness. Upper genital tract infections
often arise from ascending lower genital tract disease and their
sequelae may be serious including peritonitis, septicemia, infertility, and ectopic pregnancy. Although Pap tests are primarily
used for the diagnosis of epithelial abnormalities, many infections can be diagnosed on cervical cytology. Women of all ages
infected with microbial agents have higher rates of atypical cervical epithelial cells, including atypical squamous cells of unde-
termined significance (ASCUS) and squamous intraepithelial
lesions (SIL). This may be attributed in part to a greater predis-
position to human papillomavirus (HPV) infection, and hence the
development of cervical neoplasia in these women. This chapter
covers common and rare infections likely to be encountered on a
cervicovaginal Pap test. Infections of the vulva are covered in the
chapter with skin infections.

L. Pantanowitz et al., *Cytopathology of Infectious Diseases*,
Essentials in Cytopathology 17, DOI 10.1007/978-1-4614-0242-8_5,
© Springer Science+Business Media, LLC 2011

TABLE 5.1. Infections of the female genital tract.

Anatomical location	Infection	Microorganisms
Vulva	Viral	Human papillomavirus (HPV), Herpes simplex virus (HSV type I and II), *Molluscum contagiosum*, CMV, EBV
	Bacterial	*Treponema pallidum* (chancre, condyloma lata), *Corynebacterium minutissimum* (erthrasma), *Haemophilus ducreyi* (chancroid), *Chlamydia trachomatis* (granuloma inguinale), tuberculosis, *Bartonella henselae* (bacillary angiomatosis)
	Fungal	*Candida, Histoplasma capsulatum, Cryptococcus neoformans*, dermatophytes
	Parasites	*Enterobius vermicularis, Schistosoma haematobium*
	Infestation	*Phthirus pubis* (pubic lice), *Sarcoptes scabiei* (scabies), myiasis
Cervix and vagina	Viral	HPV, HSV, CMV
	Bacterial	*Neisseria gonorrheae, Gardnerella vaginalis, Leptothrix, C. trachomatis, Actinomyces israelii*, Mycobacterial infection, *Treponema pallidum* (syphilis), malakoplakia
	Fungal	*Candida* spp., *Fusarium, Aspergillus, Cryptococcus, Histoplasmosis, Blastomyces, Coccidioides, Paracoccidioides*
	Parasites	*Trichomonas vaginalis*, Amebiasis, *S. haematobium, E. vermuclaris, Echinococcus*, Filaria, Trypanosomes (Chagas disease), *Strongyloides, Taenia, Trichuris trichiura, Ascaris lumbricoides*
Upper genital tract	Salpingitis, pelvic inflammatory disease (PID), tubo-ovarian abscess, endometritis	*N. gonorrheae, C. trachomatis, Prevotella* spp., *Peptostreptococcus, Bacteroides, Escherichia coli, Haemophilus influenza*, group B streptococci, *Actinmycosis, Mycoplasma genitalium, Mycobacterium tuberculosis, Cryptococcus, Blastomyces, Schistosoma, Enterobius, Toxoplasma gondii, Entamoeba histolytica*, malakoplakia

Inflammatory Changes

- *Acute inflammation.* Various infectious agents may cause an acute inflammatory infiltrate comprised of abundant neutrophils. However, the presence of neutrophils alone in Pap tests does not necessarily indicate infection. If inflammatory changes are marked and obscure the epithelial cells, the specimen may be unsatisfactory for interpretation.
- *Follicular (lymphocytic) cervicitis.* The formation of reactive lymphoid follicles in the subepithelium of the cervix may occasionally be seen on a Pap test. It is more common in women who have an atrophic cervix as the epithelium is thin, allowing the underlying stroma to be sampled. Mature and immature lymphoid cells are noted in addition to a few plasma cells and tingible-body macrophages. Follicular cervicitis is associated more often with *Chlaymida trachomatis* than other infections of the cervix. The differential diagnosis includes high-grade squamous intraepithelial lesion (HSIL), endometrial cells, and non-Hodgkin lymphoma.
- *Epithelial change.* Epithelial cells may show various degrees of inflammatory and reparative change including cytoplasmic vacuolization, polychromasia, perinuclear halos, nuclear enlargement, anisonucleosis, prominent nucleoli, mitoses, as well as bi- and multinucleation. Reparative change can be distinguished from more severe (dysplastic or neoplastic) lesions by the fact that cells showing repair show good cohesion, flat monolayer sheets have a streaming appearance, maintain polarity, and while they may have prominent nucleoli their chromatin is evenly distributed within round, smooth, nuclear membranes (Fig. 5.1).

Normal Flora

Microbiology

- Lactobacillus (lactobacilli, formerly called Dőderlein bacilli) are Gram-positive, anaerobic, lactic acid producing bacteria normally found within the vagina (i.e., normal flora). Lactobacilli such as *Lactobacillus acidophilus* maintain the acid vaginal pH by converting cytoplasmic glycogen within intermediate

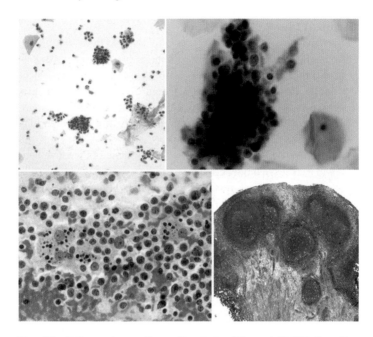

FIG. 5.1. Inflammatory cells on Pap tests. (*Upper left*) ThinPrep Pap test showing several pus balls characteristic of trichomoniasis (Pap stain, intermediate magnification). (*Bottom left*) Follicular cervicitis seen on a conventional Pap smear consists of polymorphous lymphocytes and several tingible-body macrophages (Pap stain, high magnification). (*Upper right*) This ThinPrep Pap test from a postmenopausal women with follicular cervicitis shows a loose aggregate of lymphocytes in various stages of maturation together with a tingible-body macrophage (Pap stain, high magnification). (*Bottom right*) Cervix biopsy of follicular cervicitis showing prominent subepithelial reactive lymphoid follicles with germinal centers (H&E stain, low magnification; courtesy of Dr. Christopher Otis, Tufts University School of Medicine, USA).

epithelial cells into lactic acid via proteolytic destruction (cytolysis). This renders the vaginal environment hostile for unwanted organisms. The normal vaginal flora does not extend up into the sterile endometrium.

- Loss of lactobacilli plays a role in the development of bacterial vaginosis (BV) (so-called shift in flora) (Fig. 5.2).

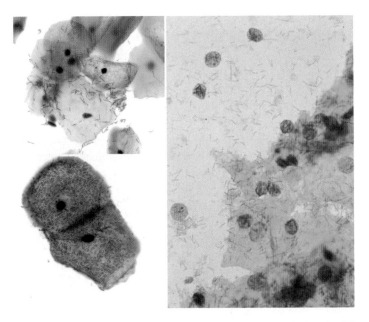

FIG. 5.2. Lactobacilli (high magnification images). (*Top left*) Thin bacilli forming part of the normal flora are shown in this routine Pap test (Pap stain, ThinPrep). (*Bottom left*) Multiple lactobacilli are seen coating these two squamous epithelial cells, not to be confused with clue cells (Pap stain). (*Right*) Long slender lactobacilli are seen associated with cytolysis and bare nuclei (Pap stain, conventional smear).

Clinical Features

- Common and normal finding in Pap tests. More common in the second half of the menstrual cycle, during pregnancy, and in patients with diabetes mellitus.
- Decreased with BV.

Cytomorphologic Features

- Slender, rod-like bacilli can be seen lying in the background and/or over the surface of cells.

- Cytolysis results in free-lying bare nuclei and cellular debris of intermediate squames mixed with lactobacilli.

Diagnostic Note

- Lactobacilli can form long chains, not to be confused with fungal hyphae.
- Free-lying nuclei following cytolysis should be distinguished from trichomonads, HSIL, endometrial cells, follicular cervicitis, small cell carcinoma, and lymphoma.
- Other sources of debris include atrophy and tumor diathesis.
- Diagnostic ancillary tests are not required.

Leptothrix vaginalis

Microbiology

- *Leptothrix* are long Gram positive anaerobic bacteria.
- They are often associated with trichomonas infection ("spaghetti and meatballs").

Clinical Features

- These bacteria are usually non-pathogenic on their own.

Cytomorphologic Features

- Long filamentous bacteria are seen that do not form spores.

Diagnostic Note

- Compared to *Actinomyces*, *Leptothrix* are much less densely clustered and are not associated with companion bacteria.
- The finding of *Leptothrix* should encourage a thorough investigation of the specimen for associated *Trichomonas*.
- Ancillary tests are not required (Fig. 5.3).

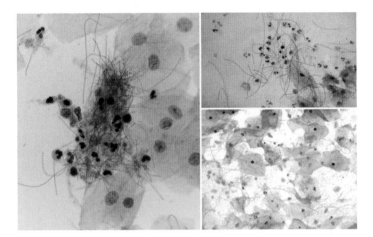

FIG. 5.3. *Leptothrix* (high magnification images). (*Left*) *Leptothrix* are shown in this ThinPrep Pap test caught up with a few inflammatory cells (Pap stain). (*Top right*) Long filamentous bacteria consistent with *Leptothrix* are shown in a conventional Pap smear (Pap stain). (*Bottom right*) *Leptothrix* are shown associated with several scattered trichomonads (Pap stain).

Viral Infections

Human Papillomavirus (HPV)

Microbiology

- Papillomaviruses are DNA viruses that belong to the family Papoviridae. They selectively infect skin and mucous membranes. Genital HPV infection is almost exclusively sexually transmitted.
- HPV is the dominant causative agent in anogenital warts, SILs, and cervical carcinoma. Most HPV infections regress spontaneously. Persistence of oncogenic HPV infection is required for progression to carcinoma.
- There are over 100 different types of HPV. The types infecting the female genital tract are divided into low- and high-risk (HR). Low-risk (LR) HPVs are associated with condylomata acuminata and LSIL, while the intermediate and HR oncogenic HPV types are associated with LSIL, HSIL, and carcinoma.

- LR HPV types include HPV 6, 11, 42–44, 53–55, 62, 66, and 70.
- Intermediate-risk HPV types include 31, 33, 35, 39, 51, 52, 54, 58, 59, 61, and 66–68.
- HR HPV types include HPV 16, 18, 45, and 56.

- HPV 16 accounts for most HPV-related vulvar cancers. HPV 18 accounts for a large proportion of cervical adenocarcinoma and adenosquamous carcinoma.
- Impaired patient immunity from HIV infection, transplantation, or immunosuppressive drugs increases HPV persistence and hence the development of CIN and cervical cancer.

Clinical Features

- Initial infection is often asymptomatic.
- *Condyloma accuminatum* (anogenital warts). In women, these lesions usually initially involve the posterior introitus and nearby labia. They can extend to other parts of the vulva, vagina, and cervix. They can occur singly or in clusters and appear as flesh-colored or pink polypoid or flat lesions.
- *SIL.* SIL are asymptomatic. Mucosal lesions can be identified after application of acetic acid and are best visualized on colposcopy. The older concept that SIL progress from low-grade (LSIL) to high-grade (HSIL) lesions has now been replaced by the concept that LSIL and many CIN2 lesions are nonprogressive lesions and that true precancerous lesions (CIN3) develop de novo in a subset of patients with persistent high-risk HPV infection.
- *Cervical carcinoma.* Early invasive carcinoma may be asymptomatic. Later stages present with watery or blood-stained discharge, postcoital bleeding, or spontaneous, irregular vaginal bleeding but may present with advanced local disease or metastases. In such cases the cervix may appear irregular, raised, reddened, or ulcerated.

Cytomorphologic Features

- HPV cytopathic effect includes koilocytosis and dyskeratosis (atypical parakeratosis). In LSIL, koilocytosis is seen in intermediate or superficial squamous cells (koilocytes) and includes

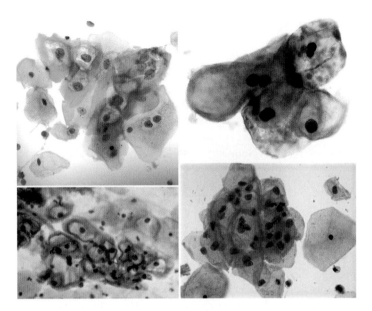

Fig. 5.4. Koilocytosis (high magnification images). (*Upper left*) Koilocytes in a ThinPrep Pap test with LSIL. Note the striking nuclear abnormalities in the koilocytes compared to the adjacent normal appearing squamous cells (Pap stain). (*Bottom left*) A group of koilocytes with prominent perinuclear halos and enlarged nuclei are shown in a conventional Pap smear (Pap stain). (*Upper right*) Polka dot cells with intracytoplasmic eosinophilic hyaline globules (Pap stain). These cells more than likely represent a degenerative process than an HPV effect associated with condylomas as previously suggested. (*Bottom right*) Glycogenated squamous cells mimicking koilocytes (Pap stain).

nuclear enlargement (3–4 times increase in size), hyperchromasia with coarse granular to smudgy chromatin, and nuclear irregularity (Fig. 5.4). Bi- and multinucleation is frequently seen, but without molding of nuclei. Nucleoli are inconspicuous. The perinuclear halo in LSIL cells tends to be well-defined.

- HSIL, squamous cell carcinoma, and adenocarcinoma cells related to HPV infection do not exhibit characteristic viral changes. HSIL and squamous cell carcinoma may be keratinizing or nonkeratinizing (Fig. 5.5).

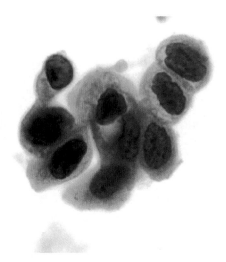

FIG. 5.5. High-grade squamous intraepithelial lesion (HSIL). This group of dysplastic squamous cells has scant cytoplasm, irregular nuclear contours, and hyperchromatic nuclei (Pap stain, high magnification).

Diagnostic Note

- Detectable HPV does not always imply the presence of clinical disease.
- Squamous cells showing inflammatory changes may demonstrate small clearings around the nucleus (perinuclear halo) and enlarged nuclei. However, the nuclei in such reactive cells tend to be more round and vesicular than in true koilocytes.
- Navicular cells are boat-shaped squamous cells with an intracytoplasmic vacuole containing glycogen. Empty vacuoles may resemble the halo seen in koilocytes, but the associated nuclear changes are not seen and the nucleus is usually eccentric.
- ASC-US is the term reserved for cells that are suggestive of, but not diagnostic of, koilocytes.
- Parakeratosis refers to small keratinized squames with pyknotic nuclei. These cells and nuclei are much smaller than koilocytes.

Ancillary Tests

- Several FDA-approved options exist for HPV testing using cervicovaginal Pap test material. Several non-FDA-approved options are also available for routine use, but caution must be exercised as clinical validation of routine non-FDA-approved routine HPV tests and for more novel HPV tests is very limited.
  - Direct probe methods include Southern, dot blot, and in situ hybridization.
  - Signal amplification systems include hybrid capture like the FDA-approved automated, qualitative Hybrid Capture 2 (HC2) assay (Qiagen, Netherlands) that detects intermediate and HR HPV types. The Cervista High Risk HPV test (Hologic Corp, Marlborough, MA, USA) is also FDA approved in the USA.
  - Emerging test methods like microarrays and genotype assays.
- Serology (e.g., anti-HPV L1 antibody) and HPV viral load have been used to predict the development of CIN lesions (prognostic markers).
- Immunocytochemistry for surrogate biomarkers of HPV infection in dysplastic and cancer cells.
  - p16^{INK4a} has high specificity for HPV transformed cells, but may also stain nondysplastic cells (e.g., tubal metaplasia, endometrial glandular cells) and, depending on the antibody clone, some microorganisms such as trichomonads (Fig. 5.6).
  - Others including ProExC and Ki-67.

Herpes Simplex Virus (HSV)

Microbiology

- Herpes simplex virus (HSV) is a double-stranded DNA virus that belongs to the Herpesviridae family. Like other herpes viruses, HSV can remain latent and re-activate. There is no difference between the cytology of primary and secondary genital herpesvirus infection.
- HSV include HSV-1 that primarily infects the oral cavity, eye, central nervous system, and HSV-2 which infects the genital tract. However, HSV-1 infection of the anogenital tract is not

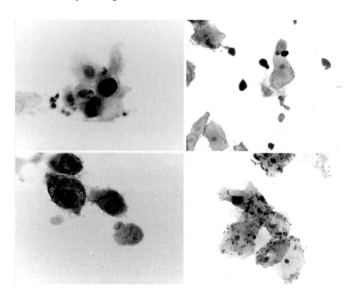

FIG. 5.6. p16 immunocytochemistry (high magnification images). Thin-Prep Pap test with (*upper left*) a group of HSIL cells (*top left*, Pap stain) that shows nuclear and cytoplasmic immunoreactivity for p16 (*bottom left*). Nonspecific staining with p16 (clone G175-405) is demonstrated with (*upper right*) *Trichomonas* trophozoites and (*bottom right*) lactobacilli.

uncommon. The cytopathic effect due to HSV-1 and HSV-2 is identical. Recurrent genital infection is mainly due to HSV-2 (Fig. 5.7).

Clinical Features

- The first episode of genital herpes usually produces fever, headache, and malaise. Genital symptoms include pain, dysuria, vaginal discharge, tender inguinal lymphadenopathy, and varying stages of vesicles, pustules, and/or ulcers on an erythematous base. Recurrent genital herpes is usually milder and shorter than the first episode. Patients may remain asymptomatic, but infectious. Complications of infection include local spread, extragenital lesions, superinfection, and CNS disease (e.g., meningitis).
- Transmission to neonates during vaginal delivery may cause serious disseminated infection. A Cesarean section may therefore

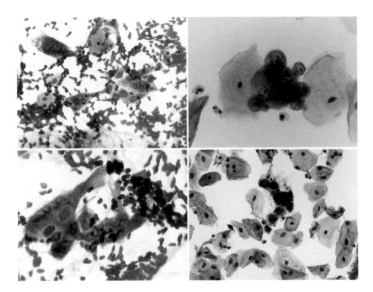

FIG. 5.7. Herpes (high magnification images). (*Upper left*) Conventional Pap smear in a 16-year-old female showing many squamous cells with Cowdry type B inclusions including nuclear molding, chromatin margination, ground glass nuclei, and (*bottom left*) prominent multinucleation (Pap stain). (*Upper right*) Squamous cells in a ThinPrep Pap test with eosinophilic intranuclear inclusions typical of Cowdry type A inclusions (Pap stain). (*Bottom right*) Single dark stained cells with herpetic changes may mimic HSIL (ThinPrep, Pap stain). Processing of liquid-based specimens often causes increased numbers of isolated herpetic cells.

be preferentially performed if a mother about to deliver has active genital herpes.

Cytomorphologic Features

- Infected squamous cells may show Cowdry type A inclusions (eosinophilic intranuclear inclusions surrounded by a clear zone) and/or Cowdry type B inclusions (nuclei molded rather than overlapped, chromatin margination beneath the nuclear membrane imparting a ground glass appearance to the nucleus, and multinucleation).
- A background acute inflammatory cell infiltrate may be marked.

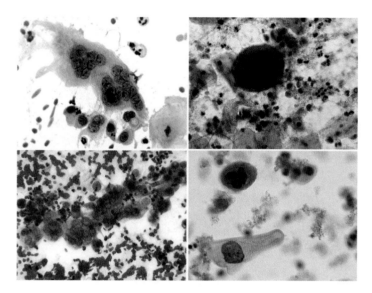

FIG. 5.8. Mimics of Herpes (high magnification images). (*Upper left*) Enlarged reactive multinucleated endocervical cell. Note the presence of small nucleoli, a feature not seen in herpes (Pap stain). (*Bottom left*) Conventional Pap smear showing neoplastic cells in a case of endocervical adenocarcinoma. Pale malignant nuclei demonstrate overlapping instead of molding (Pap stain). (*Upper right*) A syncytiotrophoblast is shown in this Pap test from a patient with a threatened abortion. The nuclei of this cell are overlapped and have coarse chromatin. The background in this case contains trichomonads and a few *Leptothrix* (Pap stain). (*Bottom right*) In this Pap test from a patient with squamous cell carcinoma of the cervix the eosinophilic degenerated tumor cell shows multinucleation and clearing of the chromatin (Pap stain).

Diagnostic Note

- The Bethesda system interpretation is "Cellular changes consistent with herpes simplex virus."
- Reactive endocervical cells with multinucleation may mimic herpetic change. Neoplastic cells with multinucleation and/or pale vesicular nuclei may also mimic herpes (Fig. 5.8). Other mimics of herpes may include reactive/repair change, air-drying artifact, cell distortion, and poor cell preservation.
- The differential diagnosis for large multinucleated cells on a Pap test includes giant cell macrophages (granulomatous

inflammation, postpartum, after surgery), syncytiotrophoblast, radiation or chemotherapy effect, macrocyte of LSIL, neoplasia (e.g., choriocarcinoma, MMMT), and B12 or folate deficiency.

- The diagnosis of herpes infection on a Pap test in a pregnant patient close to delivery should be handled precipitously, which may warrant a call to their healthcare provider so that appropriate measures can be taken if necessary to avoid vertical transmission of HSV to the neonate.

Ancillary Tests

- Immunocytochemistry
- HSV DNA detection by PCR or ISH
- Serology (type-specific assays)
- Viral culture

Cytomegalovirus (CMV)

- Detection of cytomegalovirus (CMV) cytopathic effect in cervical Pap tests or biopsy is rare. CMV typically involves endocervical glandular epithelium, and less commonly squamous cells.
- The characteristic viral cytopathic change includes cytomegaly with an intranuclear inclusion surrounded by a halo ("owl's-eye"), which can be confirmed using immunocytochemistry if necessary.

Molluscum contagiosum (Fig. 5.9)

Microbiology

- This is a contagious viral infection caused by a DNA poxvirus. Of the four types of MCV, MCV-2 is often sexually transmitted.

Clinical Features

- Infection with M. contagiosum is common in the pubic area, and infrequently affects the vagina and cervix.
- Infection occurs after trauma to the skin or mucosa. Persistent and disseminated infection occurs in immunosuppressed patients like those with HIV coinfection.

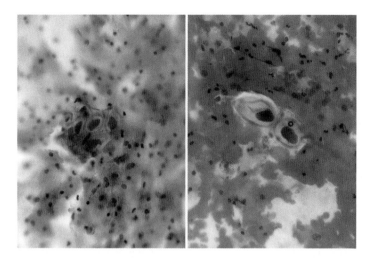

Fɪɢ. 5.9. *Molluscum contagiosum.* Conventional Pap smear showing (*left*) a group and (*right*) single infected squamous cells with typical molluscum bodies. The bloody background has only few inflammatory cells (Pap stain, high magnification).

- Lesions may be variable in number and cutaneous dome-shaped papules and nodules may appear umbilicated.

Cytomorphologic Features

- Infected squamous cells show characteristic cytoplasmic inclusions called molluscum bodies. Inclusions may be eosinophilic or basophilic in appearance. The nuclei of infected cells are pushed to the periphery and therefore often inconspicuous.
- There is usually little or no background inflammation.

Diagnostic Note

- Molluscum bodies may mimic CMV intranuclear inclusions.
- As this viral infection is recognized as being an STD, slides should be carefully screened for the presence of other STDs.
- Ancillary studies may include a confirmatory biopsy, PCR, and electron microscopy.

Bacterial Infections

Bacterial Vaginosis

Microbiology

- BV is a polymicrobial infection associated with overgrowth of several anaerobic bacteria including mainly *Gardnerella vaginalis*, but also *Mobiluncus* spp., *Mycoplasma hominis*, *Prevotella* spp., *Bacteroides* spp., *Ureaplasma* spp., and *Peptostreptococcus* spp.
- These bacteria overgrow the lactobacilli, raising the vaginal pH and produce malodorous amines.
- BV is a risk factor for HPV infection acquisition. Women with HPV-induced abnormalities in Pap tests have a higher proportion of clue cells than their HPV-negative counterparts. The exact association between BV and CIN development is unclear (Fig. 5.10).

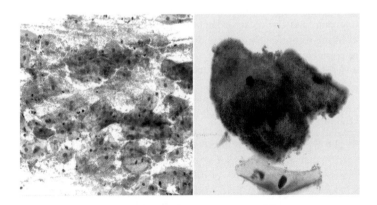

FIG. 5.10.   Shift in vaginal flora. (*Left*) Conventional Pap smear showing altered vaginal flora. The large number of bacteria in this specimen imparts a *gray color* to the background smear (Pap stain, intermediate magnification). (*Right*) Clue cells are shown with squamous cells coated by many small coccobacillary bacteria (Pap stain, ThinPrep, high magnification).

Clinical Features

- Infection in women of any age can be asymptomatic or patients may present with a vaginal discharge or offensive (fishy) odor. Clinical (Amsel) criteria for the diagnosis include vaginal pH ≥ 4.7, homogeneous milk-like discharge, amine "fishy" odor, and clue cells in a wet mount.
- Gynecologic sequelae of BV may include increased frequency of pelvic inflammatory disease (PID) and posthysterectomy vaginal cuff cellulitis.
- In pregnant women, BV can result in preterm labor, chorioamnionitis, premature rupture of membranes, postpartum endometritis, and low birth weight in newborns.

Cytomorphologic Features

- The characteristic finding is the presence of coccobacilli coating squamous cells imparting a grainy look to the cell (so-called "clue cells"). The adherence pattern of these bacteria to squamous cells between conventional smears and liquid-based Pap tests is similar.
- Coccobacilli may also form a film pattern in the background, best seen in conventional smears. In liquid samples, the background may be clean or bacteria are more clumped.
- Many erythrocytes may be observed attached to clue cells.
- Lactobacilli are absent.
- Background inflammation is variable but usually sparse.
- Epithelial cells may have inflammatory and reactive changes.

Diagnostic Note

- The Bethesda system interpretation is "shift in flora suggestive of bacterial vaginosis." The reason is that the detection of coccobacilli does not necessarily indicate clinical infection of BV.
- The presence of at least 20% clue cells on a cervical Pap test appears to be an accurate and reproducible criterion for the diagnosis of BV.

Ancillary Tests

- Although rarely used by cytologists, the "whiff test" can be performed at the bedside, whereby volatile amines are liberated when vaginal secretions are mixed with 10% potassium hydroxide.

- Gram stain
- Culture
- Multiplex PCR for both *G. vaginalis* and *Mobiluncus* spp.

Neisseria gonorrheae

Microbiology

- *Neisseria gonorrheae* is a sexually transmitted infection.
- They are Gram-negative diplococci, typically found within neutrophils.

Clinical Features

- Infected patients are often asymptomatic, but may present with pruritis, a mucopurulent vaginal discharge, dysuria, and edematous, friable cervix.
- If untreated, urethritis, endometritis, tubo-ovarian abscess, and PID may develop. Scarring from PID may result in infertility or ectopic pregnancy. Disseminated disease is possible.

Cytomorphologic Features

- Monococci or diplococci may be seen within neutrophils. However, cytolomorphology alone is not a reliable diagnostic modality and ancillary tests are required.
- Patients with chronic gonorrhea infection may show reactive epithelial change.

Diagnostic Note

- Many women are routinely screened for *N. gonorrheae* infection, along with *C. trachomatis* at the time of Pap test collection. Concomitant testing for these microorganisms does not appear to affect the adequacy of the Pap test, even if separate endocervical swabs are obtained before or after the Pap test. The type of collection device (e.g., broom, brush) also does not appear to impact the test.
- Nucleic acid amplification tests (NAATs, see below) permit testing of female patients to be performed on endocervical swabs, liquid-based Pap specimens, self-collected vaginal swabs, and urine specimens.

Ancillary Tests

- Gram stain.
- DNA for *N. gonorrheae* can be performed on liquid-based cytology of cervicovaginal specimens. Commercial kits are available that employ NAAT. These offer more rapid results than culture. Second-generation assays (e.g., APTIMA Combo 2 assay) can simultaneously detect *N. gonorrheae* and *C. trachomatis* from the same specimen.
- Culture, which needs to be performed within 24 h or less of specimen collection.
- Also available are fluorescent antibody testing, co-agglutination, and DNA probe.

Actinomyces

Microbiology

- *Actinomyces* spp. are Gram-positive, nonacid-fast bacteria that exhibit branching, filamentous growth. *Actinomyces israelii* is the species most commonly associated with the female genital tract. They are part of the normal flora of the mouth and gastrointestinal tract, and less commonly the vagina. Damage to the mucosa is required for the development of actinomycosis.
- *Actinomyces* spp. grow as colonies that can form abscesses and subsequent fibrosis. Yellow sulfur granules containing bacteria may be visible macroscopically.
- *Actinomyces* infection of the female genital tract is most often associated with intra-uterine contraceptive device (IUD) use. Around 25% of patients with an IUD will have *Actinomyces* present in their Pap test specimens. Rare cases may develop endometritis and/or PID.

Clinical Features

- Symptoms may include vaginal bleeding and discharge, fever, weight loss, and abdominal pain. Patients may present with a tubo-ovarian abscess (Fig. 5.11).

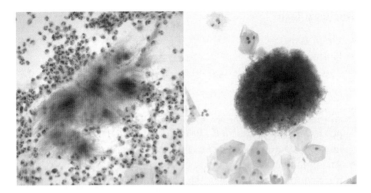

Fig. 5.11. *Actinomyces*. (*Left*) Conventional Pap smear showing dense balls of bacteria with radiating filaments consistent with *Actinomyces* spp. (Pap stain, high magnification). (*Right*) ThinPrep Pap test showing a ball of *Actinomyces* organisms (Pap stain, high magnification).

Cytomorphologic Features

- The main finding is dense basophilic balls ("dust bunnies") of bacteria with radiating filaments. Their center is often more dense and poorly stained than the surrounding delicate filaments (best visualized by focusing up and down). Occasionally the organisms may be arranged in a horizontal array. At higher magnification the filaments may be club-shaped and can be seen branching at acute angles.
- In conventional Pap smears bacteria balls are gray-blue in color, whereas with liquid-based specimens they may be more eosinophilic.
- Acute inflammatory cells are often present in the background, as well as macrophages, rare multinucleated giant cells and calcified debris, the latter of which is probably from the IUD.

Diagnostic Note

- The Bethesda system interpretation is "Bacteria morphologically consistent with *Actinomyces* spp."
- IUD removal and possible antibiotic treatment may be required in symptomatic patients if actinomycosis is diagnosed.

Ancillary Tests

- Gram stain
- Culture

Granuloma Venereum

- This STD, also known as granuloma inguinale and Donovanosis, is caused by *Klebsiella granulomatis*, an intracellular Gram-negative bacteria, sometimes referred to as *a Donovan body.*
- The organism is seen in histiocytes, enclosed within thin-walled intracytoplasmic vacuoles. The classic "safety-pin" appearance of the bacteria is not apparent in alcohol-fixed smears.
- There may be a paucity of epithelial cells present due to ulceration. As a result, the majority of the Pap test is comprised of inflammatory cells, mainly neutrophils but also macrophages. Epithelioid histiocytes may be encountered, but giant cells are not seen. Intact capillaries may be seen due to direct scraping of the stroma.
- Various ancillary tests are available including special stains (Romanowsky and Warthin-Starry stains), immunocytochemistry, PCR, serology, culture, and electron microscopy (Fig. 5.12).

Tuberculosis

Microbiology

- Tuberculosis (TB) of the female genital tract is primarily caused by *Mycobacterium tuberculosis.*
- TB involvement of the female genital tract in almost all cases is secondary to extragenital disease, and usually involves the fallopian tubes and endometrium. Infection of the cervix is rare, even where mycobacterial infection is endemic.
- The cervix is infected through direct spread from the upper genital tract or lymphatic spread. It has been suggested that occasionally cervical TB may be sexually transmitted from a partner with tuberculous epididymitis or if infected sputum is used as a sexual lubricant.

Clinical Features

- Patients may present with amenorrhea, menstrual irregularities, infertility, vaginal discharge, and postmenopausal bleeding. The

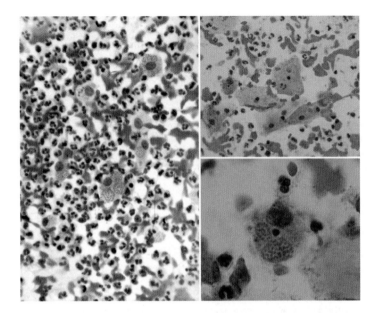

Fig. 5.12. Donovanosis (high magnification images). (*Left*) A cervical smear showing many macrophages containing intracellular organisms present in a background of predominantly acute inflammatory cells (Pap stain). (*Top right*) Conventional Pap smear showing macrophages containing bacteria scattered among benign squamous cells (Pap stain). (*Bottom right*) Epithelioid macrophage with intracytoplasmic vacuoles containing many Donovan bodies (Pap stain) (images courtesy of Prof. Gladwyn Leiman, University of Vermont, USA).

gross appearance of the tuberculous cervix is highly variable (e.g., ulcer, polyp).

- Cases of TB cervicitis are often clinically misdiagnosed as carcinoma of the cervix.

Cytomorphologic Features

- The main finding is granulomatous inflammation with or without necrosis. Epithelioid histiocytes form sheets or can be seen as single cells, along with acute and chronic inflammatory cells in the background, as well as multinucleated giant cells.

Diagnostic Note

- The presence of granulomas with multinucleated giant cells in Pap tests should raise the suspicion of tuberculosis.
- Granulomas in Pap tests can also be seen in other conditions such as syphilis, granuloma inguinale, amebiasis, schistosomiasis, foreign body (suture) granulomas, and malakoplakia.

Ancillary Tests

- Acid-fast stains for mycobacteria
- Autofluorescence
- Culture
- PCR

Chlamydia trachomatis

Microbiology

- Chlamydia (previously called TRIC agent) are obligate intracellular Gram-negative bacteria. They require growing cells to remain viable, forming intracellular inclusions as they grow.
- *C. trachomatis* is transmitted via sexual contact and during vaginal child birth. This is the most common nonulcerative STD worldwide. Coinfection with HPV, gonorrhea, syphilis, HSV-2, and HIV is common (Fig. 5.13).

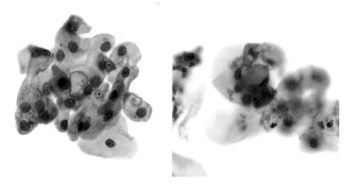

Fig. 5.13. Chlamydia inclusions. (*Left*) Squamous cells on a Pap test are shown with several small intracytoplasmic chlamydia inclusions (Pap stain, high magnification). (*Right*) Squamous cell with a nebular body, which is highly specific for chlamydial infection (Pap stain, high magnification).

Clinical Features

- Most infected patients are asymptomatic.
- Female urogenital infection may cause vaginal bleeding, discharge, pelvic pain, dyspareunia, and urinary symptoms. Patients develop cervicitis (typically follicular type), and possibly salpingitis, PID, and/or Reiter's syndrome (genital inflammation with conjunctivitis and arthritis).
- Chlamydia may also result in ophthalmic infection (trachoma) and systemic disease.

Cytomorphologic Features

- Inclusion bodies may be seen in squamous, endocervical, and/or metaplastic cells. Several different types of inclusions have been described including small elementary bodies, larger reticulate bodies, and aggregate bodies (e.g., nebular body).
- Reactive cellular changes may include cytomegaly, nuclear enlargement, nuclear irregularity, and multinucleation.
- Mixed acute and chronic inflammatory cells are often present.

Diagnostic Note

- The interpretation of Chlamydia is not included in the Bethesda System, because of the low sensitivity and reproducibility of cytologic findings and the availability of more specific detection methods.
- The finding of intracellular inclusions within epithelial cells is not diagnostic of chlamydia infection, as there are many other causes for such vacuoles (faux chlamydia inclusions) including intracellular targetoid mucin, condensed secretions, intracellular debris, degeneration, IUD effect, and radiation change. Macrophages may also show a similar vacuolated appearance.

Ancillary Tests

- Giemsa stain demonstrates chlamydial organisms
- NAAT, which facilitates screening. Swabs and liquid-based samples are both acceptable. Commercial assays (e.g., APTIMA Combo 2 assay) can simultaneously detect *N. gonorrheae* (GC) and *C. trachomatis* (CT) from the same liquid-based cytology specimen. Nucleic acid testing cannot differentiate dead from viable organisms.

- Other nucleic acid tests (e.g., PCR, transcription-mediated amplification, strand displacement amplification, ligase chain reaction).
- Immunocytochemistry.
- Antigen detection (direct immunofluorescence and ELISA).
- Serology, which is of limited value in adults. Detection of IgM in neonatal infection is useful.
- Culture using susceptible cells (e.g., McCoy cells). Culture is the test of choice (gold standard) in sexual abuse cases.

Fungal Infections

Candida

Microbiology

- *Candida* may be identified in the vaginal tract of up to 50% of asymptomatic women.
- *Candida albicans* is seen in most (90%) infections (called candidiasis or candidosis). Less common causes are *Candida glabrata* (previously called *Torulopsis glabrata*) forms small budding yeasts, but not pseudohyphae and *Candida parapsilosis*.
- Pregnancy, diabetes, and immunosuppression predispose women to the development of candidiasis.
- Candida vulvovaginitis is not considered to be an STD, and appears not to be associated with an increased risk of SIL.

Clinical Features

- Infection can be asymptomatic or patients with vulvovaginitis may experience pruritis, burning, or have a yellow-white thick ("cheesy") discharge.

Cytolomorphogic Features

- Budding yeasts and/or pseudohyphae are noted ("sticks and stones" or "spaghetti and meatballs"). Yeast are 3–7 μm in size, round to oval, and sharply defined. Pseudohyphae are formed by budding, have parallel side walls, and show constriction along their length (like a string of sausages).

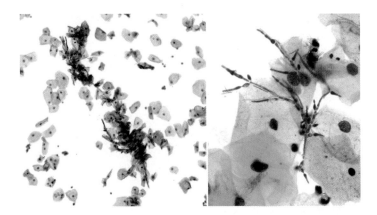

FIG. 5.14. *Candida*. (*Left*) *Candida* hyphae in this ThinPrep Pap test appear to have skewered the surrounding squamous cells forming a shish kebab-like structure (Pap stain, intermediate magnification). (*Right*) Higher magnification shows characteristic pseudohyphae with distinct constrictions along their length (Pap stain).

- *C. glabrata* presents with budding yeast only. The yeasts are often surrounded by halos and may cluster.
- Fungal elements may appear to "skewer" surrounding squamous cells (making "shish kebabs").
- Candida-associated nonspecific changes that may be observed in squamous cells include perinuclear halos, keratotic change (intense orangeophilia and anucleate squames), and vacuolated ("moth-eaten") cytoplasm (Figs. 5.14 and 5.15).

Diagnostic Note

- The Bethesda System recommends reporting these organisms as "Fungal organisms morphologically consistent with *Candida* spp."
- The identification of Candida on a Pap test does not necessarily indicate infection.
- Nonspecific reactive changes in squamous cells may be interpreted as ASC-US or pseudokoilocytosis. True dysplastic cells have larger and more hyperchromatic nuclei.

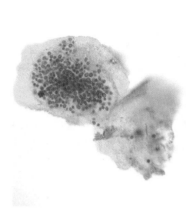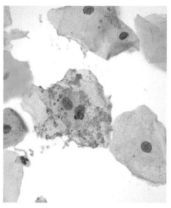

FIG. 5.15. *Candida glabrata.* With *C. glabrata* the only finding in a Pap test is rare to many yeasts (*left* and *right* images Pap stain, high magnification).

- The diagnosis of well-formed pseudohyphae and/or spores is needed to make a diagnosis of Candida. Other fungi like *Geotrichum*, which have true hyphae and contaminating fibers, are included in the differential.

Ancillary Tests

- Special stains (PAS and GMS)
- Fungal culture

Parasitic Infections

Trichomonas vaginalis

Microbiology

- *Trichomonas vaginalis* is a parasitic protozoan that causes trichomonaisis.
- Trichomoniasis is a very common sexually transmitted infection. Its prevalence is highest among those with multiple sexual partners and other sexually transmitted infections (Fig. 5.16).

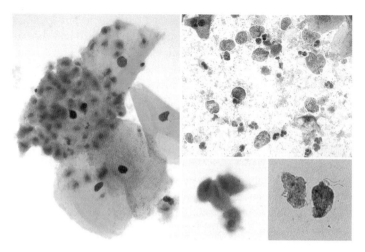

Fig. 5.16. Trichomoniasis. (*Left*). Many pear-shaped *blue-gray* trichomonads are shown attached to a squamous cell in a ThinPrep Pap test (Pap stain, high magnification). (*Upper right*) Several trichomonads are shown in this conventional Pap smear with prominent *red* cytoplasmic granules (Pap stain, high magnification). (*Middle bottom*) A *darker gray* elliptical nucleus can be seen within these protozoa (high magnification under oil). (*Bottom right*) Trichomonads demonstrate p16 immunoreactivity. Note the thin flagella of the parasite on the right (immunocytochemistry, clone G175-405, BD Biosciences Pharmingen, San Diego, CA; oil magnification).

Clinical Features

- Patients may be asymptomatic or present with burning, pruritis, a profuse yellow-green, frothy and malodorous vaginal discharge and dysuria. Males may present with urethritis.
- Trichomonas may be associated with PID, infertility, and in pregnant women premature rupture of membranes and preterm birth.

Cytomorphologic Features

- Round to oval or pear-shaped extracellular organisms are seen usually just slightly larger than inflammatory cells and parabasal cells. They range in size from 15 to 30 μm. In liquid-based preparations the organisms are often smaller due to rounding. On

Pap stain their cytoplasm is gray and red cytoplasmic granules may be noted. The nucleus is eccentrically situated and appears a darker gray than the cytoplasm, but is still pale and vesicular. Flagella are not usually seen on conventional smears, but may be noted in liquid-based preparations.

- Trichomonads may be present singly or aggregate in small colonies ("Trich parties") scattered around the slide. They may also attach in large numbers to squamous cells.
- *Leptothrix* may be associated with *Trichomonas*.
- Associated inflammatory reactive changes ("Trich change") include neutrophils present in ball-like arrangements (poly cannonballs), squamous cells with small perinuclear (trich) halos, mild nuclear hyperchromasia, slight nuclear enlargement, pseudokeratinization, increased numbers of anucleate (ghost) squames, erythrophagocytosis by trichomonads, and dirty background.

Diagnostic Note

- Diagnosis made by the identification of trichomonads on wet mount preparation and Pap test has lower sensitivity (50–80%) compared to culture (70–100%).
- The morphologic identification of *T. vaginalis* on a Pap test is highly accurate and should not require confirmatory testing.
- Degenerated inflammatory cells, cellular debris, degenerated bare epithelial nuclei in atrophic vaginitis, and small mucus aggregates may be confused with trichomonads. Trichomonads by comparison have a well-defined shape and a gray eccentrically located nucleus.

Ancillary Tests

- Immunocytochemistry. With the p16 immunostain (using clone G175-405 from BD Biosciences Pharmingen, San Diego, CA, USA) nonspecific immunoreactivity of *T. vaginalis* has been reported.
- Immunofluorescent antibody staining
- PCR
- Culture

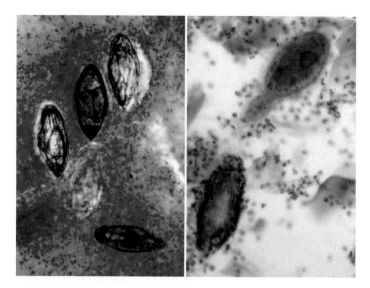

FIG. 5.17. Schistosomiasis. (*Left*) Several nonviable empty ova of *S. hae-matobium* are shown in a conventional Pap smear with a bloody background (Pap stain, high magnification). (*Right*) A miracidium (upper structure) and ovum (lower structure) of *S. haematobium* in a Pap smear are shown. The miracidium has possibly just escaped from the ovum (Pap stain, high magnification).

Schistosomiasis

Microbiology

- Schistosomiasis is due to infection by the trematodes (flukes) *Schistosoma haematobium*, *S. mansoni*, or *S. japonicum*. Cervical infections are most often due to *S. haematobium*.
- Mature ova release miracidia in moist environments. The cervix is sufficiently moist to allow this (Fig. 5.17).

Clinical Features

- Cervical symptoms of infection include vaginal discharge and bleeding. The infected cervix appears inflamed, ulcerated, nodular, and friable, which may mimic carcinoma clinically.

- Early infection causes inflammation (eosinophils, lymphocytes, and granulomas) around ova. Chronic inactive infection with calcified dead eggs leads to scarring.
- The relationship between schistosomiasis and cervical cancer is unclear. It is postulated that cervical schistosomiasis damages cervical epithelium, thereby serving as a co-factor for the transmission of viral infections such as HIV and HPV infections in endemic regions.

Cytomorphologic Features

- Viable ova are 150 μm in length and 50 μm in width and are surrounded by a thick shell. *S. haematobium* has a terminal spine while *S. mansoni* has a lateral one. *S. japonicum* is slightly oval with a rudimentary lateral spine. Sometimes the structure of a miracidium within the ovum is apparent.
- Nonviable ova are empty (have no internal structure) and may exhibit a variety of forms including calcified, black, opaque, shrunken, or collapsed eggs. Empty shells are often found in association with multinucleated histiocytes.
- Miracidia are not often seen. They usually have a pointed anterior end and round posterior end. Cilia are not seen on Pap smear. The cytoplasm containing various structures within the miracidia stain brightly eosinophilic while the nuclei are basophilic.
- There is usually an acute inflammatory infiltrate and multinucleated histiocytes present in the background.

Diagnostic Note

- Cervical infection may occur in the absence of urinary egg excretion.
- The differential diagnosis for empty ova includes collections of lubricant gel and plant cells. Lubricant gel lacks a spine and is not refractile while plant cells may be refractile but lack a spine.
- Viable ova appear different from the ova of other parasites that have been described in cervical smears including *Ascaris*, *Trichuris*, *Enterobius*, and *Taenia*. Refer to parasitic ova in Chap. 4.
- Miracidia are larger than those of *Balantidium coli*.

Ancillary Tests

- Special stains include GMS and Ziehl-Neelsen
- Serology

Enterobius vermicularis

Microbiology

- *Enterobius vermicularis* (known as the pinworm or thread-worm) is an intestinal parasite (nematode) that can occasionally migrate to the vagina, uterus, and even the peritoneal cavity via the fallopian tubes.
- The finding of an adult pinworm and/or egg on a Pap test slide likely represents contamination from perianal parasites (gravid female worms and ova), or infrequently a true genital infection.

Clinical Features

- Symptoms of intestinal infection (enterobiasis) mainly include perianal pruritis.
- Vaginal discharge may occur with infestation of the lower genital tract.

Cytomorphologic Features

- An *Enterobius* ovum is oval, measures $50–60 \times 20–30$ μm in size, and has a thick double-walled shell that is flattened on one side. Occasionally, larvae may be seen in the ova or free-lying. One may find one or many ova in a Pap test specimen.
- The adult pinworm is cylindrical and has a sharply pointed posterior end. Female worms measure 8–13 mm long and males are only 2–5 mm in length. Both are ~0.5 mm thick.
- With contamination there will be no associated inflammation. With a true genital infection the background inflammatory response varies and includes granulomatous inflammation.

Diagnostic Note

- Psammoma bodies and pollen grain may mimic parasitic ova.

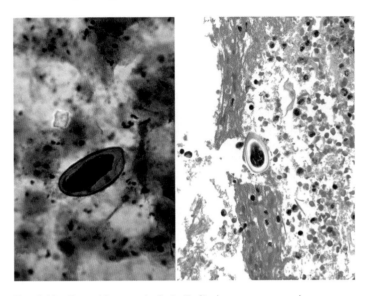

FIG. 5.18. *Enterobius vermicularis* (*Left*) pinworm egg seen in a conventional pap smear, which is flat on one end (pap stain, high magnification) (courtesy of Dr. Gladwyn Leiman, University of Vermont, USA). (*Right*) Pinworm egg shown in cell block material from a cervicovaginal specimen (H&E stain, high magnification).

- *Enterobius* ova need to be distinguished from *Ascaris*, *Trichuris*, and *Taenia* eggs.
- Plant and synthetic fibers may mimic pinworms.
- The *Strongyloides stercoralis* adult worm is 180–350 μm long, also has a curved pointed tail, but one can often also find a short buccal canal. Microfilariae can be distinguished because they have a sheath and contain many nuclei along their length.

Ancillary Tests

- Microbiology consultation
- Examination of stool for parasites and/or cellulose (Scotch/ sticky) tape applied to the perianal skin for microscopic examination (Fig. 5.18).

Insects

Phthirus pubis

- *Phthirus pubis*, also known as pubic or crab lice, are wingless parasitic insects usually found on pubic hair, but may also be seen on other hairy parts of the body including the eyelashes.
- Lice have three distinct body segments, in addition to crab-like claws on the legs for climbing hairs. They have an overall "crab-like" appearance. They measure between 1 and 2.5 mm in size.
- The presence of a pubic louse on a Pap test represents a contaminant. The clinician should be alerted to the possible infestation of the pubic hair.
- *Pediculus humanus capitis* (head lice) and *Pediculus humanus human* (body lice) are morphologically distinct (Fig. 5.19).

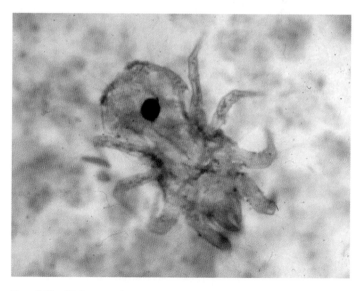

Fig. 5.19. *Phthirus pubis* seen on a conventional Pap smear (Pap stain, medium magnification).

Suggested Reading

Aslan DL, McKeon DM, Stelow EB, Gulbahce HE, Kjeldahl K, Pambuccian SE. The diagnosis of trichomonas vaginalis in liquid-based Pap tests: morphological characteristics. Diagn Cytopathol. 2005;32:253–9.

Discacciati M, Simoes J, Amaral R, Brolazo E, Rabelo-Santos S, Westin M, et al. Presence of 20% or more clue cells: an accurate criterion for the diagnosis of bacterial vaginosis in Papanicolaou cervical smears. Diagn Cytopathol. 2006;34:272–6.

Giacomini G. Permanent diagnosis of bacterial vaginosis: gram stain or Papanicolaou stain? Diagn Cytopathol. 2000;23:292–3.

Gupta R, Dey P, Jain V, Gupta N. Cervical tuberculosis detection in Papanicolaou-stained smear: case report with review of literature. Diagn Cytopathol. 2009;37:592–5.

Huang JC, Naylor B. Cytomegalovirus infection of the cervix detected by cytology and histology: a report of five cases. Cytopathology. 1993; 4:237–41.

Leiman G, Markowitz S, Margolius KA. Cytologic detection of cervical granuloma inguinale. Diagn Cytopathol. 1986;2:138–43.

McMillan A. The detection of genital tract infection by Papanicolaou-stained tests. Cytopathology. 2006;17:317–22.

Noël JC, Engohan-Aloghe C. Morphologic criteria associated with *Trichomonas vaginalis* in liquid-based cytology. Acta Cytol. 2010;54:582–6.

Pantanowitz L, Florence RR, Goulart RA, Otis CN. *Trichomonas vaginalis* p16 immunoreactivity in cervicovaginal Pap tests: a diagnostic pitfall. Diagn Cytopathol. 2005;33:210–3.

Tambouret R. Gynecologic infections. In: Kradin RL, editor. Diagnostic pathology of infectious disease. Philadelphia: Saunders Elsevier; 2010. p. 443–63.

6
Pulmonary Infections

Walid E. Khalbuss[1], Rodolfo Laucirica[2], and Liron Pantanowitz[1]

[1]Department of Pathology, University of Pittsburgh Medical Center, 5150 Centre Avenue, Suite 201, Pittsburgh, PA 15232, USA

[2]Department of Pathology and Immunology, Baylor College of Medicine, Ben Taub General Hospital, Houston, TX, USA

The lungs are a frequent site of infectious diseases. An accurate diagnosis of infection by means of cytology can be lifesaving. Sputum, lung FNA, bronchoscopic brushing, washing, and BAL are useful procedures that can help provide a fast, cost-effective, and noninvasive diagnosis of pulmonary infection. Pleuropulmonary infections include bronchitis and bronchiolitis, pneumonia (inflammation of the lung parenchyma), lung abscess, cavity formation, allergic bronchopulmonary reaction, as well as pleural effusion and empyema (pus in the pleural cavity).

A variety of microorganisms can infect the lungs including viruses, bacteria, fungi, and parasites. The implicated pathogen depends in part on the clinical setting. For example, microorganisms responsible for community-acquired pneumonia include *Streptococcus pneumoniae*, *Haemophilus influenzae*, and *Staphylococcus aureus*. Atypical community-acquired pneumonia is caused by *Mycoplasma pneumoniae*, *Chlamydia* spp. and several viruses including respiratory syncytial virus (RSV) and parainfluenza virus in children and influenza A and B in adults. Nosocomial infections may be caused by *Klebsiella* spp., *Escherichia coli*, *Pseudomonas* spp., and penicillin resistant *S. aureus*. Finally, there are certain pathogens responsible for infections in the immunocompromised host like cytomegalovirus (CMV), *Pneumocystis jirovecii*, and *Mycobacterium avium-intracellulare* (MAI). This chapter discusses

L. Pantanowitz et al., *Cytopathology of Infectious Diseases*, Essentials in Cytopathology 17, DOI 10.1007/978-1-4614-0242-8_6, © Springer Science+Business Media, LLC 2011

the cytologic features of a variety of pathogens that infect the respiratory tract.

The optimal diagnostic method depends on the location of the lesion and radiologic findings. Sputum samples, and bronchial brushings and washings yield diagnostic material for centrally located lesions that involve major airways, while a BAL is useful for assessing inflammatory and infectious processes in the peripheral regions of the lung. Transbronchial or ultrasound guided FNA permits endobronchial lesions or hilar lymph nodes to be sampled, and radiologically guided FNA is used when subpleural regions need to be aspirated that cannot be assessed by bronchoscopy. Given that cytologic examination of the respiratory tract is less invasive compared to open surgical biopsies, cytology is often the initial and only means by which patients are evaluated for infectious diseases. This is especially true in immunocompromised patients who need to be followed over a given period of time to rule out opportunistic infections. In fact, BAL remains the diagnostic procedure of choice for detecting opportunistic infections in immunocompromised hosts.

Viral Infections

Viruses are one of the most common causes of infection of the respiratory tract. Not all viral infections have cytopathic changes (e.g., influenza, swine flu, severe acute respiratory syndrome/ SARS, EBV). However, in many cases the cytologic features of viral infection are fairly specific as to the etiology (Table 6.1). Ancillary studies such as immunohistochemistry, viral culture, and molecular tests are often necessary to accurately identify the cause of certain infections.

Herpes Simplex Virus (HSV)

Microbiology

- Herpesvirus types 1 and 2 (HSV 1 and 2) can both infect the lungs.

TABLE 6.1. Cytologic featuwres of common pulmonary viral pathogens.

Virus	Cytologic finding
Herpes simplex / herpes zoster virus	Cowdry type A and B inclusions
Cytomegalovirus	Large intranuclear and small cytoplasmic inclusions
Adenovirus	Intranuclear inclusions (smudge cells) and ciliocytophthoria
Respiratory syncytial virus	Syncytial giant cells
Parainfluenza	Syncytial giant cells with large cytoplasmic inclusions and ciliocytophthoria
Measles	Multinucleated giant cells with cytoplasmic and intranuclear Cowdry type A inclusions

Clinical Features

- HSV infection of the upper respiratory tract can lead to pharyngitis, laryngotracheitis, and pneumonia. HSV infection of the lung may cause a necrotizing pneumonia or diffuse interstitial pneumonia.
- HSV commonly infects neonates and immunocompromised patients.

Cytomorphologic Features

- Herpetic inclusions can be found within metaplastic squamous cells when the inflammation is centered around airways or in multinucleated giant cells within necroinflammatory debris in the interstitial form of disease.
- Infected cells often display prominent nuclear molding.
- Two forms of characteristic herpes inclusions may be seen, including Cowdry type A inclusions (distinct eosinophilic intranuclear inclusions surrounded by a clear halo due to margination of chromatin material) and Cowdry type B inclusions (eosinophilic ground glass "smudge nuclei" with margination of the chromatin material) (Fig. 6.1).
- The background may have associated acute inflammatory cells and necrosis.

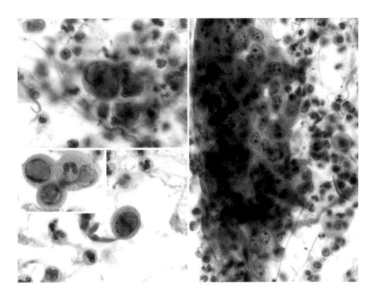

FIG. 6.1. BAL specimen from a patient with a history of colon adeno-carcinoma who presented with respiratory distress. The *left photos* show characteristic of *Cowdry type B* herpes inclusions. The *right photo* shows accompanying reactive reparative change with prominent and multiple nucleoli that mimics malignancy in this case (Pap stain, high magnification).

Differential Diagnosis

- Nonspecific reactive bronchial cells and alveolar macrophages (multinucleated bronchial cells and cells with clearing/washed out nuclei).
- Squamous dysplasia in metaplastic cells or in a squamous papilloma lesion.
- The cytopathic features are identical to those of herpes zoster (clinical history and/or ancillary studies are required to resolve this differential diagnosis).
- CMV infection (rarely causes multinucleation, see Fig. 6.2 (see next page)).

Ancillary Studies

- Most cases do not need ancillary studies to confirm the diagnosis.

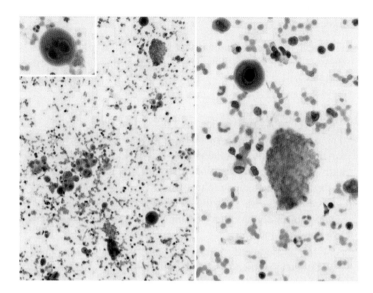

FIG. 6.2. Co-infection with CMV and *P. jirovecii* is shown in this BAL specimen from an immunocompromised patient. Characteristic "owl eye" inclusions are seen. Multinucleation is rare in CMV infection, but can occur (see *inset*). Pneumocystis infection resulted in the cast of frothy material; each *circlet* with a central dot is an organism (Pap stain, intermediate magnification *left* and high magnification *right*).

- Immunostains are available for HSV infection and can be performed on cell block material or smears.
- Viral culture.
- HSV DNA detection by in situ hybridization or PCR.
- Serology (type-specific assays).
- Electron microscopy.

Cytomegalovirus (CMV)

Microbiology

- CMV is one of the most common causes of opportunistic infections involving the respiratory tract. In the respiratory tract, CMV mainly targets pulmonary macrophages, endothelial cells and fibroblasts, but virtually any cell can be infected by this virus.

Clinical Features

- CMV pneumonia is frequently seen in patients with HIV/AIDS, those receiving organ transplants, or individuals at the extremes of age.

Cytomorphologic Features

- The diagnostic features of CMV infection include cytomegaly, large amphophilic intranuclear inclusions with perinuclear halos and chromatin margination ("owl eye" inclusion), and small basophilic cytoplasmic inclusions.
- The number of cells showing cytopathic changes varies with the severity of infection or as a result of patients receiving prophylactic antiviral therapy.
- As CMV is frequently found in immunosuppressed patients, it may be seen together with other opportunistic pathogens such as fungi including *P. jirovecii* (Fig. 6.2).

Differential Diagnosis

- Herpes simplex infection.
- Neoplastic cells.
- Reactive epithelial cells or macrophages with karyomegaly.
- Other viral infections including adenovirus and RSV infection.

Ancillary Studies

- Most cases do not need ancillary studies to confirm the diagnosis.
- Immunocytochemistry or in situ hybridization for CMV.
- Molecular testing (PCR).
- Viral culture.

Adenovirus

Microbiology

- Adenovirus is a DNA virus that can cause ulcerative bronchiolitis, acute pneumonia, or diffuse alveolar damage (DAD).

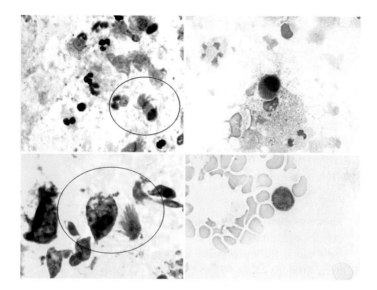

FIG. 6.3. Adenovirus pneumonia. The images on the *left* are of a smear prepared from sputum showing an infected cell (*circled*) with a degenerated nucleus (*top left*, Pap stain, intermediate magnification) and a detached ciliary tuft (*bottom left*, Pap stain, high magnification). The images on the *right* are of a BAL from a child with adenovirus pneumonia showing a smudgy appearing nucleus of an infected cell (*top right*, Pap stain, cytospin, high magnification) with positive immunocytochemistry confirming this is due to adenovirus infection (*bottom right*, high magnification) (BAL images courtesy of Dr. S. Ranganathan, Pittsburgh Children's Hospital, USA).

Clinical Features

- Pulmonary adenovirus infections may occur in healthy subjects living in close quarters (e.g., military recruits), but can also cause severe and potentially fatal infections in immunocompromised patients.

Cytomorphologic Features

- Infected cells exhibit two types of nuclear inclusions: amphophilic intranuclear inclusions with perinuclear clearing that mimic herpes simplex infection, or "smudge cells" where large basophilic inclusions fill the entire nucleus and obscure the chromatin detail (Fig. 6.3).

- Another finding is the presence of decapitated ciliated respiratory epithelial cells, so-called ciliocytophthoria.
- There may be an associated neutrophilic pneumonia, marked hemorrhage, or evidence of necrosis.

Differential Diagnosis

- Other viral infections such as herpes infection.
- Reactive epithelial cells.
- Cytotoxic drug injury.

Ancillary Studies

- Immunocytochemistry for adenovirus.
- Monoclonal antibody-based enzyme immunoassay can be performed on a fresh specimen.
- Immunofluorescence assay.
- Microbiology tissue culture.
- PCR.
- Electron microscopy.

Respiratory Syncytial Virus (RSV)

Microbiology

- RSV is an RNA virus (a member of the paramyxovidae subfamily Pneumovirinae) that targets the respiratory lining epithelium.
- Infection produces syncytial giant cells with inconspicuous eosinophilic cytoplasmic inclusions.

Clinical Features

- RSV is a major cause of lower respiratory tract infection (bronchiolitis and pneumonia) during infancy and childhood.
- RSV causes benign respiratory infections in older children and has been linked to more severe adult community-acquired pneumonia, acute bronchiolitis, and diffuse alveolar disease (DAD) in the immunocompromised host or in lung allograft recipients.

Cytomorphologic Features

- Syncytial giant cells with cytoplasmic inclusions surrounded by clear halos.

Differential Diagnosis

- Other viral infections such as human metapneumonia virus and measles.
- Benign noninfectious entities with giant cells.

Ancillary Studies

- Binax NOW® RSV (BN) used on cytology specimens.
- Microbiology tissue culture.
- Shell vial culture.
- PCR.

Parainfluenza

Microbiology

- Human parainfluenza viruses are RNA viruses belonging to the *paramyxovidae* family that cause upper respiratory tract infections.

Clinical Features

- In children, upper respiratory tract infections (e.g., croup) usually follow a benign course.
- Severe disease may occur in immunocompromised patients.

Cytomorphologic Features

- As with RSV, this infection is associated with syncytial giant cells and epithelial cells with intracytoplasmic inclusions. However, these inclusions tend to be more frequent and larger than those seen with RSV.
- Ciliocytophthoria may be prominent.

Differential Diagnosis

- Other viral infections such as RSV.
- Benign noninfectious entities with giant cells (e.g., hard metal pneumoconiosis).

Ancillary Studies

- Immunocytochemistry for parainfluenza virus.
- Rapid real-time multiplex PCR assay.
- Multiplex nucleic acid sequence-based amplification (NASBA) assay.
- Viral culture.

Measles

Microbiology

- Measles (also known as rubeola) is an infection of the respiratory system caused by the RNA rubeola virus of the genus Morbillivirus.
- Measles pneumonia is a rare and serious complication of the viral exanthem, especially in immunocompromised patients.

Clinical Features

- Measles pneumonia can range from mild (bronchiolitis) to severe (DAD) disease.

Cytomorphologic Features

- Cytology specimens show large multinucleated giant cells with cytoplasmic and intranuclear inclusions. The intranuclear inclusion has a glassy, eosinophilic appearance reminiscent of Cowdry types A inclusions (Fig. 6.4).
- There may be associated acute inflammation.

Differential Diagnosis

- Other viral infections such as RSV.
- Benign noninfectious entities with giant cells morphology (e.g., hard metal pneumoconiosis).

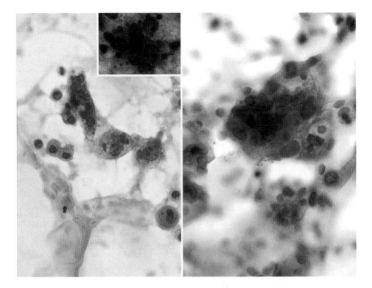

FIG. 6.4. Measles pneumonia in a 42-year-old woman showing giant cell pneumonia with enormous multinucleated giant cells that have cytoplasmic and intranuclear inclusions (Pap stain, high magnification). The *inset* shows a cell stained with Phloxine Tartrazine that highlights the *bright red* cytoplasmic inclusions (images courtesy of Dr. Pawel Schubert, South Africa).

Ancillary Studies

- Phloxine tartrazine special stain, which stains viral inclusions bright red.
- Serology: IgM (acute infection); IgG (immunity).
- PCR (from a swab).
- Viral culture.

Bacterial Infections

Bacterial pneumonia may be lobar, lobular, or present in an atypical manner (e.g., mass-like or interstitial appearance). Gram-positive and negative-bacteria are a common cause of pulmonary

infection. Most bacteria cause a nonspecific acute necroinflammatory reaction associated with a variable fibrohistiocytic response
(organization). Necrotizing pyogenic infections may result in
abscess formation. Mycobacteria may evoke a granulomatous
process. The etiology of infectious pneumonia is best established
by correlating clinical and radiologic findings with microbiology
studies.

Actinomyces

Microbiology

- *Actinomyces* are Gram-positive filamentous bacteria that cause
  suppurative and granulomatous inflammation. Infections may
  also result in bronchiectasis and abscesses containing sulfur
  granules.
- Pulmonary infections occur via aspiration of oral organisms and
  are seen most often in persons with poor oral hygiene, immunocompromised patients, or from direct extension of cervicofacial
  or subdiaphragmatic infection.
- Secondary actinomycotic infection can involve devitalized lung
  tissue damaged by other infections.

Clinical Features

- The clinical manifestations of pulmonary actinomycosis are
  fever, productive cough, and hemoptysis. Chronic infection may
  cause sinus tracts.
- Lung imaging findings may include consolidation, necrosis,
  abscess, or an aspirated broncholith.

Cytomorphologic Features

- Specimens contain acute inflammation and bacterial colonies
  composed of thin beaded and delicate branching filaments
  that are cyanophilic with a Pap stain (so-called "cotton ball"
  appearance).
- Some cases may have sulfur granules which are colonies
  of tangled Gram-positive bacilli, often coated with an eosi-

nophilic matrix of exudate plasma proteins (Splendore-Hoeppli reaction).

Differential Diagnosis

- Actinomyces are commonly found in tonsillar crypts, and therefore may be seen (associated with squamous cells) contaminating sputum and bronchial specimens. Their presence on FNA is unlikely to be due to contamination. True infection is associated with abundant neutrophils.
- Nocardia (less beading, no sulfur granules).
- Botryomycosis (may also form sulfur granules, but contains cocci).
- Mycobacteria.
- Fungal infection.

Ancillary Studies

- Special stains (*Actinomyces* are positive with Gram and GMS stains, but negative with an AFB/Fite stain).
- Microbiology culture.

Nocardia

Microbiology

- *Nocardia* are weakly staining Gram-positive, partially acid-fast, rod-shaped, aerobic bacteria. They form beaded branching filaments. The majority of infections (80%) are due to *Nocardia asteroides*.
- Pulmonary infection occurs via inhalation. Pre-existing pulmonary disease, particularly pulmonary alveolar protienosis, increases the risk of contracting *Nocardia* pneumonia.

Clinical Features

- Patients commonly present with slowly progressive pneumonia. In immuncompromised patients, infection may be associated with cavitary lung nodules. Infection can also spread to the pleura or to chest wall.

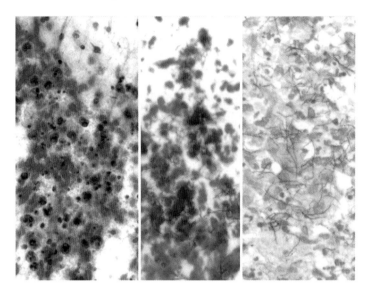

FIG. 6.5. FNA of Nocardia pneumonia with numerous PMNs and necrotic material (*left image* Pap stain, high magnification) associated with thin filamentous branching bacteria (*middle image* Gram stain and *right image* AFB stain, both high magnification).

Cytomorphologic Features

- Cytology findings include those of acute pneumonia (numerous neutrophils and necrotic material) together with the presence of thin filamentous, beaded bacteria with right angle branching that resembles Chinese letters (Fig. 6.5).

Differential Diagnosis

- Actinomyces (more beading and more commonly have sulfur granules).
- Mycobacteria.

Ancillary Studies

- Special stains (*Nocardia* are positive with Gram and GMS stains, and weakly positive with an AFB/Fite stain).
- Microbiology culture.

Tuberculosis

Microbiology

- Pulmonary tuberculosis (TB) is caused by the bacterium *Mycobacterium tuberculosis*. Pulmonary TB may be due to primary or reactivation (chronic) infection. Pulmonary manifestations of TB include bronchopneumonia, caseating pneumonia, nodular disease (tuberculoma), tracheobronchitis, milliary disease, hilar lymphadenopathy, and pleural disease.
- Individuals at risk for infection are those who are immunosuppressed, the elderly, and infants.
- Nontuberculous mycobacteria (NTM), such as *Mycobacterium avium complex* (MAC) and *Mycobacterium kansasii*, may also cause pulmonary infections.
- Infections are often associated with granulomatous inflammation. In NTM infection, particularly in immunocompromised patients, granulomas tend to be nonnecrotizing and incompletely formed.

Clinical Features

- Patients usually present with night sweats, fever, weight loss, fatigue, chronic cough, chest pain, hemoptysis, and possibly extrapulmonary TB that may involve the pleura and mediastinal lymph nodes.
- Thoracic imaging studies may show infiltrates or cavities (especially of the upper lobes), solitary or milliary nodules, pleural effusion, pneumothorax, and/or hilar lymphadenopathy.

Cytomorphologic Features

- The main finding is granulomas that show clusters of epithelioid histiocytes that may be mixed with lymphocytes, Langhans, and/or foreign body-type multinucleated giant cells with/without a necrotic background (Fig. 6.6).
- In NTM infections, macrophages laden with abundant mycobacteria may show abundant foamy cytoplasm (referred to as pseudo-Gaucher cells).
- A negative image of extracellular mycobacteria may be notable with Diff-Quik, Giemsa, or other Romanowsky-type stains (Fig. 6.7). In NTM infection, these unstained mycobacteria (especially within macrophages) are usually more numerous.

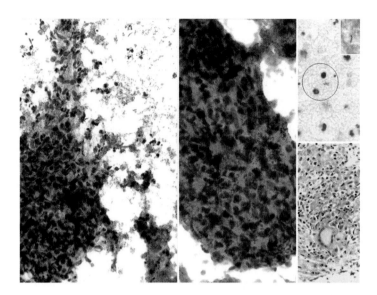

FIG. 6.6. Necrotizing granulomatous pneumonia caused by *M. tuberculosis* shown on Pap stained smears at high magnification (*left* and *middle images*) and cell block (H&E stain, high magnification). Rare mycobacteria are seen with an AFB stain (*upper right image* and *inset*, high magnification).

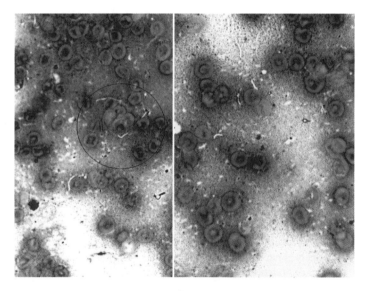

FIG. 6.7. Tuberculosis pneumonia with numerous mycobacteria seen as negative images on Diff-Quik stain (high magnification).

Differential Diagnosis

- Other microorganisms that cause necrotizing granulomatous inflammation and are AFB positive (*Nocardia*, *Rhodococcus*, and *Legionella micdadei*).
- Noninfectious causes of granulomatous lung disease (e.g., sarcoidosis).

Ancillary Studies

- Acid-fast stains (Ziehl-Neelsen or Kinyoun stains). The diagnosis of mycobacterial infection can be on the basis of the identification of microorganisms with acid-fast (AFB) stains. Mycobacteria with *M. tuberculosis* compared to NTM may be rare and require careful and lengthy scrutiny of slides. Some mycobacteria have a distinct morphology; for example *M. kansasii* resembles a shepherd's crook or candy cane and *Mycobacterium fortuitum* closely resembles *Nocardia* spp.
- Mycobacteria may be weakly Gram-positive and will stain with GMS.
- Fluorescence microscopy with fluorochrome dyes such as auramine O or auramine–rhodamine are more sensitive and specific than AFB stains.
- Autofluorescence.
- PCR for diagnosis and subclassification (can be done on cell block material).
- Culture for diagnosis and subclassification, although mycobacteria are slow growing and culture can take weeks (6–8 weeks with conventional Lowenstein-Jensen medium and 3 weeks with Middlebrook liquid and solid media).

Legionella

- Pneumonia is the predominant manifestation of *Legionella* infection (Legionnaire's disease).
- Bacteria (Gram-negative coccobacilli) can be identified with silver stains (Steiner, Warthin-Starry, or Diertrle stains), and are often abundant prior to therapy. *Legionella micdadei* stains with modified Ziehl-Neelsen stains.

- Immunocytochemistry (for *Legionella pneumophilia*) can be performed if needed.

Fungal Infections

Pulmonary fungal infections can be readily diagnosed by means of exfoliative cytology or FNA. Infections are often associated with a granulomatous or necroinflammatory reaction. Fungal morphology varies with the stage of the disease and fungal organism. Table 6.2 summarizes the cytologic features of common fungal pathogens that infect the respiratory tract.

Candidiasis

Microbiology

- Candidiasis, infection caused by *Candida* spp., can involve the lungs. *Candida albicans* is the primary causative agent. They are yeast-like fungi that can form true hyphae and pseudohyphae.
- Most cases of candida pneumonia are secondary to hematological dissemination of organisms from a distant mucocutaneous site.
- The respiratory tract is often colonized with *Candida* spp., especially in hospitalized patients. Patients at particular risk of

TABLE 6.2. Morphology of pulmonary fungal organisms.

Species	Morphology
Candida	Pseudohyphae (elongated yeasts joined together)
	Narrow neck "teardrop" shaped budding yeast (2–10 μm)
Histoplasma	Narrow neck budding yeast (3–5 μm)
Blastomyces	Broad neck budding yeast with a thick cell wall (5–15 μm)
Cryptococcus	Yeast with thick capsules (5–20 μm)
Coccidioides	Thick walled spherules (10–80 μm) filled with endospores (2–5 μm)
Aspergillus	Regular septate hyphae with 45° branching (3–6 μm wide)
	Fruiting bodies (conidiophores)
Mucor	Ribbon-like, nonseptate hyphae with 90° branching (6–50 μm wide)

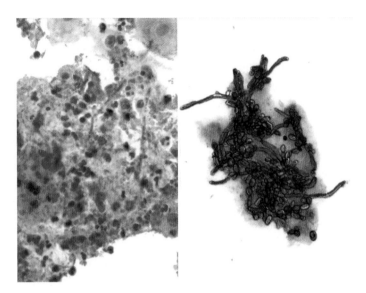

FIG. 6.8. Candidiasis in a BAL specimen with pseudohyphae (elongated yeast joined together) and budding yeast (*left* Pap stain and *right* GMS stain, high magnification).

acquiring a candida lung infection include those with impaired immunity (e.g., transplant recipients, HIV positive individuals, those using corticosteroids, burn victims, and patients with a hematologic neoplasm).

Clinical Features

- Infection of the airways (laryngeal candidiasis and tracheobronchitis) may present with a sore throat, hoarseness, fever, productive cough, and possibly dyspnea. Candida pneumonia is usually associated with disseminated candidiasis. The most common form of infection is multiple lung abscesses.

Cytomorphologic Features

- Specimens containing candida elements may contain pseudohyphae (elongated yeast joined together), true hyphae, and/or budding yeast (blastoconidia) with/without background inflammatory cells (Fig. 6.8).

Differential Diagnosis

- Contamination from oropharyngeal sites (e.g., oral thrush)
- Other fungal organisms (e.g., *Aspergillus*, *cryptococcus*)
- Fungal mimics (e.g., synthetic fibers, pollen grains, etc.)

Ancillary Studies

- Fungal stains (GMS and PAS are positive)
- Gram stain: Positive
- Fungal culture

Histoplasmosis

Microbiology

- Histoplasmosis, caused by the dimorphic fungus *Histoplasma capsulatum*, infection is acquired through inhalation of infective spores (microconidia), which primarily target macrophages in the respiratory system.
- Pulmonary infection may be acute or chronic and present with localized or diffuse pulmonary disease.

Clinical Features

- Pulmonary histoplasmosis can present clinically with pneumonia, lung nodule, cavitary lung disease, mediastinal or hilar lymphadenopathy, and even superior vena cava syndrome or obstruction of other mediastinal structures.
- It is not uncommon for localized infections to mimic cancer.

Cytomorphologic Features

- There are numerous intracellular yeasts measuring 3–5 μm, with narrow based budding, within macrophages. When cells are disrupted they may also be extracellularly located (Fig. 6.9).

Differential Diagnosis

- Candida
- *Cryptococcus neoformans* (microform)

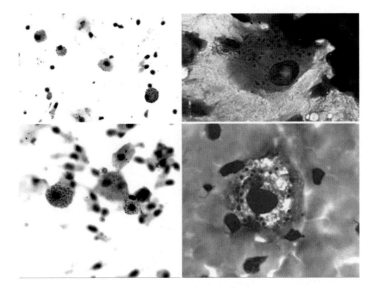

Fig. 6.9. Histoplasmosis. (*Left images*) Macrophages are shown in this ThinPrep specimen of a bronchoalveolar lavage specimen from an AIDS patient with multiple intracellular yeast (Pap stain, *top image* intermediate and *bottom image* high magnification). (*Right images*). Macrophages containing *H. capsulatum* microorganisms are shown at high magnification in these direct smears from lung specimens (Diff-Quik stain).

- *Blastomyces dermatitidis*
- *P. jiroveci*
- Microcalcifications (especially in the cell block)
- Platelets (extracellular only)

Ancillary Studies

- Special stains (GMS and PAS stains are positive)
- Fungal culture
- Antigen detection (enzyme immunoassay using urine, blood, or bronchoalveolar lavage fluid).
- Serology

Blastomycosis

Microbiology

- This is a systemic infection caused by inhaling the conidia of the dimorphic fungus *B. dermatitidis*.
- Infections primarily involve the lung, usually associated with the formation of microabscesses, but may disseminate to cause extrapulmonary disease.

Clinical Features

- Blastomycosis of the lung can be asymptomatic or manifest as acute or chronic pneumonia. In the lungs, this organism usually infects the upper lobes.

Cytomorphologic Features

- One finds round large yeast (5–15 μm) that have a characteristic double contoured thick cell wall, and show broad-base budding.
- There is often associated granulomatous inflammation present.

Differential Diagnosis

- Other fungal organisms (e.g., the microform of *H. capsulatum* and giant form of *Coccidioides immitis*).

Ancillary Studies

- Fungal stains (GMS and PAS are positive)
- Mucicarmine stain (negative, to exclude cryptococcus)
- Immunocytochemistry
- Fungal culture

Cryptococcosis

Microbiology

- Humans are infected with cryptococcus by inhaling basidiospores or yeast. The important human pathogens are *Cryptococcus neoformans* and *Cryptococcus gattii*.

- The course of disease depends on whether yeast are encapsulated (encapsulated yeast may cause a granulomatous reaction) and the patient's immune status. Invasive cryptococcus has become increasingly common among HIV positive and transplant patients.

Clinical Features

- Cryptococcal pulmonary disease varies from asymptomatic airway colonization to a slowly progressive lung mass (cryptococcoma), pneumonia, acute respiratory distress syndrome (ARDS), and pleural effusion.

Cytomorphologic Features

- Round to oval yeasts measuring 5–20 μm are seen with narrow-based buds.
- Yeasts are surrounded by thick capsules that are positive with mucicarmine, alcian blue, and colloidal iron stains (Figs. 6.10 and 6.11).

Differential Diagnosis

- Other fungal organisms (e.g., candida, blastomycosis)
- Fungal mimics

Ancillary Studies

- Fungal stains (GMS and PAS are positive)
- Mucicarmine stain is positive in encapsulated forms
- Fontana-Masson stain may stain the yeast wall
- India ink (requires live organisms)
- Immunocytochemistry
- Serum cryptococcal antigen
- Fungal culture

Coccidioidomycosis

Microbiology

- *C. immitis* infection typically causes a necrotizing granulomatous inflammation. The major pulmonary manifestations include

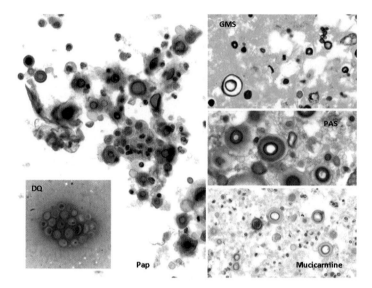

Fig. 6.10. *Cryptococcus* pneumonia. Yeasts are round to oval and have narrow-based buds (Pap stain *left image*, high magnification). Yeasts may resemble pneumocystis cysts, but tend to be more variable and often larger in size (*left inset*, DQ stain, high magnification). Encapsulated cryptococcal organisms are surrounded by a thick capsule that stains with GMS (*top right*), PAS (*middle right*), and mucicarmine (*bottom right*) stains (high magnification).

pulmonary nodules, cavities, diffuse reticulonodular pneumonia, and rarely pleural disease.

• Fungemia can also produce multiple septic pulmonary emboli, especially in patients with immune deficiency.

Clinical Features

• Most people are asymptomatic following initial respiratory exposure to arthroconidia. Those who become ill typically develop respiratory symptoms, such as cough, pleurisy, fever, and weight loss.

Cytomorphologic Features

• The common morphologic forms of *C. immitis* seen in cytology specimens are thick walled spherules (measuring

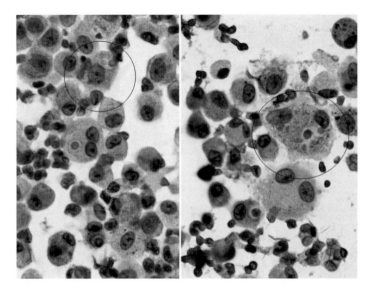

Fɪɢ. 6.11. In cryptococcus pneumonia, organisms may be intracellular. The halo around the organism indicates the presence of a thick capsule (Pap stain, high magnification).

10–80 μm) that contain endospores (measuring 2–5 μm). There are generally very few spherules present in most specimens (Fig. 6.12).

- Sometimes the spherules may be collapsed and appear as empty structures, surrounded by scattered endospores all over the slide.
- Mycelial elements may rarely be present, but these have no distinguishing morphologic characteristics.
- An inflammatory background with/without granulomas may be present.

Differential Diagnosis

- Other large fungal organisms (e.g., *Rhinosporidium* and *Prototheca wickerhamii*).
- Fungal mimics.

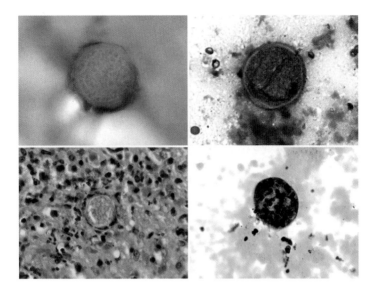

FIG. 6.12. Coccidioidomycosis. (*Left images*) The images shown on the *left* are from a patient who presented with a lung mass that was thought to be a malignancy. An intraoperative touch preparation (*top left*) revealed a spherule with endospores (H&E stain, high magnification). The lung resection in this case confirmed an infection due to Coccidioidomycosis. A spherule is shown (*bottom left*) surrounded by granulomatous inflammation and eosinophils (H&E stain, high magnification). (*Right images*) The images on the *right* are from a lung FNA of a 33-year-old nonsmoking man who presented with a 3 cm lung nodule. Present among the necrotic acellular material were many large round spherules, some of which were empty (*top right*) as they were disrupted after being smeared on the slide (DQ stain, high magnification). A GMS stain in this case shows a spherule filled with endospores and many dispersed free spores in the background (high magnification).

Ancillary Studies

- Fungal stains (GMS, PAS).
- Gram stain is negative.
- Mucicarmine stain is positive.
- Wet preparation of fresh samples using saline or potassium hydroxide solution can be utilized to demonstrate spherules.
- Calcofluor staining is positive.

- Immunocytochemistry using a specific fungal antibody
- Serology and antigen tests
- Skin test
- Fungal culture

Aspergillosis

Microbiology

- Aspergillosis is caused by the fungus *Aspergillus*. Transmission occurs via inhalation of airborne conidial forms.
- Although most people are exposed to this fungus, infections mainly occur in individuals with underlying lung disease (e.g., cystic fibrosis) or impaired immunity (e.g., transplant or AIDS patients).
- There are four types of lung disease caused by *Aspergillus*:
  - Allergic bronchopulmonary aspergillosis.
  - Aspergilloma (fungus ball or mycetoma), which develops in a preexisting lung cavity.
  - Chronic necrotizing pneumonia.
  - Invasive pulmonary aspergillosis, which may cause lung infarction and dissemination to other organs.

Clinical Features

- Symptoms depend on the type of infection, and range from cough to hemoptysis or manifestations from extrapulmonary infection.
- Chest imaging findings are also variable and may include pulmonary infiltrates or a lung cavity with a fungus ball.

Cytomorphologic Features

- Usually only the hyphal form is seen, characterized by septate hyphae with relatively straight walls and 45° (dichotomous) branching (Fig. 6.13).
- Conidial forms of this organism (fruiting bodies) are seen when this organism is exposed to air (e.g., abscess cavity or involvement of large airways).

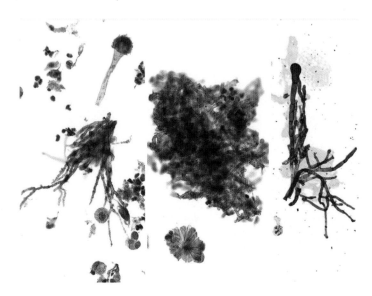

FIG. 6.13. Aspergillosis shown in a ThinPrep preparation of a bronchial washing. Hyphae have relatively straight walls with 45° (dichotomous) branching. The hyphal form of the organism is also septated, best seen with the GMS stain (*right image*, high magnification). A conidial form (fruiting body) was observed in this specimen (*left image*, Pap stain, high magnification), as well as calcium oxalate crystals (*lower part of the middle image*, Pap stain, high magnification).

- A necroinflammatory background is often present.
- Calcium oxalate crystals, which are strongly birefringent under polarized light, may be seen and are highly suggestive of aspergillosis (Fig. 6.13).

Differential Diagnosis

- Other fungal organisms (e.g., mucormycosis, candida, blasto-mycosis).
- Fungal mimics.

Ancillary Studies

- Fungal stains (GMS and PAS are positive).
- Mucicarmine stain is positive.

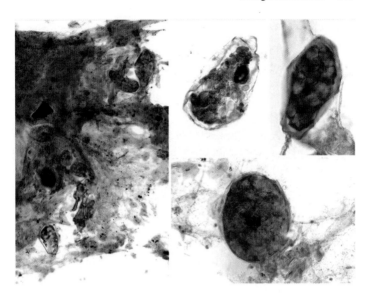

FIG. 6.14. Pulmonary mucormycosis (zygomycosis). Sputum showing terminal chlamydoconidia that are spherical and have thick walls (Pap stain, intermediate magnification on the *left*, and high magnification for *right images*).

- Immunocytochemistry using an immunostain specific to the *Aspergillus* genus (but not species specific).
- Aspergillosis antibody test.
- Galactomannan (a molecule from the fungus sometimes found in blood).
- Fungal culture.

Mucormycosis (Zygomycosis)

Microbiology

- This invasive fungal infection is caused by mycelia-forming fungi of the *Mucorales* (e.g., *Rhizopus*, *Mucor* spp.) and Entomophthorales (e.g., *Conidiobolus* and *Basidiobolus* spp.) orders.
- Primary pulmonary zygomycosis tends to occur in patients with immunosuppression such as patients with neutropenia, transplant recipients, and in those persons receiving high-dose corticosteroid therapy (Fig. 6.14).

Clinical Features

- Patients with pulmonary infection typically present with respiratory symptoms like cough, hemoptysis, chest pain, and dyspnea.

Cytomorphologic Features

- Specimens contain broad, ribbon-like, nonseptate, irregularly shaped hyphae with right-angle branching.
- One may only find a terminal chlamydoconidium that is spherical with thick walls.
- A necroinflammatory background is often present.

Differential Diagnosis

- Other fungal organisms (e.g., candida, blastomycosis).
- Fungal mimics.

Ancillary Studies

- Fungal stains (GMS and PAS are positive).
- Mucicarmine stain is positive.
- Immunocytochemistry using a specific fungal antibody.
- Direct immunofluorescence.
- No serologic tests are available.
- Fungal culture (3–5 days).

Pneumocystis

Microbiology

- Pneumocystis pneumonia (or pneumocystosis) is caused by the yeast-like fungus *P. jirovecii* (formerly called *Pneumocystis carinii*).
- Infection typically involves the distal airspaces and is associated with a foamy or frothy exudate.
- Immunocompromised patients including persons with AIDS and those receiving immunosuppressive therapy are at increased risk of infection.

Clinical Features

- Symptoms include fever, nonproductive cough, shortness of breath, weight loss, and night sweats.
- Complications may include pneumothorax and extrapulmonary disease. Pleural effusion and intrathoracic adenopathy are rare.
- Specimens used to diagnose pulmonary infection include sputum (induced sputum is more sensitive than expectorated samples), BAL (more invasive but has a greater diagnostic yield), and for intubated patients tracheal aspirates.

Cytomorphologic Features

- The typical finding is circumscribed foamy alveolar foamy casts that contain cysts. In some cases, casts may be absent, with organisms present only within macrophages.
- The background inflammatory infiltrate is variable, and may rarely include granulomas.
- Organisms are not well stained but are still visible with a Papanicolaou stain, seen mainly as multiple clear spaces within casts. Cysts are best visualized with silver stains (e.g., GMS).
- Cysts measure 4–8 μm, resemble crushed ping-pong balls (cup-shaped), and with a GMS stain a central dot-like area may be seen representing a focus of cell membrane condensation (Fig. 6.15).
- Cysts tend to be present in aggregates of 2–8, and should not be confused with *Histoplasma* or *Cryptococcus* which typically do not aggregate.
- Budding does not occur. However, adjacent or overlapping cysts may mimic budding organisms.

Differential Diagnosis

- Other fungal organisms (e.g., Candida, cryptococcus, blastomycosis).
- Alveolar proteinosis.
- Amyloidosis.
- Lysed red blood cells.

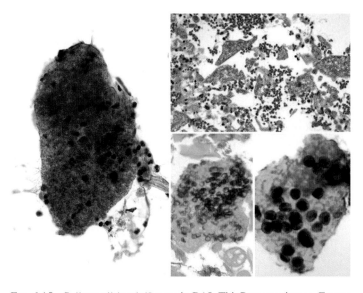

FIG. 6.15. *P. jirovecii* (*carinii*) seen in BAL ThinPrep specimens. Foamy casts are shown containing "empty spaces" that represent cysts entrapped in alveolar exudates (Pap stain, *top left* intermediate magnification, *bottom left* high magnification). Numerous alveolar casts are also present in the cell block (*top right*, H&E stain, intermediate magnification). The cysts tend to aggregate together (*bottom middle*, GMS stain, high magnification), and often have a central dot-like area in the cyst (*right lower*, GMS stain, high magnification).

- Other potential mimics including mucus, lubricant, bacterial clumps, talc, neutrophils, hemosiderin filled macrophages, and epithelial cells.

Ancillary Studies

- Cyst wall stains with GMS, PAS, and mucicarmine stains.
- Intracystic or free sporozoites (not cyst walls) stain with Giemsa.
- Immunocytochemistry using a specific *Pneumocystis* immunostain.
- Calcofluor white.
- Direct immunofluorescence.
- PCR.

TABLE 6.3. Pulmonary parasitic organisms.

Protozoa
  Toxoplasma gondii
  Entamoeba histolytica
  Cryptosporidium
  Microsporidium

Nematoda (roundworms)
  Dirofilaria immitis
  Filaria spp. (*Wuchereria bancrofti*, *Onchocerca volulus*, etc.)
  Strongyloides stercoralis

Cestoda (tapeworms)
  Echinococcus granulosus, *Echinococcus multilocularis*

Trematoda (flukes)
  Paragonimus spp. (*westermani*, *africanus*, *mexicanus*, etc.)
  Schistosoma spp. (*mansoni*, *japonicum*, *haematobium*)

Parasitic Infections

Parasites are rare in most developed countries, but may be endemic in other parts of the world. Pulmonary involvement often occurs because the lungs represent a site of infection during the life cycle of some parasites. Infection is often associated with eosinophilia in the blood and pulmonary tissue. Table 6.3 lists parasitic organisms likely to infect the respiratory tract.

Dirofilariasis

- Humans may acquire *Dirofilaria immitis* (dog heartworm) through insect vectors (mosquitoes) from dogs. Parasites that become entrapped within pulmonary vessels may result in pulmonary infarction.
- FNA of infarcted nodules demonstrate worm fragments mixed with necrotic lung tissue and an inflammatory and granulomatous response.
- Worms measure 120–310 mm in length depending on the sex (females are larger than males). *Dirofilaria* are distinguished from other nematodes by their prominent muscular lateral cords and striated cuticle.

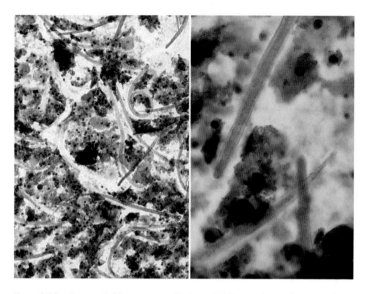

FIG. 6.16. *Strongyloides stercoralis* in a BAL specimen from an HIV positive patient. The specimen shows many filariform larvae with rounded ends and notched (coiled) tails (Pap stain, intermediate magnification *left*, high magnification *right*).

Strongyloidiasis

- *Strongyloides stercoralis* involves the respiratory tract via hematogenous spread of the infective form (filariform larvae), especially in those who are immunosuppressed.
- Sputum, tracheal aspirates, and BAL samples are all useful for establishing the diagnosis.
- Filariform larvae are large (400–500 µm), and possess notched tails and a short buccal cavity. They need to be distinguished from the larval forms of *Ascaris lumbricoides* and hookworms (Fig. 6.16).

Paragonimiasis

- The species that commonly causes human infection is *Paragonimus westermani*.

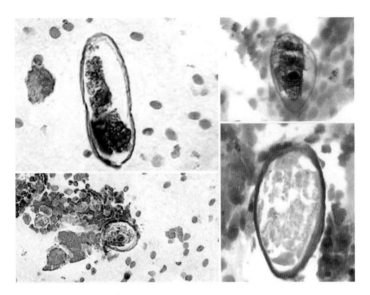

FIG. 6.17. Paragonimus eggs identified in this FNA cell block from a lung nodule. The eggs have a thick, double contour shell (H&E stain, low and high magnification, *left* and *right* respectively).

- Mature worms in the lung shed eggs that may be visible in exfoliated samples (sputum or bronchial washings) or FNA specimens.
- Eggs have a thick, double contour shell with an operculated end that has a flattened appearance, and, depending upon the species, measure approximately 80–118 µm (Fig. 6.17).

Toxoplasma gondii

- Lung involvement occurs with severe disseminated infection (toxoplasmosis), especially in neonates (via congenital trans-placental infection) and immunocompromised patients.
- Respiratory specimens like BAL require close inspection for crescent or arc-shaped free (extracellular) trophozoites, as they measure only around 5–7 µm in length. Macrophages may be seen containing several parasites. Parasites contain a prominent

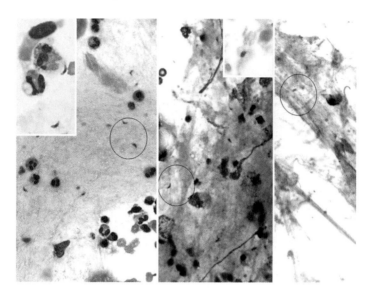

FIG. 6.18. Toxoplasmosis in a BAL specimen from a transplant patient. The extracellular trophozoites caught up in the mucus are banana-shaped organisms with a prominent central nucleus (Giemsa stain, high magnification). The parasites are barely visible with a Pap stain (*right image*, high magnification). The *inset* in the *middle* shows an immunoreactive parasite (immunocytochemical stain, high magnification).

central nucleus, and need to be distinguished from similar sized *Histoplasma* (which exhibit narrow-neck budding) and *Leishmania* (which also contain a kinetoplast).
- Parasitic organisms are best identified using a Giemsa-stained preparation.
- An immunohistochemical stain for Toxoplasma is available (Fig. 6.18).

Entamoeba

- With *Entamoeba histolytica* infection, the lungs may be involved by extension from an amebic liver abscess or via hematogenous spread.

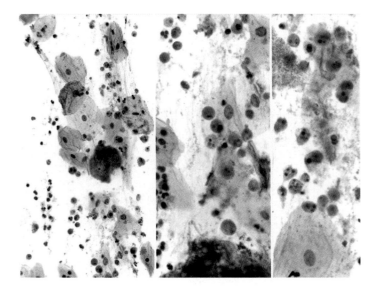

FIG. 6.19. A sputum specimen from a 32-year-old man is shown with *E. gingivalis*. The amebae are larger than histocytes, have amphophilic bubbly cytoplasm, and a sharply defined nuclear karyosome (Pap stains, intermediate magnification on the *left*, high magnification *middle* and *right*).

- *E. gingivalis* is a parasitic protozoan of the oral cavity. In patients with poor oral hygiene, aspiration can result in a lung infection.
- Amebae have a histiocyte-like morphology and typically contain ingested RBCs in their cytoplasm. Trophozoites are, however, slightly larger than macrophages and have smaller nuclei with coarser chromatin than histiocytes.
- The morphologic appearances of *E. histolytica* and *E. gingivalis* are quite similar, although the trophozoites of *E. gingivalis* tend to be comparably larger (10–35 vs. 15–20 μm) and, unlike with *E. histolytica*, there is no associated cyst stage. *E. gingivalis* is also the only species of amebae that can phagocytose white and red blood cells as well as ingest bacteria (Fig. 6.19).

Echinococcosis (Hydatid Disease)

- The most common cestode pathologic to the lung is *Echinococcus granulosus*, which manifests as an echinococcal (hydatid) cyst.

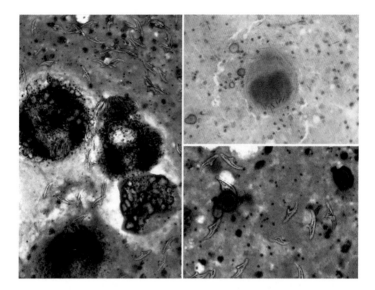

Fig. 6.20. Echinococcosis (hydatid disease of the lung). This lung FNA from a 38-year-old woman yielded 20 mL of clear fluid that contained numerous intact protoscoleces containing radially arranged hooklets shown with a DQ stain (*left*, intermediate magnification) and Pap stain (*upper right*, intermediate magnification). Detached hooklets resembling shark's teeth are also seen (DQ stain, *lower right*, high magnification) (images courtesy of Dr. Pawel Schubert, South Africa).

- Patients may be asymptomatic for many years. A primary hydatid cyst of the chest may mimic a neoplasm.
- FNA usually contains hydatid sand consisting of variable numbers of intact protoscoleces containing radially arranged hooklets and detached (free) refractile hooklets (resembling shark's teeth) present in a background of thick granular material (Fig. 6.20).
- Cell blocks may contain portions of a cyst wall that consists of three layers: (1) host layer with giant cells, fibroblasts, and eosinophils; (2) middle acellular laminated membrane; and (3) inner germinal layer.
- It is controversial whether suspected hydatid cysts should be aspirated as fluid leakage could result in anaphylaxis or disseminated disease.

Pleural Infections and Empyema

- Pleural (parapneumonic) effusion occurs in 20–40% of hospitalized patients with bacterial pneumonia, and has three stages: exudative (early culture negative), fibrinopurulent (infected), and pleural rind stage. Empyema is defined as pus in the pleural space.
- Pleural infection can also occur following trauma, surgery, esophageal rupture, or as a result of direct extension (from the lung or subdiaphragmatic disease).
- Infectious causes of pleural disease include bacteria (e.g., *Streptococcus*, *H. influenza*, anaerobes, actinomycosis, *Legionella*), mycobacteria, fungi (*Candida*, Pneumocystis), and parasites (*E. histolytica*).
- A predominance of neutrophils indicates an acute infection, while many mononuclear inflammatory cells usually indicate a more indolent process (e.g., TB or fungal infection).
- Pleural fluid eosinophilia (>10%) may be caused by infection (fungal, parasitic) and noninfectious causes (e.g., air, blood, drugs).

Suggested Reading

Lemos LB, Baliga M, Taylor BD, Cason ZJ, Lucia HL. Bronchoalveolar lavage for diagnosis of fungal disease. Five years' experience in a southern United States rural area with many blastomycosis cases. Acta Cytol. 1995;39:1101–11.

Moriarty AT, Darragh TM, Fatheree LA, Souers R, Wilbur DC. Performance of Candida – fungal-induced atypia and proficiency testing: observations from the College of American Pathologists proficiency testing program. Arch Pathol Lab Med. 2009;133:1272–5.

Naimey GL, Wuerker RB. Comparison of histologic stains in the diagnosis of *Pneumocystis carinii*. Acta Cytol. 1995;39:1124–7.

Pisani RJ, Wright AJ. Clinical utility of bronchoalveolar lavage in immunocompromised hosts. Mayo Clin Proc. 1992;67:221–7.

Raab SS, Cheville JC, Bottles K, Cohen MB. Utility of Gomori methenamine silver stains in bronchoalveolar lavage specimens. Mod Pathol. 1994;7:599–604.

Saad RS, Silverman JF. Respiratory cytology: differential diagnosis and pitfalls. Diagn Cytopathol. 2010;38:297–307.

Sheehan MM, Coker R, Coleman DV. Detection of cytomegalovirus (CMV) in HIV+ patients: comparison of cytomorphology, immunocytochemistry and in situ hybridization. Cytopathology. 1998;9:29–37.

7
Gastrointestinal and Hepatobiliary Infections

Robert M. Najarian and Helen H. Wang
Department of Pathology, Beth Israel Deaconess Medical Center/Harvard
Medical School, 330 Brookline Avenue, Boston, MA 02215, USA

The diagnosis of gastrointestinal and hepatobiliary infections can be effectively made by the use of endoscopic brushings, touch imprints of endoscopic mucosal biopsies, as well as fine needle aspiration (FNA), or a combination of the above modalities with concomitant histologic evaluation, microbiologic culture, and relevant laboratory data (e.g., stool examination). This chapter discusses characteristic infections of the gastrointestinal and hepatobiliary tracts and focuses on their cytomorphology, differential diagnosis, and ancillary studies.

Gastrointestinal Infections

Fungal Esophagitis

- Fungal esophagitis in both immunocompetent and immunocompromised patients results mainly from infection by *Candida* spp.
- More rare forms of fungal esophagitis in immunocompromised patients include those caused by dimorphic fungi, *Aspergillus* spp., and the zygomycetes.
- Infection typically presents in the mid to lower esophagus with symptoms of dysphagia or odynophagia. However, patients can be asymptomatic, especially those who are immunocompetent.

L. Pantanowitz et al., *Cytopathology of Infectious Diseases*,
Essentials in Cytopathology 17, DOI 10.1007/978-1-4614-0242-8_7,
© Springer Science+Business Media, LLC 2011

- Predisposing factors include damage to the esophageal mucosal barrier (chemotherapy, antibiotic use, indwelling devices such as naso- or orogastric tubes) and a compromise of the host defense mechanism (such as neutropenia).
- Sensitivity for diagnosis via brushing closely approximates and, in some studies, exceeds that of the mucosal biopsy.

Cytomorphologic Features

- Infection with *Candida* spp. manifests with pseudohyphae or budding yeast forms that stain blue to pink with the Papanicolaou stain.
- In contrast, true branching hyphae forming 45° angles in the setting of a severely debilitated patient confirms the diagnosis of *Aspergillus* infection.
- Predominance of admixed neutrophils with reactive squamous cells and focal necrosis may be seen in the background (Fig. 7.1).

Differential Diagnosis

- Squamous epithelial reactive changes and an associated neutrophilic infiltrate can mimic those seen in viral esophagitis or ulcers due to direct chemical injuries to the mucosa.
- Flattened, desquamated anucleate squames, or ingested food can approximate the appearance of fungal pseudohyphae, but can be definitively ruled out by lack of staining of these elements with a PAS plus diastase stain.
- Oral flora in coccoid forms can be mistaken for yeast forms; however, no budding will be demonstrated and deployment of the brushing device in the tubular esophagus below the level of the oral cavity should eliminate the risk of such bacterial contamination.
- Filamentous (*leptothrix*-type) organisms may be associated with esophageal malignancies. These may resemble *actinomyces* clumps.

Ancillary Studies

- PAS plus diastase or methanamine silver stains will outline hyphae, pseudohyphae, as well as budding yeast forms.

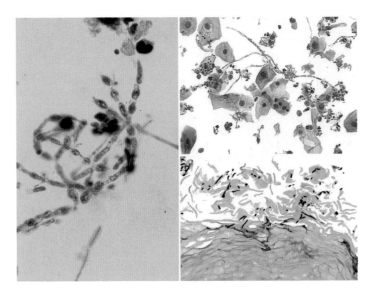

Fig. 7.1. (*Left*) Brushing preparation of *Candida* esophagitis with blue-staining pseudohyphae and purple-staining budding yeast forms (Pap stain, high magnification). Rare inflammatory cells are seen in the background. (*Right upper*) Candida esophagitis is shown in association with reactive squamous cells (Pap stain, high magnification). (*Bottom right*) Superficial esophageal mucosal biopsy showing colonization by Candida (GMS stain, high magnification).

- Fungal culture, while not time efficient for diagnosis, can help to guide antimicrobial therapy and to identify species with resistance to standard antifungal agents.

Herpes Simplex Viruses

- HSV infection occurs in both immunocompromised and immunocompetent individuals, presenting clinically with acute onset of odynophagia, fever, and atypical chest pain.
- In most cases, active infection represents reactivation of latent infection in immunocompetent individuals.
- Endoscopically there may be discrete, punched-out ulcers with an exudative base and erythematous margins. The edge of the

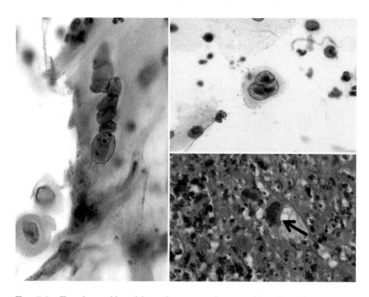

FIG. 7.2. Esophageal brushings demonstrating a multinucleated squamous cell (*left*) with nuclear molding as well as nuclear chromatin margination and (*top right*) typical Cowdry A inclusions (Pap stain, high magnification). (*Bottom right*) An image from an esophageal mucosal biopsy is shown demonstrating similar multinucleated squamous cells (*arrow*) with nuclear molding and ground glass cytoplasmic change in a background of necrotic and exudative material characteristic of herpes viral infection (H&E stain, intermediate magnification).

ulcer should be brushed to identify herpetic changes within squamous cells and not the ulcer base with granulation tissue.

- Diffuse and sometimes confluent ulceration is more common in an immunocompromised patient (Fig. 7.2).

Cytomorphologic Features

- Esophageal brushings demonstrate large, glassy, eosinophilic (Cowdry A) inclusions of the squamous epithelial cell nucleus, with peripherally condensed margin of chromatin.
- Multinucleation of squamous cells with molding of the nuclei to each other and ground glass cytoplasmic change (Cowdry B) are also characteristically seen.
- Background neutrophils and necrotic debris may also be present.

Differential Diagnosis

- Reactive cytologic changes seen adjacent to ulcers of varying etiologies, as well as other infectious conditions, can mimic those of herpes esophagitis. However, the presence of multinucleated squamous cells with intracellular inclusions is fairly characteristic.
- Carcinoma, since viral inclusions may be misinterpreted as macronucleoli of malignant cells.
- Radiation esophagitis can produce enlarged squamous cells with degenerative changes that can simulate ground-glass type viral inclusions.
- Cytomegalovirus infection.

Ancillary Studies

- Immunohistochemical stains for HSV 1 and 2 can increase the sensitivity for detection of viral cytopathic effect.
- Viral culture samples, while being highly sensitive for the diagnosis of HSV, also have the limitation of requiring days to weeks for the characteristic cytopathic effect to develop in vitro.
- Detection of viral DNA by PCR on blood samples is sensitive, but not specific, for esophageal infection by herpes viruses.

Cytomegalovirus

- CMV infection of the gastrointestinal tract occurs primarily in the immunosuppressed patient population, including solid organ and stem cell transplant recipients, as well as in patients receiving immunosuppression therapy.
- Patients may present clinically with nonspecific symptoms such as epigastric or abdominal pain, nausea, vomiting, and diarrhea. CMV infection of endothelial cells may also result in ischemic necrosis with subsequent ulceration and/or pseudotumor formation causing bowel obstruction.
- Endoscopy shows punched-out ulcers in the esophagus, stomach, and/or colon with surrounding erythema (Fig. 7.3).

Cytomorphologic Features

- Mucosal brushings and biopsies demonstrate enlargement of infected endothelial or mesenchymal cells with a characteristic

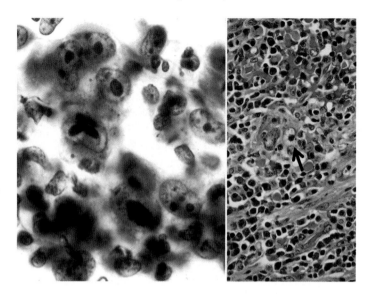

Fig. 7.3. (*Left*) Esophageal brushing demonstrating marked enlargement of esophageal endothelial cells with a prominent eosinophilic nuclear inclusion and surrounding cleared-out halo (Pap stain, high magnification). (*Right*) A characteristic endothelial cell infected by cytomegalovirus is shown (*arrow*) within the colonic submucosa. The eosinophilic nuclear inclusion in this case could be mistaken for an enlarged, oval-shaped nucleolus but was immunoreactive for antibodies to CMV (H&E stain, high magnification).

    single, eosinophilic, intranuclear inclusion, often with a circumferential clear halo surrounding it.

- Infected cells of mesenchymal origin can also demonstrate intracytoplasmic, basophilic granules.
- Focal necrotic debris, scattered neutrophils, fibrinopurulent exudate, and reactive squamous cells or glandular cells are often seen in the background.

Differential Diagnosis

- Nucleoli of reactive squamous cells or adenocarcinoma
- Enlarged endothelial cells within granulation tissue of an ulcer
- Herpes simplex virus Cowdry A inclusions

- Immunoblasts or follicular dendritic cells associated with a reactive lymphoid aggregate or mucosa-associated lymphoid tissue

Ancillary Studies

- Immunocytochemical stain for cytomegalovirus can increase sensitivity for detection of viral cytopathic effect from about 50 to 70% based on H&E evaluation alone to approximately 85%.
- CMV DNA viral load performed on a blood specimen is extremely sensitive for detecting infection, but is not predictive of systemic disease, which requires demonstration of the organism in a mucosal biopsy or sampling.

Helicobacter pylori Gastritis

- This bacterial infection is the most common cause of gastritis in the developing world, with up to 75% of individuals infected by the age of 25 years, and the most common cause of infectious gastritis in the developed world.
- Clinically, patients may present with nonspecific symptoms such as abdominal or epigastric pain, dyspepsia, and nausea, while others remain asymptomatic carriers of infection.
- Gastric infection with *Helicobacter pylori* has been linked to the development of the majority of gastric and duodenal ulcers, as well as to extranodal marginal zone lymphomas of the stomach, and the intestinal type of gastric adenocarcinoma (Fig. 7.4).

Cytomorphologic Features

- Specimens obtained via touch imprints of endoscopic mucosal biopsies reveal a flagellated, curved, or spiral bacterium (S or C shaped) measuring 0.3 μm in width and 3–5 μm in length, often in a background of mucus with superficial gastric foveolar epithelial cells.
- The presence of associated lymphoplasmacytic inflammation (chronic gastritis) with scattered neutrophils (active gastritis) is variable.
- Glandular epithelial cells may show reparative atypia and intestinal metaplasia.
- *Candida* spp. may also be present if they have colonized an associated peptic ulcer.

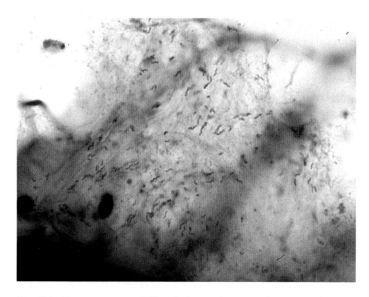

FIG. 7.4. Numerous curved *H. pylori* organisms are demonstrated in this imprint obtained from a gastric mucosal biopsy. Note the abundant mucus layer within which the organisms are seen (Pap stain, high magnification).

Differential Diagnosis

- Infection with other related spiral-shaped bacteria, such as *Helicobacter heilmanii* can be excluded based upon morphology alone, in that the latter bacterium is both larger in size (up to 7.5 μm) and more tightly coiled.
- Debris caught in the superficial gastric mucin layer can often cause diagnostic difficulty. This can be definitively resolved with ancillary studies.
- Contamination of slides with oral flora or environmental bacteria, some of which may stain using nonspecific ancillary methods noted below, are chiefly excluded by the presence of a polymorphous bacterial population.

Ancillary Studies

- Special stains that increase the sensitivity of *Helicobacter* detection such as the silver-based Steiner, Warthin-Starry, Diff-Quik, and Giemsa stains will nonspecifically also stain bacterial contaminants and debris. The bacteria are Gram-negative.

- Immunocytochemical stains for *Helicobacter* spp. are sensitive and specific for organism detection, but stain both *H. pylori* and atypical *Helicobacter* spp.
- Urease breath tests and the CLO slide test for the urease enzyme are utilized for detection of infection with fair rates of sensitivity.
- Serologic tests for *H. pylori* can aid in documenting a patient's history of past infection and guide future ancillary tests performed on mucosal samples.
- PCR
- Microbiologic culture

Cryptosporidiosis

- This gastrointestinal infection, caused by the intracellular protozoal parasite *Cryptosporidium parvum*, is most frequently acquired through the ingestion of contaminated water or by fecal–oral route.
- While seen as a rare, self-limited infection in immunocompetent individuals, systemic infection in those who are immunocompromised, especially patients with AIDS, may involve the entire length of the gastrointestinal tract, including the gallbladder.
- Clinically, immunocompetent patients present with a short duration of diarrheal illness including abdominal cramps and mild malabsorption. Those with impaired immune function may have a protracted course with severe weight loss, cholera-like watery diarrhea, and frequent rates of relapse (Fig. 7.5).

Cytomorphologic Features

- Specimens obtained via stool sampling or endoscopic brushings/mucosal biopsies demonstrate spherical organisms measuring 2–5 µm that irregularly protrude from the apical aspect of the surface epithelium. The microorganisms appear to be adherent to the epithelial cells.
- Background inflammation is typically not present, but may be seen in the setting of intense infections.

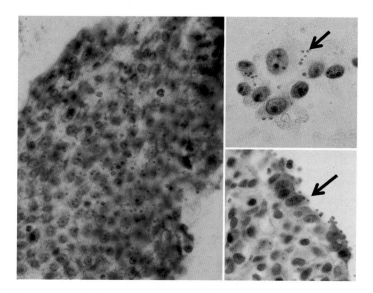

FIG. 7.5. (*Left*) Gastric brushing specimen demonstrating many small spherical organisms adherent to the apical surface of epithelial cells (Pap stain, high magnification). (*Top right*) Similar gastric brushing specimen demonstrating the small spherical organisms (*arrow*) in a background of reactive appearing glandular epithelial cells and lack of significant inflammation (Pap stain, high magnification). (*Bottom right*) Mucosal biopsy with evidence of Cryptosporidium infection. Note that these small organisms (*arrow*) are located at the apical surface of the mucosal cells (i.e., intracellular but "extracytoplasmic") (H&E stain, high magnification).

Differential Diagnosis

- Cellular debris and apical mucin adherent to epithelial surfaces can mimic cryptosporidial infection and sometimes require the use of ancillary detection techniques.
- *Cyclospora cayetanensis* are also located apically within enterocytes, but are larger (8–10 μm) and GMS negative.
- Microsporidiosis, where multiple microorganisms are collectively located within a supranuclear intracytoplasmic vacuole.
- *Isospora belli* are located within deeper intracytoplasmic vacuoles, and are oval and larger (20 μm).

Ancillary Studies

- Modified acid fast and silver-based stains (such as Steiner or Warthin-Starry stains) are of benefit in the detection of cryptosporidial infection. They are GMS negative.
- Immunocytochemical stain for *Cryptosporidia.*
- Stool examination (modified acid fast stain).
- Direct and indirect immunofluorescence microscopy can increase the detection rate of oocysts in stool samples.
- Transmission electron microscopy.

Giardiasis

- This is the most commonly diagnosed intestinal parasitic infection in both the United States and worldwide.
- Infection caused by the extracellular protozoal parasite *Giardia lamblia* (*Giardia intestinalis*) is most frequently acquired through the ingestion of contaminated water, typically untreated water from springs or lakes or via the fecal–oral route in child care settings.
- In the acute phase, a self-limited, but severe diarrheal illness can result in volume depletion while chronic infection can result in a severe malabsorptive state with iron and folate deficiency.
- Commonly associated symptoms include abdominal pain, cramping, nausea, and vomiting with acute illness and weight loss, malabsorption, and malnutrition in chronic illness (Fig. 7.6).

Cytomorphologic Features

- Specimens obtained via stool sampling, endoscopic brushings, or mucosal biopsy imprints demonstrate flagellated, pear-shaped organisms similar in size to the nuclei of intestinal epithelial cells (12–15 μm in greatest dimension).
- Parasites have a centrally placed nucleus that is gray to lightly basophilic with the most common cytologic staining preparations.

Differential Diagnosis

- Extracellular debris can rarely mimic giardial infection.

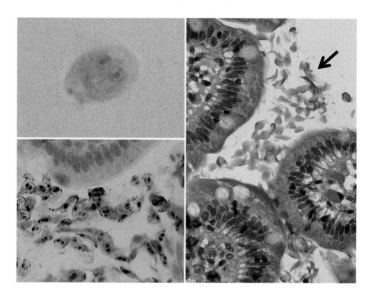

FIG. 7.6. (*Top left*) Single, pear-shaped Giardia trophozoite is present in a duodenal brushing specimen with two prominent, centrally placed nuclei (Pap stain, high magnification). (*Right*) Multiple organisms are seen (*arrow*) overlying the villous epithelial surface in a duodenal mucosal biopsy (H&E stain, high magnification). (*Bottom left*) Immunostaining of a duodenal mucosal biopsy with antibodies to c-kit demonstrates positive staining of Giardia organisms (high magnification).

Ancillary Studies

- Stool examination for ova and parasites, while reasonably sensitive for organism detection in the setting of active infection, often requires multiple samples to achieve high levels of diagnostic sensitivity.
- Fecal antigen detection and stool PCR tests are available for sensitive and specific organism detection.
- An immunostain for c-kit (CD117) can be used to highlight trophozoites and distinguish them from extracellular debris.

Microsporidiosis

- This is one of the most common gastrointestinal opportunistic infections in the setting of HIV/AIDS.

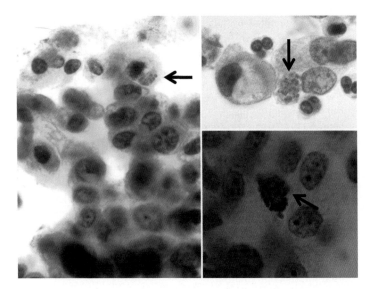

FIG. 7.7. (*Left and top right*) Brushing from the biliary epithelium demonstrates glandular epithelial cells with an intracellular cluster (*arrow*) of numerous round spores with a purple color on Papanicolaou stain. Nearby epithelial cells display a mild increase in nuclear to cytoplasmic ratio and prominent nucleoli (Pap stain, high magnification). (*Bottom right*) Microsporidia spores within an intestinal epithelial cell (*arrow*) are readily visible with a Brown-Brenn Gram stain (high magnification).

- Microsporidia include the obligate intracellular parasites *Enterocytozoon bieneusi* and *Encephalitozoon intestinalis*.
- Despite clinical symptoms of watery diarrhea that are mild relative to other opportunistic organisms, the propensity for systemic dissemination is great with biliary tract, colonic, respiratory tract and pancreatic infection.
- Mild infection presents with a normal endoscopic appearance, while severe cases can have extensive ulcers (Fig. 7.7).

Cytomorphologic Features

- Specimens obtained via mucosal biopsy demonstrate intestinal epithelial cells with oval-shaped, supranuclear spores measuring approximately 1 μm in diameter.

- Special care must be taken to examine sampled degenerating enterocytes for organisms, as there is a greater likelihood of detection of these microorganisms in the setting of degeneration.

Differential Diagnosis

- Supranuclear mucin vacuoles of oval shape can mimic microsporidia organisms. Problematic cases can be stained with mucicarmine to demonstrate intracytoplasmic mucin.

Ancillary Studies

- Acid fast, silver-based, Gram, and PAS stains can all help with organism detection, as its small size and intracellular location can easily lead to a false negative diagnosis.
- Ultrastructural examination is useful in cases in which a particular species of organism must be isolated or for confirmation of light microscopic findings.

Mycobacterium avium Complex

- Extrapulmonary disseminated infection due to atypical mycobacteria occurs almost exclusively in the HIV/AIDS population, especially those with very low CD4 cell counts. Involvement of the gastrointestinal tract is nearly twice as common as pulmonary involvement.
- Infection is mainly due to the *Mycobacterium avium complex* or MAC (also called *Mycobacterium avium intracellulare* or MAI).
- The entire tubular gastrointestinal tract may be involved in such infections, with the small intestine being the site of most pronounced disease.
- Clinical symptoms and signs are nonspecific with nausea, chronic diarrhea, abdominal pain, and malabsorption being most commonly reported (Fig. 7.8).

Cytomorphologic Features

- Specimens obtained via brushings or mucosal biopsies demonstrate organisms with a characteristic "beaded rod" shape measuring 4–6 μm in length contained either within foamy histiocytes or seen lying free in the background.

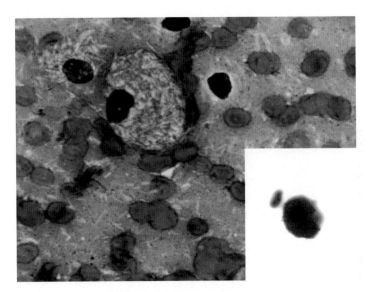

FIG. 7.8. Duodenal brushing specimen demonstrating infected macrophages with copious foamy cytoplasm (due to negative images of mycobacterial organisms within the cytoplasm of macrophages). Note the many free scattered unstained mycobacteria in the background (Diff-Quik stain, high magnification). The *bottom right inset* shows a macrophage stained with an acid fast stain that demonstrates the mycobacteria (high magnification).

- The negative (clear or unstained) image of these mycobacteria may be apparent with a Diff-Quik stain.
- Rarely, poorly formed granulomas comprised of aggregates of organism-laden histiocytes can be observed, but much less frequently than in cases of *Mycobacterium tuberculosis* infection.

Differential Diagnosis

- Whipple's disease and histoplasmosis are diagnostic considerations, which are both Periodic acid Schiff stain positive, but acid fast negative.

Ancillary Studies

- Acid fast stain of cytologic preparations or formalin fixed tissue biopsy.

- PCR analysis.
- Mycobacterial culture is both sensitive and specific for organism detection, but requires weeks to months to achieve adequate organism growth.

Anal Pap Test

- The incidence of anal intraepithelial neoplasia (AIN) and invasive anal cancer is increasing, especially in the HIV population.
- Anal Pap tests have been utilized in the HIV population for the evaluation of HPV-related disease of the anus. The sensitivity (42–98%) and specificity (16–96%) of the anal Pap test for the detection of squamous intraepithelial lesions (SIL) are quite variable.
- It is recommended that anal–rectal cytologic findings be reported according to the criteria and terminology of the Bethesda System (2001) used for reporting cervical cytology.
- Cellular elements that may be encountered in an anal Pap test include:
  ○ Squamous cells, anucleate squames, and anal transformation zone components (metaplastic cells and/or rectal glandular cells).
  ○ HPV-related diseases include SIL and squamous cell carcinoma. SIL tend to, but not always, exhibit prominent keratinization.
  ○ Contamination with bacteria and fecal material, which may obscure cells, making the specimen unsatisfactory for evaluation.
  ○ Less commonly, infectious organisms other than HPV can be detected such as *Candida* spp., *herpes simplex virus*, *trichomonas*, and other parasites including ova and worms (Fig. 7.9).

Intra-Abdominal Infections

Liver Abscess

- The majority of liver abscesses are due to bacterial infections. Pyogenic abscesses are mainly due to streptococci, staphylococci, or enteric bacteria. They may occur as a result of ascending

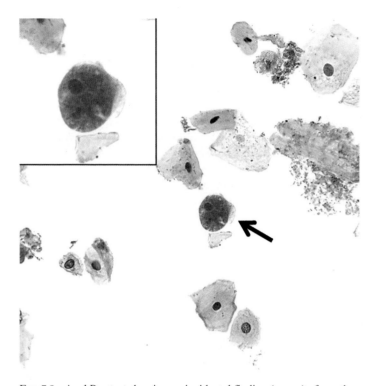

FIG. 7.9. Anal Pap test showing an incidental finding (*arrow*) of a pathogenic ameba (higher magnification shown in the *upper left inset*) containing phagocytosed erythrocytes (Pap stain, high magnification) (image courtesy of Christine Panetti CT (ASCP), Baystate Medical Center, Springfield, MA, USA).

cholangitis, sepsis, or following trauma. Not all patients have a fever or right upper quadrant tenderness. FNA contains abundant neutrophils with necrotic debris and occasionally bacteria that can be readily confirmed with a Gram stain.

- *Candida* is the most common cause of an hepatic fungal abscess, and usually encountered in patients with an impaired immunity. Other organisms that may be encountered in an FNA of a liver abscess include actinomyces, Leishmania, and *G. lamblia*.

- Hepatic amebic abscess, due mainly to infection with *Entameba histolytica*, is an uncommon complication of amebiasis involving the gastrointestinal tract. They mainly involve the right liver lobe. FNA material contains trophozites associated with abundant necrotic debris ("anchovy paste"), macrophages, degenerated hepatocytes, and only scant neutrophils. Trophozoites of *E. histolytica* resemble macrophages with their round shape, foamy cytoplasm, and single round nucleus. They typically contain phagocytosed red blood cells.
- The finding of numerous eosinophils may be related to parasites, such as the liver flukes *Clonorchis sinensis* or *Fasciola hepatica*.
- FNA material containing granulomas may be seen and due to infection (e.g., tuberculosis, fungi) or other liver disorder (e.g., primary biliary cirrhosis, sarcoidosis, drug reaction, etc.).
- The differential diagnosis of a liver abscess includes a neoplasm with marked tumor necrosis (Fig. 7.10).

Pancreatitis

- Pancreatitis (usually acute) may be caused by a variety of infections including viruses (e.g., mumps, HSV, HIV), bacteria (e.g., *mycoplasma, salmonella*), fungi (e.g., *Aspergillus*), and parasites (e.g., *Toxoplasma, cryptosporidium, Ascaris*). FNA is typically not performed in patients with acute pancreatitis, but if performed will show numerous neutrophils with fat necrosis, epithelial cells with inflammatory atypia, and a dirty background.
- Microorganisms may be detected in cytology material or can be cultured from aspirated material submitted to the microbiology laboratory.
- As pancreatitis may occur secondary to obstruction from a neoplasm, a careful search for associated neoplastic cells is important.

Hydatid Disease

- Echinococcosis (hydatid disease) is caused by ingestion of the larval forms of *Echinococcus* tapeworms, most commonly *Echinococcus granulosus*, which spread via the portal venous circulation to the liver.

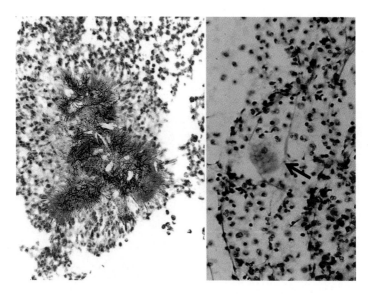

FIG. 7.10. (*Left*) Liver abscess following cholecystectomy in this case was found to be due to actinomyces on FNA. A sulfur granule is shown containing filamentous bacteria surrounded by many neutrophils (Gram stain, high magnification). (*Right*) Percutaneous liver FNA of an amebic liver abscess shows an ameba present (*arrow*) in an inflamed background (Pap stain, high magnification) (image courtesy of Dr. Pam Michelow, South Africa).

- Patients commonly present with a slowly growing hydatid cyst identified either incidentally on an imaging study or after episodes of abdominal pain, jaundice, or portal hypertension in cases of larger cysts.
- The diagnosis is often made preliminarily on abdominal imaging studies following the identification of a thin-walled cyst in the setting of positive serologic studies (Fig. 7.11).

Cytomorphologic Features

- A confirmatory diagnosis can be made by FNA of hepatic cystic lesions that demonstrate ovoid protoscoleces measuring about 100 μm in diameter that are attached to the germinal membrane of the cyst wall.

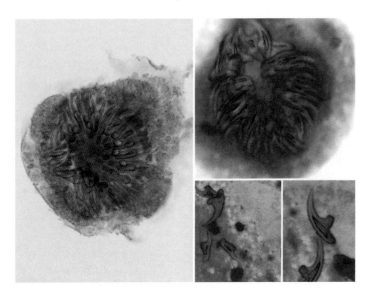

FIG. 7.11. Fine needle aspirate of hydatid cyst fluid demonstrates a protoscolex with radial array of hooklets with a (*left*) Papanicolaou stain and
(*top right*) Diff-Quik stain (high magnification). (*Lower right*) Hydatid
cyst fluid is shown to contain only scattered hooklets without an associated protoscolex. Note their characteristic scimitar shape (Diff-Quik stain,
high magnification) (image courtesy of Thomas Buck, M.D., Beth Israel
Deaconess Medical Center, Boston, MA).

- Intact protoscoleces contain two circular arrays of hooklets and
  a sucker. However, cysts often contain only shed hooklets or
  degenerated material (hydatid sand).
- Shed hooklets are said to have a characteristic scimitar (curved,
  single-edged sword) shape that may be accompanied by calcareous bodies.

Differential Diagnosis

- Differentiation of a viable hydatid cyst from simple benign
  hepatic cysts or mesothelial inclusion cysts rests on the ability
  to demonstrate any viable components of the hydatid cyst
  including the protoscoleces, hooklets, or germinal membrane.

Surgical excision with extensive sampling of tissue for histopathology is often required to demonstrate these components.

Ancillary Studies

- Serologic studies for antibodies to *E. granulosus*

Peritoneal Effusion with Infection

- Intraperitoneal infection may be diffuse (peritonitis), localized (intraperitoneal abscess), or abscess may form around diseased viscera (e.g., periappendiceal abscess).
- Secondary intra-abdominal infection may result from spillage of gastrointestinal or genitourinary microorganisms into the peritoneal cavity (e.g., trauma, abdominal surgery, perforated appendicitis, or diverticulitis). These infections are typically polymicrobial.
- Primary peritonitis (also called spontaneous bacterial peritonitis) occurs in patients of all ages and may be associated with ascites, cirrhosis, or nephrotic syndrome.
  - ○ Microorganisms that cause primary peritonitis include bacteria of enteric origin (e.g., *Escherichia coli*, *Klebsiella*) and streptococci. Culture negative cases have also been described.
  - ○ Peritoneal fluid or ascites contain many neutrophils (>250 cells/mm^3 is diagnostic of primary peritonitis irrespective of the culture results). A Gram stain along with cultures is also diagnostic.
- Effusions with fungal infections are usually the result of disseminated infection in an immunocompromised host. Fungi that may be identified include *Candida* spp., *Aspergillus*, *Cryptococcus*, and several of the dimorphic fungi.
- Infection is usually associated with a significant inflammatory background. Depending on the host, evolution of the infection and treatment there may be mainly acute or chronic inflammatory cells present.
- Parasitic infections are often accompanied by many eosinophils. Other causes of increased eosinophils in peritoneal fluid include peritoneal dialysis, allergy, eosinophilic gastroenteritis, collagen vascular disease, and neoplasia (leukemia/lymphoma) including hypereosinophilic syndrome.

Suggested Reading

Bean SM, Chhieng DC. Anal-rectal cytology: a review. Diagn Cytopathol. 2010;38:538–46.

Huppmann AR, Orenstein JM. Opportunistic disorders of the gastrointestinal tract in the age of highly active antiretroviral therapy. Hum Pathol. 2010;41:1777–87.

Kotler DP, Giang TT, Garro ML, Orenstein JM. Light microscopic diagnosis of microsporidiosis in patients with AIDS. Am J Gastroenterol. 1994;89:540–4.

Marshall JB, Kelley DH, Vogele KA. Giardiasis: diagnosis by endoscopic brush biopsy of the duodenum. Am J Gastroenterol. 1984;79:517–9.

Muir SW, Murray J, Farquharson MA, Wheatley DJ, MCPhaden AR. Detection of cytomegalovirus in upper gastrointestinal biopsies from heart transplant recipients: comparison of light microscopy, immunocytochemistry, in situ hybridization, and nested PCR. J Clin Pathol. 1998;51:807–11.

Ramanathan J, Rammouni M, Baran J, Khatib R. Herpes simplex esophagitis in the immunocompetent host: an overview. Am J Gastroenterol. 2000;95:2171–6.

Senturk O, Canturk Z, Ercin C, et al. Comparison of five detection methods for *Helicobacter pylori*. Acta Cytol. 2000;44:1010–4.

8
Urinary Tract Infections

Walid E. Khalbuss, Liron Pantanowitz, and Anil V. Parwani
Department of Pathology, University of Pittsburgh Medical Center,
5150 Centre Avenue, Suite 201, Pittsburgh, PA 15232, USA

Infections of the urinary tract can be classified into upper (pyelonephritis) and lower tract infections (ureteritis, urethritis, and cystitis). This chapter also covers male genitourinary infections. Urologic specimens submitted for cytologic examination mainly include urine cytology, but specimen procurement may involve FNA. Apart from detecting infections (viral, bacterial, fungal, or parasitic), cytology can diagnose malignancy masquerading as an infection. Transplant related infections of the kidney are covered in Chap. 13.

Kidney Infections

In general, the morphologic characteristics of infectious agents that affect the kidney are similar to those present in other organs.

Acute Pyelonephritis

- Acute infection of the renal parenchyma and pelvis usually results from a bacterial infection of the kidney, most commonly with *Escherichia coli* ascent via the urethra. Other etiological agents include *Staphylococcus* and *Enterococci*. Hematogenous spread of microorganisms to the kidney can cause a renal abscess that presents as a kidney mass.

- Infections in diabetic patients may be due to *Klebsiella*, *Enterobacter*, *Clostridium*, *Candida* and are rarely of viral etiology.
- Risk factors include abnormal kidneys (e.g., polycystic or horseshoe kidney), vesicoureteric reflux, foreign body, instrumentation, and immunosuppression.
- Infected kidneys are infiltrated with neutrophils and may result in abscess formation, ischemic necrosis, and cystic change.

Cytomorphologic Features

- White blood cell (WBC) casts in urine samples are characteristic of acute bacterial pyelonephritis, but are not always seen.
- FNA of a renal or perirenal abscess contains mainly neutrophils as well as chronic inflammatory cells and necrosis.
- Viral inclusions (cytomegalovirus [CMV], polyoma (BK) virus, adenovirus) may be seen in renal tubular cells.
- Fungal casts may be identified. However, filamentous fungi may not be present in voided urine specimens, and their diagnosis may require direct ureteral or renal pelvis catheterization.

Differential Diagnosis

- Overgrowth of bacteria or yeast (no inflammation is present).

Ancillary Studies

- Urinalysis: >5 WBCs/HPF
- Positive leukocyte esterase and nitrite tests
- Gram stain for bacterial infection
- GMS stain for fungal infection
- Urine microbiology culture

Chronic Pyelonephritis

- Chronic pyelonephritis is the result of a persistent renal infection that may lead to chronic renal failure and small scarred kidneys.
- Such chronic infections occur in patients with major anatomical anomalies, renal stones, obstructive uropathy, or vesicoureteral reflux. Obstruction leads to urine stasis which in turn results in infection.

Cytomorphologic Features

- The urine cytology of chronic pyelonephritis is nonspecific and may include variable numbers of inflammatory cells, a granular background (amorphous debris) indicative of tissue damage, and casts (broad waxy, hyaline, and granular casts).

Differential Diagnosis and Ancillary Studies

- Same as acute pyelonephritis

Xanthogranulomatous Pyelonephritis (XPN)

- Xanthogranulomatous pyelonephritis (XPN) is a chronic destructive granulomatous inflammatory process of the kidney associated with obstruction due to infected renal stones.
- Positive urine cultures frequently show *E. coli* and *Proteus mirabilis*, and less often *Pseudomonas, Streptococcus faecalis,* and *Klebsiella*. In approximately 25% of cases urine cultures may be sterile.
- Patients are typically middle-aged women with a history of recurrent urinary tract infections. They may present with flank pain, fever, hematuria, pyuria, calculi, and a unilateral mass that mimics cancer. Imaging of the kidney often shows multiple nodules, calculi (often staghorn type), and perirenal extension.
- The histopathology is characterized by a focal or diffuse granulomatous mixed inflammatory infiltrate (neutrophils, lymphocytes, plasma cells, and multinucleated giant cells) associated with xanthomatous histiocytes (foamy cytoplasm), spindle cell proliferation, microabscesses, fibrosis, renal tubular atrophy, and squamous metaplasia of the urothelium (Fig. 8.1).

Cytomorphologic Features

- FNA specimens contain vacuolated histiocytes admixed with acute and chronic inflammatory cells, as well as occasional multinucleated giant cells.
- The findings in urine are nonspecific and may show an intense inflammatory and/or hemorrhagic background.

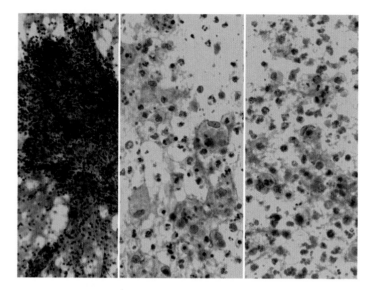

FIG. 8.1. Xanthogranulomatous pyelonephritis (XPN). The images shown are from an FNA of XPN presenting as a renal mass in a 70-year old female. The specimen is cellular and shows numerous clusters of inflammatory cells (*left image*, Pap stain, low magnification) that consist largely of histiocytes with vacuolated cytoplasm (foam cells) present in a background of granular debris, neutrophils, and lymphocytes (*middle* and *right images*, Pap stain, high magnification).

- Squamous metaplastic cells may be numerous in FNA and urine samples.
- A predominant spindle cell component may be mistaken for sarcomatous renal cell carcinoma. Fat necrosis may mimic lipoblasts.
- Bacteria are usually not identified, although basophilic intracytoplasmic PAS-negative inclusions have been reported.

Differential Diagnosis

- Nonspecific inflammatory response (requires clinical and radiologic correlation)
- Inflammatory diseases with giant cells such as tuberculosis

- Other entities with foamy histiocytes such as malakoplakia. (XPN does not contain Michaelis-Gutmann bodies).
- Clear cell renal cell carcinoma involving the renal pelvis may exfoliate malignant cells in urine. Unlike foamy histiocytes of XPN, carcinoma cells have cytological atypia, higher N:C ratio, mitoses, and a prominent nucleolus. The stroma in XPN resembles granulation tissue, whereas the vascular network in renal cell carcinoma tends to be more delicate. XPN may be associated with urologic tumors in up to 4% of cases.

Ancillary Studies

- Gram stain for associated bacteria.
- Immunostains to characterize macrophages (cytokeratin and EMA negative, S100 and CD68 positive) in difficult cases.

Renal Tuberculosis

- *Mycobacterium tuberculosis* seeding of the kidney usually follows hematogenous spread from another infected site (e.g., pulmonary TB).
- Atypical mycobacteria may also cause renal disease (e.g., *Mycobacterium avium-intracellulare* and *M. bovis*).
- Infection is characterized by caseating granulomatous inflammation, chronic interstitial inflammation, thyroidization of tubules, glomerulosclerosis, fibrosis, calcification, and stricture formation resulting in obstruction.

Cytomorphologic Features

- Urine specimens usually show sterile pyuria.
- FNA material contains epithelioid granulomas, multinucleated Langhans-type giant cells, and a granular necrotic background.

Differential Diagnosis

- Other necrotizing granulomatous infections (e.g., fungal infection).
- Benign non-necrotizing granulomatous conditions (e.g., sarcoidosis).
- Granulomas associated with malignancy (e.g., lymphoma, seminoma).

- XPN
- Malakoplakia
- Malignancy that mimics granulomas (e.g., renal cell carcinoma)

Ancillary Studies

- Special stains for acid-fast mycobacteria
- PCR to confirm the diagnosis and identify species
- Microbiology cultures

Fungal Kidney Infections

- Common fungal infections of the kidney include *Candida* (*C. albicans* and *C. glabrata*), *Aspergillus*, *Cryptococcus*, *Coccidioides*, *Histoplasma*, *Blastomyces,* and *Mucor* spp.
- Infection typically arises from hematogenous spread. Candida may originate from the gastrointestinal tract, particularly in patients with nephrostomy tubes.
- Patients at increased risk of fungal infection are immunosuppressed individuals.
- Fungi may evoke a granulomatous inflammatory reaction with or without necrosis, cause abscesses, and even manifest with renal infarcts.

Cytomorphologic Features

- Urine usually shows nonspecific findings (e.g., neutrophils, reactive urothelial cells, RBCs). Necrotizing granulomatous inflammation is more likely to be observed in renal pelvic washings.
- FNA of a fungal mass will show necrotizing granulomatous inflammation.
- Fungi including fungal casts may be seen. Depending on the type of fungal infection specimens may include budding yeast (e.g., narrow-based budding of *Cryptococcus* vs. broad-based budding yeast diagnostic of balstomycosis), pseudohyphae (*Candida* spp.), or true hyphae. Fungal organisms may be intracellular within macrophages.

Differential Diagnosis

- Overgrowth of fungi in urine (inflammation is usually absent)
- Fungal mimics (e.g., contaminants)

Ancillary Studies

- Urinalysis: >5 WBCs/HPF
- Positive leukocyte esterase and nitrite tests
- GMS or PAS stains for fungal elements
- Mucicarmine stain for *Cryptococcus*
- Calcofluor stain
- Microbiology culture

Urinary Bladder Infections

Bacterial Cystitis

- Bacterial cystitis is commonly caused by Gram-negative bacteria (*E. coli*, *Klebsiella*, *Enterobacter*, *Serratia*, *Pseudomonas*, *P. mirabilis*) and is infrequently due to Gram-positive bacteria (*Staphylococcus aureus*, *Staphylococcus saprophyticus*, and *Enterococci*).
- Infection occurs from ascending bacterial infection via the distal urethra, and mostly affects women of reproductive age. Patients with structural bladder abnormalities and systemic disease such as diabetes are more susceptible to infection.
- Symptoms include increased frequency, urgency, dysuria, hematuria, and suprapubic pain.
- Infection typically presents with prominent acute inflammation in the urine, and sometimes with chronic inflammatory cells in more long-standing infections.

Cytomorphologic Features

- Bacterial colonies may be present. Bacterial morphology is often altered (e.g., filamentous appearance) following antibiotic therapy (Figs. 8.2–8.3).
- Apart from acute inflammatory cells, urine specimens also demonstrate nonspecific findings (reactive and degenerated urothelial cells, RBCs, and cellular debris). In chronic infections there are many more lymphocytes present (Fig. 8.4).
- Bacterial cystitis may be superimposed on malignancy. Therefore, admixed atypical or neoplastic urothelial cells should not be overlooked.

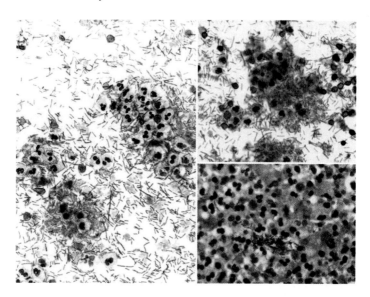

Fig. 8.2. Acute bacterial cystitis. The urine specimen shows a predominance of neutrophils with bacteria and occasional red blood cells. There were very few urothelial cells present in this case (*left* and *upper right images*: Pap stain, ThinPrep, high magnification; *bottom right image*: H&E stain, cell block, high magnification).

Differential Diagnosis

- Bacterial overgrowth (no inflammatory reaction is present)
- Bacterial contamination from a neobladder urine specimen
- Pyelonephritis (which often has associated WBC casts)

Ancillary Studies

- Urinalysis: >5 WBCs/HPF
- Positive leukocyte esterase and nitrite tests
- Gram stain for bacteria
- Microbiology culture

Malakoplakia

- This is a rare chronic granulomatous disease that primarily affects the urinary tract, particularly the bladder and ureters.
- Urine culture often isolates *E. coli*.

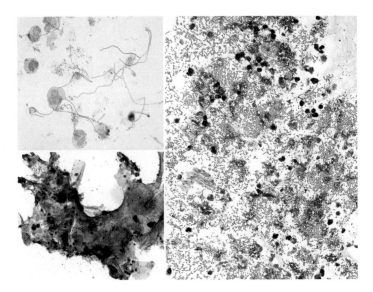

FIG. 8.3. (*Top left image*) Bacteria in urine exposed to excreted antibiotics may assume unusual forms, such as these elongated *Pseudomonas* bacteria identified in this treated patient (Pap stain, high magnification). Variable numbers of bacteria in urine may be encountered (*bottom left image*) due to fecal contamination or (*right image*) in degenerated ileal conduit samples without associated acute inflammation (Pap stain, intermediate magnification).

- The condition is characterized histologically by aggregates of large histiocytes (von Hansemann cells) containing round cytoplasmic and extracellular laminated Michaelis-Gutmann bodies, thought to contain mineralized bacterial fragments.
- The cytomorphology in FNA or urine samples shows many large, foamy, granular macrophages with large, eccentric nuclei, and prominent nucleoli. Cells containing Michaelis-Gutmann bodies may be identified, which can be highlighted with the use of a PAS stain (Fig. 8.5).

Viral Infections

- Viruses are a rare cause of cystitis, but may be seen in immunosuppressed patients. Immunocytochemistry can be used for confirmation.

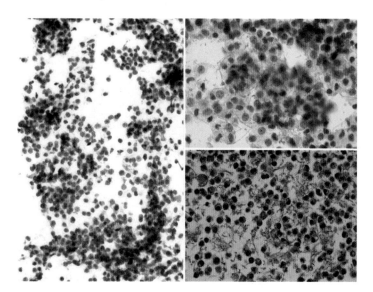

FIG. 8.4. Follicular cystitis. This voided urine specimen shows a predominance of lymphocytes associated with bacteria (*left image*; Pap stain, intermediate magnification; *upper right image*; high magnification, Pap stain; *lower right image*, H&E stain on cell block).

- *Human papillomavirus* (*HPV*) effect of squamous cells (e.g., koilocytosis) in urine may be due to contamination from genital infection or from bladder and/or urethral condylomas. Bladder condyloma is more common in women than men. Cytological features are basically the same as those seen in cervicovaginal Pap tests (Fig. 8.6). HPV has been reported to occur in the bladder, and may play a role in urethral carcinoma.
- *Herpes simplex virus* (*HSV*) causes hemorrhagic cystitis, particularly in patients with genital herpes. Infected cells are enlarged, multinucleated, exhibit nuclear molding, and margination of chromatin. Cells with ground glass nuclei and Cowdry A nuclear inclusions may also be present. Background acute inflammation is often present.
- *Adenovirus* causes hemorrhagic cystitis, especially in children. Infected cells have large, homogeneous basophilic intranuclear inclusion bodies.

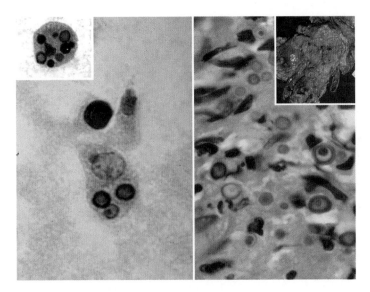

FIG. 8.5. Malakoplakia of the bladder with large histiocytes containing cytoplasmic lamellated structures of Michaelis-Gutmann bodies shown in urine (Pap stain, high magnification). The resection specimen showed that malakoplakia involved almost the entire bladder with a markedly thickened mucosa (gross pathology, *right inset*). Michaelis-Guttman bodies are highlighted by a PAS stain on histological section (*right image*, H&E stain, high magnification).

- *CMV* can cause hemorrhagic cystitis in immunosuppressed patients. Infected cells may have intracytoplasmic and nuclear inclusions, but multinucleation is rare.

BK Polyomavirus

Microbiology

- BK virus is a member of the polyomavirus family.
- Infection is usually acquired at an early age. Up to 80% of the population are likely to have had prior infection.
- Polyomavirus remains latent within urothelium and kidney tubular epithelial cells. Changes in host immune status can lead

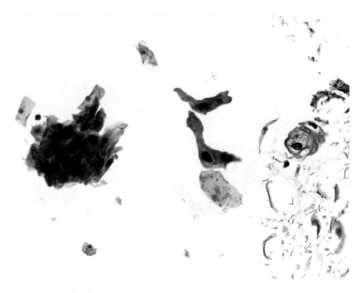

FIG. 8.6.   HPV-related koilocytes are shown in this voided urine specimen from a 31-year old male. He had a history of known anal condylomas (Pap stain, high magnification).

to viral reactivation, causing viral particles and infected cells (so-called "decoy cells") to be shed into the urine.

- As decoy cells contain BK virus antigens, in renal allograft recipients the examination of urine cytology specimens for cells with polyomavirus inclusions is often used to assess for viral reactivation, and hence the risk for BK nephropathy. The sensitivity (99%) and specificity (95%) of decoy cells for diagnosing BK nephropathy is high. While the positive predictive value varies (27–90%), the negative predictive value is high (99%) (Figs. 8.7 and 8.8).

Clinical Features

- BK virus in immunocompetent individuals rarely causes disease. Those people who are infected with this virus are usually asymptomatic, or may manifest with a transient hematuria.
- Infection in immunocompromised individuals may cause hemorrhagic cystitis, ureteral stenosis, and/or progressive renal dysfunction (nephritis).

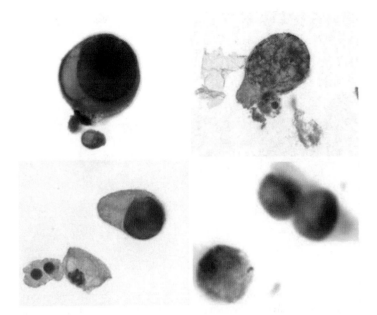

FIG. 8.7. Decoy cells are shown with viral changes in the (*top left*) inclusion and (*top right*) postinclusion stages of BK polyomavirus infection (Pap stain, high magnification). (*Bottom left*) A comet cell is shown with an eccentrically placed glassy appearing nucleus (Pap stain, high magnification). Cells infected with polyomavirus are shown to exhibit nuclear immunoreactivity with a BK virus immunocytochemical stain (high magnification).

- Approximately 1–10% of infected renal transplant patients progress to BK virus nephropathy, causing many (up to 80%) of these patients to lose their renal grafts. This may occur within a few days posttransplant to 5 years later.
- Other infected patients that may shed slightly increased numbers of decoy cells include the elderly, pregnant women, and those with cancer or diabetes mellitus.

Cytomorphologic Features

- The detection of decoy cells is easily identified (and even quantifiable) in routine Papanicolaou stained urine cytology specimens.

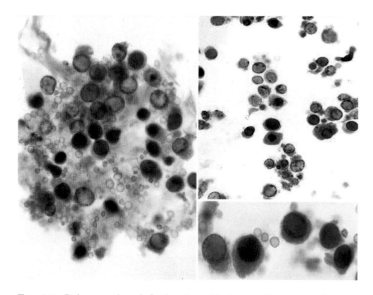

Fig. 8.8. Polyoma virus infection in voided urine from a renal transplant patient. Two types of inclusions in decoy cells can be appreciated including cells with large homogenous, basophilic, glassy intranuclear inclusions and those with vesicular nuclei containing clearing of their chromatin. Note that these cells have no nuclear contour irregularity, an important distinction from cells of high-grade urothelial carcinoma (Pap stain, high magnification).

- There are two types of infected epithelial cells:
  - Cells with large homogenous (ground-glass like) basophilic intranuclear inclusions, a condensed rim of chromatin, and that show some degree of degenerative changes (early stage of infection).
  - Cells with vesicular nuclei that have so-called "fish-net stocking" clearing of their chromatin (late or "empty" stage of infection).
- Many decoy cells may have eccentric cytoplasm resembling the tail of a comet (termed "comet cells").
- Decoy cells typically are present as single cells, and clustering of these cells is a rare finding.
- Occasionally, multinucleated decoy cells may be detected.

- Decoy cells do not show nuclear contour irregularity and there is no necrosis, as may be encountered with carcinoma in situ or high-grade urothelial carcinoma.
- Polyomavirus infection can coexist with high-grade urothelial carcinoma.
- Cytomorphologic changes in urine may persist for several months after cessation of symptoms.

Differential Diagnosis

- High-grade urothelial carcinoma
- Degenerated (urothelial) cells. To avoid high levels of cellular degeneration, it is best to avoid examining the first morning urine specimen and promptly fix or transport urine to the cytology laboratory for immediate processing
- Radiation or chemotherapy effect
- Other viral cytopathic change (e.g., adenovirus, herpes, CMV)

Ancillary Studies

- Immunocytochemistry with Simian virus 40 (SV40) antibody for BK virus
- Serology is unhelpful as many people will demonstrate past infection
- PCR (quantitative analysis is possible measuring BK virus DNA loads in serum samples)
- Electron microscopy
- Kidney tissue biopsy (gold standard test)

Fungal Infections

Microbiology

- Bladder fungal infections are mostly caused by *C. albicans*.
- Infection may also be due to invasive fungi such as *Aspergillus*, *Blastomyces*, *Mucor*, *Histoplasma*, *Cryptococcus,* and *Coccidioides*.
- Candidal and bacterial infections frequently occur simultaneously.

Clinical Features

- Fungal infection of the bladder mostly affects women. Risk factors include immunosuppression, indwelling devices, obstruction, diabetes, or antibiotic therapy.
- Most patients with candiduria are asymptomatic. Patients may also present with urinary symptoms (nocturia, suprapubic pain, frequency, and hematuria), complications (emphysematous cystitis, pyelonephritis, bezoars, abscess, rarely renal failure), and/or disseminated disease.
- Infections may cause cystitis with ulceration.

Cytomorphologic Features

- Fungal elements are identified in urine. Candida is the most common fungus seen in urine specimens, and it is also the most common contaminant.
- True fungal cystitis should be only suggested if there is associated acute inflammation and reactive cellular changes. Final diagnosis requires clinical and microbiology correlation (Fig. 8.9).
- Budding yeast and pseudohyphal forms are characteristic of *Candida* spp., larger yeasts with narrow-based budding surrounded by clear capsule are characteristic of *Cryptococcus*, broad-based budding yeast is diagnostic of blastomycosis, and intracellular microorganisms are characteristic of histoplasmosis.
- Nonspecific changes like hematuria may be present.
- Fungal cystitis may be superimposed on malignancy. Therefore, a careful search should be carried out for atypical or neoplastic urothelial cells.

Differential Diagnosis

- Fungal contaminants (usually have no inflammatory reaction)
- Fungal infection of the kidney (casts are typically present)
- Fungal mimics

Ancillary Studies

- Urinalysis: >5 WBCs/HPF
- Positive leukocyte esterase and nitrite tests

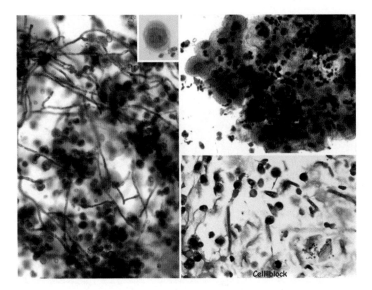

FIG. 8.9. Acute candida cystitis. This voided urine specimen shows many acute inflammatory cells and fungal microorganisms. The fungal organisms include budding yeasts and pseudohyphal forms characteristic of *Candida* spp. (*left and upper right images*: Pap stain, high magnification; *bottom right image*: H&E cell block, high magnification). The specimen contains atypical urothelial cells attributed to reactive changes associated with this fungal infection (*left upper inset*: Pap stain, high magnification).

- GMS or PAS stain for identification of fungal forms
- Mucicarmine stain for *Cryptococcus*
- Microbiology culture

Parasites

Schistosomiasis

Microbiology

- Schistosomiasis (also known as bilharzia) is caused by trematodes (flukes) of the genus Schistosoma. *Schistosoma hematobium* causes urinary schistosomiasis.

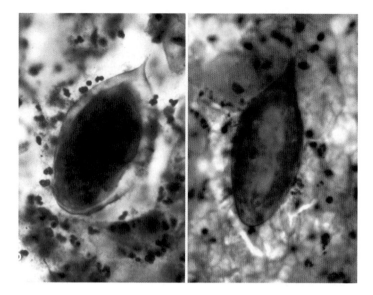

Fig. 8.10. Bladder schistosomiasis. The images show the ova of *Schistosoma hematobium* recognized by their terminal spine (DQ *left*, Pap stain *right*, high magnification).

- Worms residing in the urinary bladder venous plexus excrete eggs in the urine. Eggs that embed in tissue may calcify and cause urothelial squamous metaplasia, intestinal metaplasia, granulomas, and eosinophilia.
- Eggs can also be found in the urine with infections from *S. japonicum* and *S. intercalatum*. *S. mansoni* eggs are more common in stools and rarely seen in urine (Fig. 8.10).

Clinical Features

- Patients develop chronic cystitis and may present with hematuria.
- Chronic infection can lead to fibrosis, urinary obstruction, and rarely urothelial squamous cell carcinoma.

Cytomorphologic Features

- Microscopic identification of eggs in urine is the most practical method for diagnosis of urinary schistosomiasis.

- *S. hematobium* eggs are elliptical and recognized by a terminal spine, whereas *S. japonicum* eggs are spheroidal with a small knob. *S. mansoni* eggs are identified by their characteristic lateral spines.
- Adult worms may be recognized, but are rare. They are small (12–26 mm long and 0.3–0.6 mm wide) and their size varies with the different species.
- Urine specimens may show squamous and intestinal metaplasia, granulomas, and/or eosinophilia.
- Squamous cell carcinoma may be present in rare cases.

Differential Diagnosis

- Other parasitic ova
- Mimics of parasite eggs

Ancillary Studies

- Microbiology consultation
- Serum antibody detection
- Tissue biopsy

Trichomoniasis

- Trichomoniasis is a sexually transmitted infection caused by the protozoan *Trichomonas vaginalis*.
- Parasites may cause urethritis and cystitis in both women and men, particularly if there is a coexisting genital infection.
- The cytomorphology of trichomonads in urine cytology is the same as in Pap test (refer to Chap. 5). However, when in urine, trichomonads may assume variable shapes (smaller and more round in shape).
- Trichomonas infection can cause an inflammatory reaction, with a large number of neutrophils usually present in urine specimens.
- Immunocytochemistry with p16 (clone G175-405, BD Biosciences Pharmingen, San Diego, CA, USA) and microbiology culture can help establish the diagnosis of trichomonas in urine (Fig. 8.11).

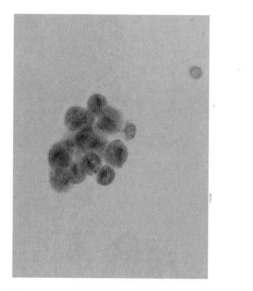

Fig. 8.11.   Urine trichomoniasis. (*Left image*) A group of trichomonads, round in shape and slightly variable in size, is shown in a urine specimen from an 80-year-old man (Thin Prep, Pap stain, high magnification). (*Right image*) These parasites were p16 positive (immunocytochemical stain, high magnification) (reprinted from Pantanowitz et al. Diagnostic utility of p16 immunocytochemistry for Trichomonas in urine cytology. Cytojournal. 2005;2:11, with permission from Biomed Central Ltd.).

Male Genital Tract Infections

- Infections of the penis may be localized (e.g., condyloma accuminatum) or widespread (e.g., Fournier gangrene). Cytologic diagnoses of these infections may be obtained by Tzanck preparation of ulcers, characteristic cells or organisms contaminating urine samples, or FNA of lesions.
- Epididymitis is the most common source of intrascrotal infection, and may extend to involve the testis. Infection of the testes may be due to viruses (e.g., mumps), bacteria (including syphilis), malakoplakia, mycobacteria (TB orchitis and leprosy), or fungi (*Candida*, *Blastomyces*, *Aspergillus*, *Histoplasma capsulatum*, *Trichophyton mentagrophytes*, and *Coccidioides immitis*).

- In general, acute bacterial infections show suppurative inflammation, whereas the cytomorphology of viral, mycobacterial, and fungal infections as well as malakoplakia is similar to that seen in other sites.

Urethritis

- Urethral infections are typically sexually transmitted and may be classified as gonococcal uretheritis (GU) or nongonococcal uretheritis (NGU).
- GU is caused by the Gram-negative intracellular diplococcus *Neisseria gonorrheae*. NGU is due to infection with *Chlamydia trachomatis*, *Ureaplasma urealyticum*, *Mycoplasma hominis*, *Mycoplasma genitalium*, or *T. vaginalis*.
- The cytomorphological features in urine include acute and/or chronic inflammatory cells. NGU typically does not present with a purulent discharge as with gonorrhea. Intracellular diplococci may rarely be detected with a Gram stain.

Suggested Reading

Cimbaluk D, Pitelka L, Kluskens L, Gattuso P. Update on human polyomavirus BK nephropathy. Diagn Cytopathol. 2009;37:773–9.

Gupta M, Venkatesh SK, Kumar A, Pandey R. Fine-needle aspiration cytology of bilateral renal malakoplakia. Diagn Cytopathol. 2004;31:116–7.

Kumar N, Jain S. Aspiration cytology of focal xanthogranulomatous pyelonephritis: a diagnostic challenge. Diagn Cytopathol. 2004;30:111–4.

Pantanowitz L, Cao QJ, Goulart RA, Otis CN. Diagnostic utility of p16 immunocytochemistry for Trichomonas in urine cytology. Cytojournal. 2005;2:11.

Waugh MS, Perfect JR, Dash RC. *Schistosoma haematobium* in urine: morphology with ThinPrep method. Diagn Cytopathol. 2007;35:649–50.

9
Central Nervous System Infections

Walid E. Khalbuss[1], Pam Michelow[2], Sara E. Monaco[1], and Liron Pantanowitz[1]

[1]Department of Pathology, University of Pittsburgh Medical Center, 5150 Centre Avenue, Suite 201, Pittsburgh, PA 15232, USA

[2]Cytology Unit, Department of Anatomical Pathology, University of the Witwatersrand and National Health Laboratory Service, Corner Hospital Hill and De Korte Streets, Braamfontein, Johannesburg, Gauteng 2000, South Africa

Infections of the central nervous system (CNS) may involve the meninges (meningitis), brain matter (encephalitis), or both (meningoencephalitis). Additionally, infections can be acute or chronic. Cerebrospinal fluid (CSF) analysis can be used to diagnose a wide variety of neoplastic and non-neoplastic conditions including infectious diseases affecting the CNS. Brain infections can also be diagnosed by cytology using touch or squash preparations of brain tissue, often performed at the time of an intraoperative consultation. Microorganisms that cause CNS infection may be bacterial (Table 9.1), fungal, parasitic, or viral. Furthermore, prions represent an unusual class of infectious agent that can damage the brain, but usually these are not diagnosed using cytology.

A slight increase in the number of leukocytes and macrophages in CSF is always pathological and should suggest that an infectious or inflammatory process may be present. Polymorphonuclear leukocytes normally do not cross the blood–brain barrier. Hence, their presence in CSF is considered pathological. Pleocytosis refers to an increased number of cells in the CSF (Table 9.2). The type of pleocytosis is usually based on the dominant cell population.

L. Pantanowitz et al., *Cytopathology of Infectious Diseases*, Essentials in Cytopathology 17, DOI 10.1007/978-1-4614-0242-8_9, © Springer Science+Business Media, LLC 2011

TABLE 9.1. Common bacterial infections of the central nervous system (CNS).

Neonatal meningitis
- Group B beta-hemolytic *Streptococcus*
- Enteric bacilli (*Escherichia coli, Proteus, Klebsiella*)
- *Listeria* (also seen in the elderly)

Meningitis in children and adults
- *Haemophilus influenzae*
- *Neisseria meningitidis* (or meningococcus)
- *Streptococcus pneumoniae* (or pneumococcus)

Less common meningitides
- *Staphylococcus*
- *Pseudomonas*
- Gram-negative meningitis
- Tuberculous meningitis
- Neurosyphilis

Brain abscess
- Staphylococci
- *Norcardia*

Changes in protein and glucose content of CSF often accompany an increase in cellularity (Table 9.3):

- *Neutrophilic pleocytosis.* This is seen in bacterial, early viral, tuberculous and fungal meningitis, cerebral abscesses, CNS hemorrhage, cerebral infarct, and high-grade malignancy (tumor necrosis).
- *Lymphocytic pleocytosis* (Fig. 9.4). This is seen in aseptic, viral, tuberculous, or fungal meningitis, partially treated bacterial meningitis, parasitic disease, polyneuritis, and Guillain–Barre syndrome. (Table 9.4) The CSF sample usually contains numerous monomorphic small lymphocytes. The differential diagnosis includes reactive lymphocytosis vs. small lymphocytic lymphoma (rarely seen in the CSF). An adequate history and/or flow cytometry will help resolve this differential diagnosis.
- *Monocytic pleocytosis.* This is seen in patients with viral meningoencephalitis, Mollaret meningitis, tuberculosis, neurosyphilis, amebic infections, fungal disease, as well as multiple sclerosis and reactions to foreign material.

TABLE 9.2. Common causes of CSF pleocytosis.

Neutrophilic pleocytosis
- Bacterial infection
- Early viral infection
- Tuberculosis infection
- Fungal meningitis
- Cerebral abscess
- CNS hemorrhage
- Cerebral infarct
- High-grade malignancy

Lymphocytic pleocytosis
- Viral (aseptic) meningitis
- Tuberculosis meningitis
- Fungal meningitis
- Partially treated bacterial meningitis
- Parasitic disease
- Polyneuritis
- Guillain–Barre syndrome

Monocytic pleocytosis
- Tuberculosis infection
- Syphilis infection
- Amebic infection
- Fungal infection
- Viral meningoencephalitis
- Multiple sclerosis
- Reaction to foreign material

Eosinophilic pleocytosis
- Parasitic infection
- Fungal infection
- Foreign material reaction (drugs, shunts)
- Idiopathic conditions
- Acute polyneuritis
- Meningioencephalitis (bacterial, viral, and fungal)
- Lymphoma
- Primary brain tumors

- *Eosinophilic pleocytosis.* This is seen in parasitic and fungal infections, reactions to foreign material (shunts) and drug induced or idiopathic conditions, acute polyneuritis, infections (bacterial, viral, and fungal meningoencephalitis), lymphoma, as well as primary brain tumors.

TABLE 9.3. CSF parameters with various infections.

Condition	Color	Glucose	Protein	Leukocytes
Normal	Clear and colorless	50–80 mg/dL	20–45 mg/dL	Fewer than six lymphocytes, no neutrophils
Bacterial meningitis	Cloudy	Low to very low	High to very high	Markedly increased neutrophils
Viral meningitis	Clear to cloudy	Normal	High	Increased lymphocytes and monocytes
Fungal meningitis	Clear to cloudy	Low	High	Variable from no inflammation to increased neutrophils and/or lymphocytes
Tuberculous meningitis	Clear to cloudy	Low	High	Increased neutrophils early, increased lymphocytes and monocytes later
Neurosyphilis	Clear to cloudy	Normal	High	Increased lymphocytes and monocytes and/or plasma cells
Parasitic meningitis	Clear to cloudy	Low or normal	High	Normal or increased neutrophils, eosinophils, lymphocytes and/or monocytes
Intracranial hemorrhage	Clear to pink-red to xanthochromic (yellow-orange)	Normal to low	High	Normal or increased neutrophils and/or lymphocytes
Neoplastic	Clear to cloudy, pink-red or xanthochromic if associated with hemorrhage	Normal to low	Normal to increased	Normal or increased neutrophils and/or lymphocytes

TABLE 9.4. Common causes of lymphocytic meningitis.

- Viral meningitis or encephalitis
- Partially treated purulent meningitis
- Tuberculous meningitis
- *Listeria* meningitis
- Brucella meningitis
- Syphilitic meningitis
- Lyme disease
- Fungal meningitis
- Sarcoidosis
- Various protozoal or helminthic infections
- Lymphoma
- Demyelinating disease
- Vascular disease (vasculitis, stroke, subarachnoid hemorrhage)

There are a variety of ancillary tests that can be performed on CSF to help make a diagnosis of infection such as protein and glucose levels, special stains (e.g., Gram stain, India ink preparation), culture and sensitivity, serology for antigens and antibodies (e.g., Venereal Disease Research Laboratory test or VDRL test for neurosyphilis), and detection of viral genetic material (DNA, RNA) by PCR. The presence of an increase of antibodies over time indicates a recent infection.

Acute Bacterial Meningitis

Microbiology

- The etiology varies with age. *Neisseria meningitidis* infection is most common in childhood, *Haemophilus influenzae* commonly affects children under 5 years of age (and may rarely be seen due to vaccination) and *Streptococcus pneumoniae* affects individuals of all ages. In the elderly and infants, the diagnosis may be challenging.
- Bacteria can reach the subarachnoid space via the bloodstream or by extension from contiguous structures such as the sinuses or ears.
- Bacterial infection usually affects the subarachnoid space. However, toxins (from bacteria or leukocytes) can cause edema and damage blood vessels, causing additional cellular damage. Cerebral edema causes an increase in intracranial pressure (Fig. 9.1).

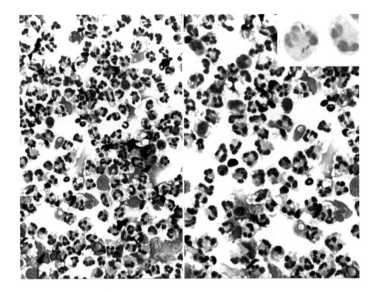

FIG. 9.1. Acute bacterial meningitis. The cytospin shows marked neutrophils (PMNs) and cellular debris. Some lymphocytes and monocytes are also present (Diff-Quik stain, intermediate magnification, *left* and high magnification *right*). The Gram stain (*inset*) shows intracellular Gram negative bacilli (high magnification).

Clinical Features

- The classic clinical trial of acute meningitis is fever, meningismus (stiff neck resistant to flexion), and a change in mental status.

Cytomorphologic Features

- The cytologic features include CSF with a marked pleocytosis (particularly neutrophils), cloudy turbid appearance, fibrin, and cellular debris.
- Very early disease may show very few cells or a predominance of lymphocytes.
- Occasionally intracellular bacteria may be identified.

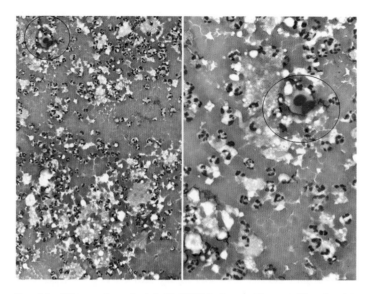

Fig. 9.2. This cerebrospinal fluid (CSF) is from a 73 year old male with no prior history of malignancy. His CSF specimen shows numerous neutrophils with very rare large atypical cells (see circle, *right*) suspicious for carcinoma (Diff-Quik stain; low magnification, *left*; and high magnification, *right*). On follow up of this case, the patient was found to have a large neuroendocrine carcinoma of the colon.

Differential Diagnosis

- Early viral meningitis/encephalitis
- Brain, subdural, and epidural abscess
- Tuberculosis meningitis
- Fungal infection
- Traumatic tap
- Toxoplasmosis
- Brain tumor. Some high-grade brain tumors may show marked necrosis and increased neutrophils, due to a paraneoplastic syndrome. Therefore, cases with neutrophilic pleocytosis should be screened carefully for any atypical cells to exclude a neoplastic process (Fig. 9.2)
- Leukemia

Ancillary Studies

- Gram stain
- High protein levels in CSF
- Low CSF glucose level (less than 50% of the serum level)
- Microbiology bacterial culture (aerobic and anaerobic)
- Bacterial antigens in CSF offer rapid testing
- Molecular testing: PCR assays for specific organisms; amplification of 16S rRNA gene; and ribosomal DNA assay

Viral Meningitis

Microbiology

- Viral meningitis is also called "aseptic meningitis," since there are no bacteria grown on culture.
- Early HIV infection (at the initial seroconversion stage) may present as aseptic meningitis.

Clinical Features

- Patients present with the clinical trial of acute meningitis that includes fever, meningismus (stiff neck resistant to flexion), and a change in mental status. They typically have no focal neurological disease or seizures.
- CSF is usually under normal pressure and contains a moderate number of white blood cells (<500/mm^3). CSF may show a marked pleocytosis for weeks.
- The CSF initially may contain predominantly neutrophils (PMNs), but after a day or two shows lymphocytosis.
- CSF protein and glucose are within normal range or may show minimal changes.
- Viral meningitis is usually a self-limited disease and complications are infrequent (Fig. 9.3).

Cytomorphologic Features

- CSF is hypercellular with a predominance of lymphocytes.
- Some atypical immature lymphocytes may be seen. Flow cytometry may be necessary in such cases to exclude lymphoma.

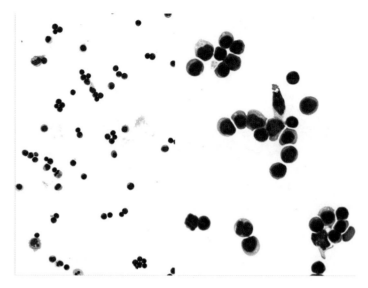

FIG. 9.3.   This CSF is from a patient with viral meningitis showing marked lymphocytosis. The CSF specimen shows numerous mature lymphocytes. The microbiology cultures were negative (Diff-Quik stain, low magnification *left*, and high magnification *right*).

- There is no necrosis or cellular debris and bacteria are not found.
- Viral inclusions are rarely identified in CSF.

Differential Diagnosis

- Bacterial meningitis (late stage or partially treated)
- Fungal infection
- Lyme disease (comprised of polytypic B-cells)
- Brain abscess
- Parameningeal sepsis

Ancillary Studies

- Stains for bacteria (Gram) and mycobacteria are negative
- Glucose is normal and protein levels may be slightly high or normal
- Viral cultures can be performed

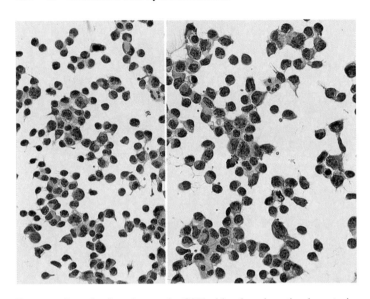

Fig. 9.4. Reactive lymphocytosis. CSF with a lymphocytic pleocytosis. This CSF specimen shows numerous lymphocytes including immature forms (Pap stain, intermediate magnification, *left*; and high magnification, *right*). It was initially considered suspicious for lymphoma. Flow cytometry was negative for lymphoma and the follow up in this patient showed no evidence of malignancy. Subsequent CSF showed a decrease in cellularity and return to normal.

- PCR testing for specific viruses (such as enterovirus, HSV, CMV, HIV)
- The intensity of lymphocytosis (leukemoid reaction) and the presence of immature or atypical appearing lymphocytes may cause an erroneous diagnosis of leukemia or lymphoma (Fig. 9.4). Flow cytometry is recommended in these conditions

Mollaret Meningitis

Microbiology

- This is a rare form of recurrent, aseptic, chronic meningitis that may be related to Herpes simplex type 1 and 2 or West Nile virus infection.

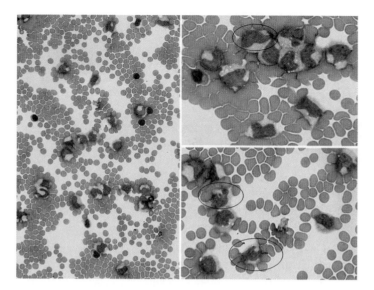

FIG. 9.5. CSF from a 31 year old female with chronic Mollaret meningitis. The specimen shows marked monocytosis present in a background of scant mature lymphocytes. Monocytes exhibit a variety of nuclear morphologies (see circles) including bean shaped and bilobed nuclei, as well as cells with nuclear clefting and cerebriform nuclear contours (Diff-Quik stain, intermediate magnification, *left*; and high magnification, *right*).

Clinical Features

- Meningitis is usually mild and self-limiting. Patients experience recurrent episodes of headache, fever, and photophobia separated by symptom-free episodes.

Cytomorphologic Features

- CSF shows marked monocytosis with characteristic Mollaret cells (activated monocytes).
- Mollaret cells are somewhat bean shaped, have enlarged nuclei and cerebriform nuclei with deep nuclear clefts, leading to their characteristic "footprint" appearance. These cells are usually seen within the first 24 h of the onset of symptoms.
- There are often background lymphocytes and some degenerated monocytes ("ghost cells") present (Fig. 9.5).

Differential Diagnosis

- Other inflammatory and infectious diseases of the CNS
- Lymphoproliferative disorder

Ancillary Studies

- PCR assays for viral agents such as HSV-2 or West Nile virus (not all cases test positive)

Tuberculous Meningitis

Microbiology

- Meningitis caused by *Mycobacterium tuberculosis* usually results from seeding of a tuberculoma (benign mass caused by tuberculosis) in the brain or meninges. Tuberculomas arise largely as a result of hematogenous spread from distant disease (typically in the lung) (Fig. 9.6).

Clinical Features

- Children, debilitated and immune incompetent adults are at greatest risk for TB meningitis.
- Infected patients present with a headache, malaise, fever, and weight loss.
- The level of CSF protein is high and glucose is low.

Cytomorphologic Features

- CSF shows a moderate pleocytosis with a predominance of lymphocytes.

Differential Diagnosis

- Bacterial meningitis
- Fungal meningitis
- Lyme disease
- Brain abscess

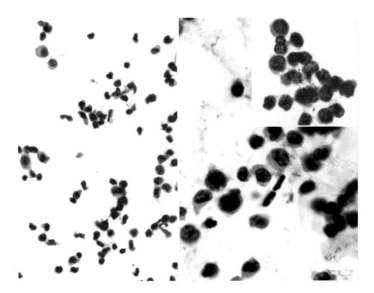

FIG. 9.6. TB meningitis. This CSF specimen from a 2-month-old male infant shows numerous neutrophils and lymphocytes, as well as some monocytes (Pap stain, high magnification, *right* and lower magnification, *left*). Microbiology culture confirmed *Mycobacterium tuberculosis*. The *upper right inset* shows a higher magnification of the polymorphous lymphocytes seen in this case.

Ancillary Studies

- AFB stain, which is only occasionally positive (low sensitivity)
- Culture for mycobacteria (takes 2–8 weeks to grow)
- Chest X-ray, sputum, skull X-ray, and a tuberculin test may indicate a distant source of infection
- PCR for diagnostic confirmation and typing

Cryptococcal Meningitis

Microbiology

- Meningitis occurs following CNS infection by the fungus *Cryptococcus neoformans*, and less of *C. gattii*.
- *Cryptococcus* is the most common mycosis of the CNS.

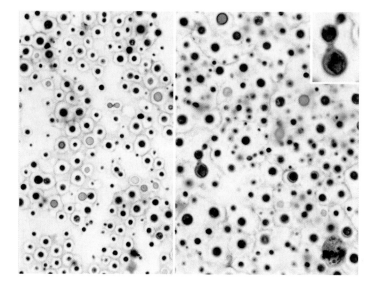

FIG. 9.7. Cryptococcal meningitis. This CSF specimen shows numerous pink/red round yeasts with thick capsules and narrow-based, asymmetric budding, highlighted in the upper right *inset* (Pap stain, high magnification). Note that there is an absence of an inflammatory reaction in the background.

Clinical Features

- Meningitis may occur in healthy and immunocompromised patients. Predisposing factors include a debilitated state, immune incompetence, and diabetes mellitus.
- Infection is indolent and symptoms may extend over a long period before the diagnosis is confirmed.
- Symptoms include headache and mental deterioration. Other symptoms may include cranial nerve palsies and focal brain stem dysfunction secondary to arteritis (Fig. 9.7).

Cytomorphologic Features

- Cryptococcal yeast may be variable in number, ranging from rare to abundant organisms. Yeast (5–15 μm) are round, but can be indented and trap air under the coverslip, resulting in a crystal-like refractile artifact. They are pink or purple with a Pap stain.

- Budding is narrow-based and asymmetric.
- Typically there are no associated inflammatory cells. However, one may also encounter a granulomatous response or variable inflammatory background composed of lymphocytes and monocytes. Organisms are harder to find when there are many inflammatory cells present.

Differential Diagnosis

- Other fungal microorganisms
- Mimics of fungus (such as talc)

Ancillary Studies

- GMS and PAS stains
- Mucicarmine stain to demonstrate mucin-positive capsules
- India ink (requires a fresh specimen)
- CSF antigen test
- Immunocytochemistry using a specific antibody to *C. neoformans*

Blastomycosis

Microbiology

- Blastomycosis is a chronic systemic fungal infection due to *Blastomyces dermatitidis* that characteristically affects the skin and lungs.
- Involvement of the CSF (meningitis) or other CNS location (intracranial mass lesion) is rare. Approximately 2.5% of patients with pulmonary or systemic blastomycosis develop CNS involvement (Fig. 9.8).

Clinical Features

- Patients may present with clinical features typical of meningitis or with signs and symptoms related to a brain mass.
- The CSF protein level is usually elevated and CSF glucose level typically normal or decreased.

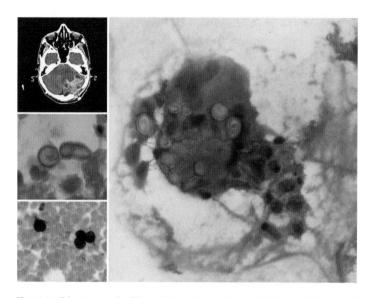

FIG. 9.8. Blastomycosis. The radiology image (*upper left*) from a 52-year-old man shows a large posterior cerebellar brain mass due to blastomycosis infection destroying the skull bone. The Pap stained imprint cytology specimen shows numerous large budding yeasts (*right image*), with broad based buds (*middle left*). A GMS stain is positive (*bottom left*). A brain biopsy confirmed blastomycosis infection. All images are shown with high magnification (images courtesy of Dr. Pawel Schubert, University of Stellenbosch, Cape Town, South Africa).

Cytomorphologic Features

- There is a CSF pleocytosis which may demonstrate a lymphocytic or neutrophilic predominance. Patients may also present with granulomatous meningitis.
- The finding of large (8–15 μm) budding yeasts with broad based buds is necessary to help establish the diagnosis. Yeasts are usually found within macrophages.

Differential Diagnosis

- Other fungal microorganisms
- Neoplastic lesions in the case of a brain mass
- Mimics of fungus (such as talc)

Ancillary Studies

- Microbiology culture. This has low sensitivity for CSF obtained via lumbar puncture. However, culture of ventricular fluid is associated with greater sensitivity.

Brain Abscess

Microbiology

- Bacteria are the most common organisms recovered from cultures of brain abscesses, including *Streptococcus cocci, Pseudomonas, Neisseria, Haemophilus, Nocardia,* and *Mycobacterium.* Most brain abscesses are caused by infections with mixed flora.
- Other organisms that may cause a brain abscess include fungi and parasites (e.g., *Toxoplasma gondii,* amebae), especially in immunocompromised patients.
- The source of a brain abscess may be a local (skull fracture, ear, dental, paranasal sinuses, epidural) or remote (lung, heart, etc.) infection. Spread of microorganisms is by hematogenous or direct extension.
- Aerobic bacteria are frequently cultured from abscesses that have sinus tracts connecting them to the exterior, such as middle-ear infections and skull fractures. On the other hand, areas in the brain with ischemic injury are most likely to include anaerobic or microaerophilic organisms.

Clinical Features

- Patients may experience symptoms related to increased intracranial pressure (e.g., headache, vomiting, confusion, coma), infection (e.g., fever) and focal tissue damage (e.g., palsy).
- An untreated brain abscess may cause cerebral herniation or rupture into the ventricles, causing severe fatal meningitis.

Cytomorphologic Features

- Examination of the CSF shows no abnormalities or may be similar to acute bacterial meningitis.

- Stereotactic biopsy may occasionally be required for the diagnosis. Procured abscess material includes many neutrophils and associated cellular debris.

Differential Diagnosis

- Bacterial meningitis
- Tuberculosis meningitis
- Fungal infection
- Brain tumor with acute inflammation
- Leukemia

Ancillary Studies

- Gram stain for bacteria
- GMS and PAS stain for fungi
- Acid-fast stain for mycobacteria and *Norcardia*
- Microbiology culture
- Immunocytochemistry for specific microorganisms (e.g., *Toxoplasma*)

Shunt Infections

Microbiology

- Ventriculoperitoneal (VP) shunts are used for intracranial pressure management and temporary CSF drainage.
- An Ommaya reservoir is an intraventricular catheter system used for the aspiration of CSF or for intrathecal delivery of drugs (e.g., chemotherapy for brain tumors) into the CSF.
- These foreign devices may introduce infections into the CNS. Typical infections are caused by bacteria (e.g., *Staphylococcus epidermidis*, *S. aureus*, *Acinetobacter* spp.) and rarely from fungi (e.g., *Candida* spp.). Shunts terminating in the peritoneal cavity have a greater risk of infection with Gram-negative organisms.
- In patients with infected ventricular shunts, cultures of CSF from the shunt or ventricles are more likely to be positive than CSF obtained via lumbar puncture.

Clinical Features

- Infection of the CNS is a major cause of morbidity and mortality in patients with CSF shunts. They may cause seizures and shunt malfunction.

Cytomorphologic Features

- CSF shows a pleocytosis and depending on the chronicity of infection will have a lymphocytic or neutrophilic predominance.
- Microorganisms (e.g., bacteria, *Candida*) may be observed. Intracellular organisms are indicative of true infection, and not just colonization.

Differential Diagnosis

- Leukemoid reaction
- Brain tumor with inflammation

Ancillary Studies

- Special stains (Gram, GMS and PAS) for microorganisms
- Microbiology culture

Neurosyphilis

Microbiology

- Neurosyphilis is caused by infection with the spirochetal bacterium *Treponema pallidum*.

Clinical Features

- Syphilis can produce a variety of CNS disorders which may mimic other infections as well as vascular, neoplastic, or degenerative disease.
- The most common presentation of neurosyphilis is meningitis (28%), followed by systemic features and dementia.

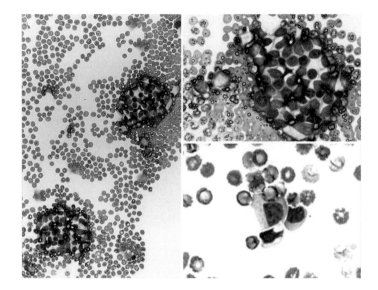

FIG. 9.9.   Neurosyphilis. This CSF specimen from a 48 year old HIV positive male shows numerous lymphocytes and plasma cells (Diff-Quik stain, Intermediate magnification, *left*; and high magnification, *right*). Serological testing supported a diagnosis of neurosyphilis.

- Meningitis may occur within 5 years of a person first contracting this infection. From 7 to 15 years after contact, inflammatory meningovascular syphilis can produce brain infarction in any area of the CNS. Tertiary syphilis (15–20 years after contact) has two classic presentations: tabes dorsalis (spinal cord degeneration) and paretic neurosyphilis (general paresis) (Fig. 9.9).

Cytomorphologic Features

- The cytological features of neurosyphilis are nonspecific, and include pleocytosis with a marked increase in lymphocytes and plasma cells.

Differential Diagnosis

- Other infectious agents
- Other conditions with increased plasma cells such as plasma cell neoplasia, late bacterial infection, and multiple sclerosis

Ancillary Studies

- CSF chemistry (high protein level and positive IgG oligoclonal bands)
- Serology using (1) nonspecific (reagin) tests such as rapid plasma reagin (RPR) or the VDRL, or (2) specific treponemal antibody tests such as the fluorescent treponemal antibody (FTA) test. A false positive CSF VDRL occurs only when positive blood is inadvertently introduced into the CSF by a traumatic lumbar puncture. Occasionally all these tests are negative.

Toxoplasmosis

Microbiology

- Toxoplasmosis is caused by infection with the obligate intracellular protozoal parasite *T. gondii*.
- Ingested oocysts transform into tachyzoites which localize in neural and muscle tissue where they subsequently develop into tissue cyst bradyzoites (Fig. 9.10).

Clinical Features

- In the CNS, toxoplasmosis may present with meningoencephalitis or with multiple small abscesses.
- Toxoplasmosis infection is more common in immunosuppressed persons, and is a common opportunistic infection in AIDS patients. It is the most common cause of a focal brain lesion in patients with AIDS.
- Congenital infection may cause underdevelopment of the cerebrum resulting in microcephaly and mental retardation.
- Ocular disease from *Toxoplasma* infection can result from congenital infection or infection after birth.

Cytomorphologic Features

- CSF in these cases shows neutrophils mixed with mononuclear cells, and only rarely tachyzoites.
- In cytology specimens from brain lesions, microorganisms are usually sparse. Typical cysts containing oval- or crescent -shaped

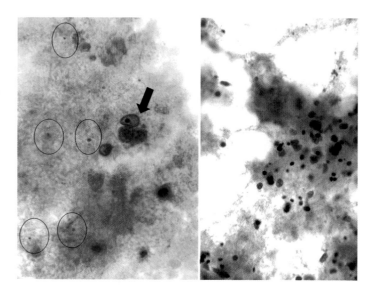

FIG. 9.10. Toxoplasmosis infection. These images are from imprint cytology of a brain biopsy in an HIV+man. (*Left*) A small oval cyst with intracellular parasites is shown (*arrow*) as well as several small scattered parasites (*circles*) in the background (Pap stain, high magnification). (*Right*) An immunostain confirms the presence of toxoplasmosis (high magnification).

bradyzoites are best seen in air-dried Romanowsky stained (e.g., Diff-Quik) preparations. The background contains associated abundant macrophages, polymorphous lymphoid cells, and occasional reactive astrocytosis.

Differential Diagnosis

- Cerebral vasculitis
- CNS lymphoma
- HIV encephalopathy
- HIV dementia
- Other (non-HIV) forms of dementia
- Cerebrovascular disease
- Neurosyphilis

Ancillary Studies

- Special stains (Giemsa stain)
- Immunocytochemistry using antibodies for *T. gondii*
- Serology

Neurocysticercosis

Microbiology

- Neurocysticercosis is an infection of the brain or spinal cord due to the pork tapeworm *Taenia solium*.
- In the CNS, larvae cannot grow to adult worms. Hence, they remain as cysts indefinitely. When they die the cyst ruptures which evokes an inflammatory response.
- *T. solium* is the most common helminthic infestation to affect the CNS worldwide.

Clinical Features

- Patients may present with seizures.
- Imaging studies typically reveal a focal brain lesion.

Cytomorphologic Features

- CSF contains abundant eosinophils, as well as mononuclear cells.
- Larvae are not identified.

Differential Diagnosis

- Angiostrongyliasis
- Schistosomiasis
- Other causes of CSF eosinophilic pleocytosis

Ancillary Studies

- Serology

Primary Amebic Meningoencephalitis

Microbiology

- Primary amebic meningoencephalitis (PAM) is caused by infection from *Naegleria fowleri.*
- These parasites live in warm, unchlorinated, stagnant bodies of freshwater. While swimming, infection is acquired through the nose, typically during the summer months. The parasites then rapidly spread into the CNS.

Clinical Features

- Patients may manifest with encephalitis and experience headache, nausea, vomiting, neck rigidity, seizures, and eventually coma.
- Death usually occurs within 14 days of exposure when the infection spreads to the brain stem.

Cytomorphologic Features

- Non-encapsulated ameba can be identified in CSF. They have a relatively large nucleus and little cytoplasm.
- CSF reveals a neutrophilic pleocytosis with early infection, and a predominant mononuclear leukocytosis with more chronic infection.

Differential Diagnosis

- Ameba may be hard to differentiate from mononuclear cells.
- Amebic brain abscess due to *Entamoeba histolytica*. These amebae are not seen in CSF.

Ancillary Studies

- Wet preparation to identify microorganism motility
- Serology (rising titers)

Angiostrongyliasis

Microbiology

- Angiostrongyliasis is an infection by a nematode from the *Angiostrongylus* genus, usually from the lungworm *Angiostrongylus cantonensis* acquired after consuming certain molluscs.
- Circulating larvae migrate to the meninges where they may develop into the adult form in the brain and CSF. However, they soon die and incite an inflammatory reaction.
- It is the most common cause of eosiniphilic meningitis.

Clinical Features

- Patients are usually from or have traveled recently to the South Pacific, Hawaii, or the Caribbean.
- Patients usually present with a headache, and occasionally neck stiffness and mild cognitive impairment.
- Infection may resolve without treatment, but with a heavy load of parasites there may be severe symptoms (paresis, coma), permanent CNS sequelae, or even death.
- Unlike cysticercosis, focal brain lesions are not identified by imaging studies.

Cytomorphologic Features

- CSF typically shows a marked eosinophilic pleocytosis (greater than 10% eosinophils).
- Larvae are only rarely identified in CSF, especially in pediatric patients.

Differential Diagnosis

- Neurocysticercosis
- Other roundworm infections that present with eosinophilic meningitis (*Gnathostoma spinigerum, Baylisascaris procyonis*)
- Other causes of CSF eosinophilic pleocytosis

Ancillary Studies

- Serology (tests are not widely available)

Suggested Reading

Brogi E, Cibas ES. Cytologic detection of *Toxoplasma gondii* tachyzoites in cerebrospinal fluid. Am J Clin Pathol. 2000;114:951–5.

Cajulis RS, Hayden R, Frias-Hidvegi D, Brody BA, Yu GH, Levy R. Role of cytology in the intraoperative diagnosis of HIV-positive patients undergoing stereotactic brain biopsy. Acta Cytol. 1997;41:481–6.

Chan TY, Parwani AV, Levi AW, Ali SZ. Mollaret's meningitis: cytopathologic analysis of fourteen cases. Diagn Cytopathol. 2003;28:227–31.

Garges HP, Moody MA, Cotten CM, Smith PB, Tiffany KF, Lenfestey R, et al. Neonatal meningitis: what is the correlation among cerebrospinal fluid cultures, blood cultures, and cerebrospinal fluid parameters? Pediatrics. 2006;117:1094–100.

Gupta PK, Gupta PC, Roy S, Banerji AK. Herpes simplex encephalitis, cerebrospinal fluid cytology studies. Two case reports. Acta Cytol. 1972;16:563–5.

Silverman JF. Cytopathology of fine-needle aspiration biopsy of the brain and spinal cord. Diagn Cytopathol. 1986;2:312–9.

Teot LA, Sexton CW. Mollaret's meningitis: case report with immunocytochemical and polymerase chain reaction amplification studies. Diagn Cytopathol. 1996;15:345–8.

van de Beek D, de Gans J, Tunkel AR, Wijdicks EF. Community-acquired bacterial meningitis in adults. N Engl J Med. 2006;354:44–53.

Verstrepen WA, Bruynseels P, Mertens AH. Evaluation of a rapid real-time RT-PCR assay for detection of enterovirus RNA in cerebrospinal fluid specimens. J Clin Virol. 2002;25 Suppl 1:S39–43.

Weller PF, Liu LX. Eosinophilic meningitis. Semin Neurol. 1993; 13:161–8.

10
Hematologic Infections

**Sara E. Monaco, Walid E. Khalbuss,
and Liron Pantanowitz**
Department of Pathology, University of Pittsburgh Medical Center,
5150 Centre Avenue, Suite 201, Pittsburgh, PA 15232, USA

Fine needle aspiration (FNA) biopsy is a rapid, safe, accurate, and cost-effective diagnostic technique that has proven to successfully diagnose hematologic infections and guide treatment decisions. The cytomorphologic findings of hematologic infections show several patterns (Table 10.1). Hematologic infections that manifest with lymphadenopathy and/or splenomegaly may mimic lymphoma. Hence, apart from obtaining a pathologic diagnosis, cytology specimens from nodes or spleen should be triaged for lymphoma work up (e.g., flow cytometry), microbiology culture in a sterile container, and other special studies (e.g., PCR). This chapter highlights key hematologic infections and focuses on their cytomorphology, differential diagnosis, and ancillary studies.

Lymph Node Infections

Acute Suppurative Lymphadenitis

- This form of lymphadenitis is characterized by acute inflammation and possible abscess formation with pus. Typical infectious causes include pyogenic bacterial organisms (e.g., *Staphylococcus*, *Streptococcus* spp., Gram-negative bacilli), less likely actinomycetes (Actinomyces and Nocardia spp.) and some fungi (Candida, Aspergillus, Zygomycetes).

L. Pantanowitz et al., *Cytopathology of Infectious Diseases*,
Essentials in Cytopathology 17, DOI 10.1007/978-1-4614-0242-8_10,
© Springer Science+Business Media, LLC 2011

TABLE 10.1. Cytomorphologic patterns of hematologic infections.

Characteristic feature	Heterogeneous lymphocytes	Suppurative lymphadenitis	Granulomatous inflammation	Necrosis	Homogeneous lymphocytes
Predominant cell type	Small polymorphous lymphocytes	Neutrophils	Macrophages	None	Atypical monotonous lymphocytes
Background	Lymphoglandular bodies	Inflammatory debris	±Inflammatory or necrotic debris	Necrotic debris	Lymphoglandular bodies
Macrophages	Tingible body macrophages	Few	Many epithelioid or spindle histiocytes	Few	Tingible body macrophages
Infectious etiology	Viral, early bacterial, or early cat scratch infection	Bacteria, early cat scratch, tuberculosis, atypical mycobacteria, actinomyces, fungi, HSV, pneumocystis	Tuberculosis, tuberculoid leprosy, fungi, atypical mycobacteria, cat scratch, LGV, leishmania	Mycobacteria, fungi	EBV (infectious mononucleosis), toxoplasmosis
Noninfectious etiology	Reactive lymphoid hyperplasia, dermatopathic lymphadenitis, low-grade lymphoma	Kikuchi's, SLE-related lymphadenopathy, infarction	Foreign body, sarcoidosis, malignancy, lipogranulomas	Metastatic tumor, infarction	Lymphoma

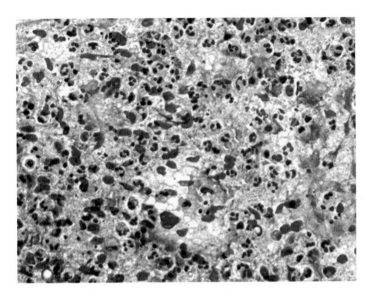

Fɪɢ. 10.1. Acute suppurative lymphadentitis (Pap stain, high magnification). This lymph node FNA shows numerous neutrophils in a background of granular inflammatory debris.

- Clinically, patients may manifest with pyrexia and enlarged, tender localized superficial lymph nodes (neck, axilla, groin) (Fig. 10.1).

Cytomorphologic Features

- Gross shows purulent aspirated material.
- Predominance of neutrophils and inflammatory debris.
- Careful examination may reveal intracellular and extracellular organisms.

Differential Diagnosis

- Abscess
- Cat Scratch disease
- Lymphogranuloma venereum
- Tularemia

- Kikuchi's lymphadenitis where karyorrhectic debris mimics neutrophils
- Inflammatory cysts (e.g., infected branchial cleft cyst)
- Metastatic tumor with superimposed acute inflammation

Ancillary Studies

- Special stains and immunostains for organisms
- Microbiology culture

Cat Scratch Lymphadenitis

- This acute self-limited acute necrotizing granulomatous lymphadenitis is caused by infection with the Gram-negative bacillus *Bartonella henselae*, and less often *Bartonella quintana.*
- Infected patients typically develop regional (localized) lymphadenopathy 1–3 weeks after a bite or scratch on the nearby skin from a cat. Low-grade fever can occur in one third of patients. Rare cases may develop more severe systemic disease (e.g., hepatosplenomegaly).
- Lymphadenopathy has three stages. The initial phase is characterized by florid reactive lymphoid hyperplasia. The second phase has loose granulomas and single histiocytes. A late phase (most characteristic) has both acute suppurative and palisading granulomatous lymphadenitis (Fig. 10.2).

Cytomorphologic Features

- Aspirates contain a variable amount of acute suppurative or granulomatous inflammatory material. Macrophages may form tight granulomas, dispersed epithelioid histiocytes, or present as suppurative granulomas.
- Bacteria are only rarely identified without special stains.

Differential Diagnosis

- Necrotizing granulomatous inflammation in Mycobacterial or fungal infection
- Acute suppurative lymphadenitis and abscess, which usually lack granulomas

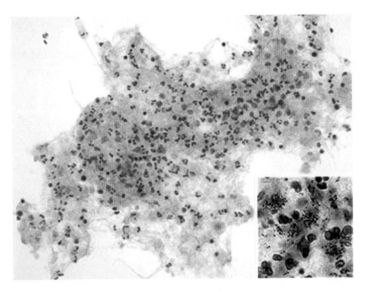

FIG. 10.2. Cat scratch lymphadentitis (Pap stain, high magnification; *inset*: Immunostain for *Bartonella henselae*, high magnification). FNA of this lymph node shows granulomatous inflammation with characteristics of acute suppurative granulomatous lymphadenitis seen in cat scratch disease. Pleomorphic bacteria are best highlighted using immunocytochemistry with a monoclonal antibody to *B. henselae* (*inset*).

- Tularemia
- Lymphogranuloma venereum

Ancillary Studies

- *B. henselae* form pleomorphic aggregates of bacilli that do not stain well with a Gram stain. Therefore, a modified silver stain (modified Steiner stain or Warthin-Starry stain) can be used for their identification. Silver positive organisms may be hard to distinguish from stained background debris.
- Immunocytochemistry with a monoclonal antibody to *B. henselae*. Immunostains are more widely available, cost-effective, and faster than molecular studies. This is the best way to identify *B. henselae*, but the antibody will not detect other strains of Bartonella.

- PCR or Southern blot for *B. henselae*. PCR is more sensitive than special stains.
- Serologic studies are of low sensitivity and specificity because some patients may never have a detectable antibody response.
- Microbiology culture, although this is a difficult and lengthy (9–45 days) procedure due to the slow growth of the organism.

Lymphogranuloma Venereum

- This sexually transmitted disease is caused by infection with *Chlamydia trachomatis*, an obligate intracellular organism.
- Clinically, patients may present with a painless ulcer at the mucosal site of entry about 7–12 days after sexual contact. Lymphadenopathy (buboes) follows 1–8 weeks later. Infected lymph nodes are usually tender and mobile, but matted nodes and sinus tracts can also occur.

Cytomorphologic Features

- FNA of involved nodes yield neutrophils, other inflammatory cells (plasma cells, lymphocytes), macrophages, and occasional multinucleated giant cells, as well as necrosis.
- Microorganisms are not readily identified without special stains.

Differential Diagnosis

- Acute suppurative lymphadenitis
- Cat Scratch disease
- Tularemia
- Kikuchi's lymphadenitis

Ancillary Studies

- Special stains can be helpful. The organisms are Gram-negative and can be identified with a Warthin-Starry stain.
- Immunocytochemistry
- Electron microscopy
- PCR for the 16S ribosomal DNA
- Microbiology culture
- Complement fixation and serologic testing

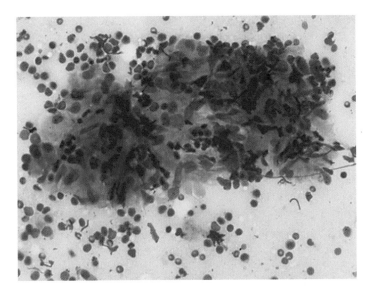

FIG. 10.3. Non-necrotizing granulomatous inflammation (Diff-Quik stain, high magnification). FNA of a lymph node contains discrete non-necrotizing granulomas in a patient with a clinical history of sarcoidosis.

Granulomatous Lymphadenitis

- This type of chronic inflammation within a lymph node is composed of aggregates of epithelioid macrophages (granulomas).
- Granulomas can occur as a result of infectious processes (e.g., tuberculosis, fungal infection) or noninfectious processes (e.g., sarcoidosis, foreign body reaction), and with certain malignancies (Figs. 10.3 and 10.4).

Cytomorphologic Features

- Granulomas are characterized by clusters of epithelioid macrophages. Reactive histiocytes have elongated, kidney bean or boomerang-shaped vesicular nuclei with nucleoli, abundant granular cytoplasm (eosinophilic on H&E and cyanophilic on Pap stain), and ill-defined cytoplasmic cell borders sometimes resulting in syncytial formation.

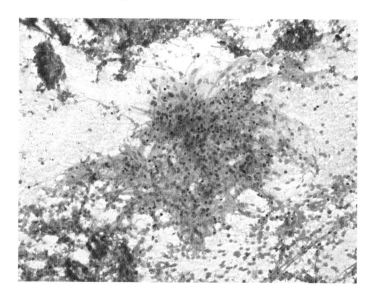

FIG. 10.4. Necrotizing granulomatous inflammation (Pap stain, low magnification). An aggregate of epithelioid histiocytes occurs within a background of granular necrotic debris in this case of tuberculosis.

- Three morphologic patterns may be encountered including suppurative, necrotizing, and non-necrotizing granulomatous inflammation (Table 10.2).
- There may be intermixed lymphocytes, plasma cells, occasionally multinucleated giant cells, and neutrophils present depending on the aforementioned inflammatory pattern.
- Close examination may identify an associated microorganism.

Differential Diagnosis

- Suppurative granulomatous inflammation may occur with dimorphic fungi (Blastomyces, Coccidioides, Paracoccidioides, Chromoblastomycosis and Phaeohyphomycosis, Sporotrichosis).
- Granulomas may be associated with malignancy (e.g., lymphoma, squamous cell carcinoma, seminoma).
- Mimics: Lymphohistiocytic aggregates in reactive lymphoid hyperplasia, sinus histiocytosis, dendritic cells, low-grade neoplasms (Table 10.2).

TABLE 10.2. Different patterns of granulomatous lymphadenitis.

Features	Acute suppurative granulomas	Necrotizing granulomas	Non-necrotizing granulomas
Predominant cell type	Neutrophils and epithelioid histiocytes	Epithelioid histiocytes	Epithelioid histiocytes
Background	Inflammatory or necrotic debris	Necrotic debris	Clean
Infection	Bacteria, cat scratch disease, tuberculosis, herpes simplex virus, dimorphic fungi	Tuberculosis, fungi, cat scratch disease	Atypical mycobacteria, histoplasmosis, leishmaniasis, schistosomiasis
Noninfectious etiology	Immunodeficiency, lymph node infarction	Kikuchi lymphadenitis, lymph node infarction	Sarcoidosis, foreign-body, lipogranulomas, lymphoma, metastatic tumor (seminoma, squamous cell carcinoma)

Ancillary Studies

- Special stains for mycobacteria (acid-fast bacilli [AFB]) and fungi (Grocott, periodic acid-Schiff [PAS]) should be routinely performed to exclude an infectious etiology.
- Immunostains with S-100 and CD68 (KP1) can be used to confirm the presence of macrophages.
- Polarization microscopy to exclude foreign polarizable material.
- Microbiology culture.

Mycobacterial Lymphadenitis

- Lymphadenitis may be caused by infection with *Mycobacterium tuberculosis* (TB) or nontuberculous (atypical) mycobacteria such as *Mycobacterium avium-intracellulare* (MAI) belonging to the group *Mycobacterium avium* complex (MAC).
- Tuberculous lymphadenitis is the most common form of mycobacterial lymphadenitis in the world, and the most common extrapulmonary manifestation of TB, predominantly in less developed countries.
- Individuals at risk for mycobacterial infection are young children, elderly adults, and those who are immunosuppressed (e.g., human immunodeficiency virus [HIV]-positive patients).
- In general, FNA detects around half of the cases of mycobacterial lymphadenitis and has a high specificity and positive predictive value. However, there is a high false negative rate due to the absence of typical granulomas and/or necrosis in cases of early tuberculous lymphadenitis. A combination of test modalities including staining for AFB and PCR can optimize sensitivity and specificity (Fig. 10.5).

Cytomorphologic Features

- Granulomas are composed of clusters of benign epithelioid histiocytes that may be mixed with lymphocytes.
- Tuberculous lymphadenitis has granulomas with Langhans and/or foreign body-type multinucleated giant cells present in a necrotic background. Mycobacteria are sparse and usually difficult to see without special stains.
- Nontuberculous lymphadenitis may show non-necrotizing granulomas and macrophages with abundant foamy cytoplasm

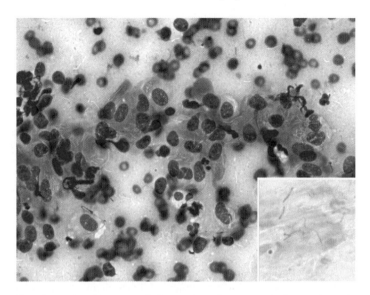

Fig. 10.5. Granulomatous inflammation due to atypical mycobacteria (Diff-Quik stain, high magnification; *inset*: AFB stain, high magnification). Numerous epithelioid histiocytes are seen along with the negative image of several long, beaded mycobacterial organisms seen on DQ stain, and highlighted with an AFB stain (*inset*).

because they contain numerous organisms. Mycobacteria-laden macrophages seen on the Pap stain have been referred to as pseudo-Gaucher cells. These mycobacteria are more numerous and this may be seen as a negative image on the Diff-Quik stain and readily highlighted with acid-fast stains. Some of these mycobacteria have distinct morphology. *Mycobacterium kansasii* resembles a shepherd's crook or candy cane and *Mycobacterium fortuitum* closely resembles *Nocardia* spp.

- Mycobacterial lymphadenitis may also present as acute suppurative lymphadenitis without typical granulomas.

Differential Diagnosis

- Bacillus Calmette-Guérin (BCG) vaccine associated lymphadenitis
- Granulomatous inflammation due to other infections (e.g., cat scratch disease, fungi)

- Noninfectious causes of granulomatous inflammation (Table 10.2)
- Acute suppurative lymphadenitis
- Necrotizing lymphadenitis unrelated to infection (e.g., infarction)
- Foamy histiocytes within lymph nodes can occur with other infections (e.g., lepromatous leprosy, Whipple disease) and metabolic storage diseases (e.g., Gaucher disease)

Ancillary Studies

- Special AFB stains for mycobacteria (Ziehl-Neelsen or Kinyoun stains)
- Fluorescence microscopy with fluorochrome dyes such as auramine O or auramine-rhodamine are more sensitive and specific than AFB stains
- Autofluorescence
- PCR for diagnosis and subclassification
- Culture for diagnosis and subclassification, although mycobacteria are slow growing and culture can take weeks (6–8 weeks with conventional Lowenstein-Jensen medium and 3 weeks with Middlebrook liquid and solid media)

Fungal Lymphadenitis

- Lymphadenitis can result from a variety of fungal infections. The most common causative agents include *Histoplasma capsulatum*, *Coccidioides immitis*, and *Cryptococcus neoformans*.
- Rare causes of fungal infection like Pneumocystis lymphadenitis usually arise in the setting of underlying HIV infection (Fig. 10.6).

Cytomorphologic Features

- Granulomatous or acute inflammation with a necrotic or inflammatory background is likely to be encountered. Fungal elements can be present in varying numbers.
- *C. neoformans* has encapsulated yeast forms measuring 5–15 μm. Their thick capsule causes a clear halo with a DQ stain. The finding of narrow based budding (tear-drop shape yeast) is very helpful.
- *H. capsulatum* is a much smaller round to oval yeast form measuring 2–4 μm. Abundant macrophages in these cases are usually

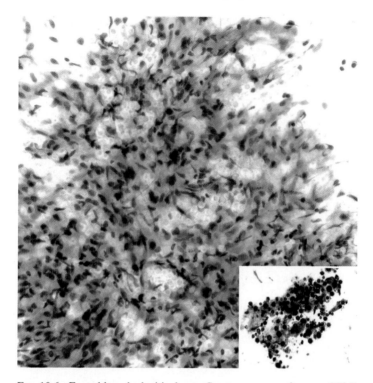

Fig. 10.6. Fungal lymphadenitis due to *Cryptococcus neoformans* (H&E stain, high magnification). Clear (unstained) yeast formation with a thick halo (capsule) are shown caught up among granulomatous inflammation in this lymph node FNA. The *inset* shows encapsulated cryptococcal yeast (Mucicarmine stain).

laden with intracytoplasmic yeast. One may also find narrow-based budding.

- *C. immitis* has larger thick-walled spherules (cysts) that measure 20–150 μm. When intact they contain 3–5 μm endospores. Endospores may also be dispersed on the slide if the spherules are ruptured.

Differential Diagnosis

- Nonfungal granulomatous lymphadenitis (e.g., tuberculosis)
- Acute suppurative lymphadenitis

- Blastomycosis, morphologically similar to Cryptococcus, is an uncommon cause of lymphadenitis; these organisms are larger, lack a capsule, and have broad-based budding

Ancillary Studies

- Histochemical stains for fungi include Grocott or Gomori methenamine silver (GMS) and PAS.
- Cryptococcus capsule also stains positive with mucicarmine and Alcian blue stains.
- A Fontana-Masson stain can be helpful to identify capsule-deficient Cryptococcus.
- Specific immunostains may be required if available (e.g., Pneumocystis).
- Fungal culture.

Toxoplasma Lymphadenitis

- Lymph node infection with the protozoan *Toxoplasma gondii* can be congenital (fetal toxoplasmosis) or acquired.
- Acquired infection causes localized lymphadenopathy, presenting mainly in the posterior cervical nodes, in normal hosts.
- Infections usually remain latent and only cause tissue damage and/or systemic disease in immunocompromised patients.

Cytomorphologic Features

- Cytology specimens characteristically show a polymorphous lymphoid population, epithelioid cell clusters (epithelioid microgranulomas), and aggregates of monocytoid B-cells with or without a necrotic background.
- Cysts with many bradyzoites ("bag of parasites") and free extracellular tachyzoites of *T. gondii* are rarely found in aspirates, but have been reported.

Differential Diagnosis

- Viral lymphadenitis
- Granulomatous lymphadenitis

TABLE 10.3. Differential diagnosis of monocytoid B-cell hyperplasia.

Early cat scratch disease
Toxoplasma lymphadenitis
EBV-related lymphadenopathy
CMV-related lymphadenopathy
Early HIV-related lymphadenopathy
Marginal zone lymphoma

- Leishmania lymphadenitis
- Brucella infection (undulant fever)
- Other causes of increased monocytoid B-cells (Table 10.3)

Ancillary Studies

- Wright-Giemsa stain for parasites
- Specific immunocytochemical stain if available
- PCR using primers designed for the ribosomal DNA of *T. gondii*
- Serology (high titers of IgG- and IgM-specific antibodies to *T. gondii* is usually necessary for the diagnosis; IgM is usually positive within 3 months of infection)

Leishmania Lymphadenitis

- This is an uncommon cause of lymphadenopathy caused by infection with the protozoan *Leishmania*, which is transmitted by sandflies.
- Infection may be associated with localized nodal infection draining a focus of cutaneous infection, or with visceral disease and widespread lymphadenopathy (kala-azar) (Fig. 10.7).

Cytomorphologic Features

- Lymph node aspirates contain a polymorphous lymphoid background, necrotizing or non-necrotizing granulomatous inflammation, and several plasma cells. Necrosis may be suppurative.
- Organisms may be detected by finding amastigotes within macrophages (Leishman-Donovan bodies), or free on the slide following rupture of cells, in routinely stained specimens. Amastigotes are round to oval in shape and range in size from 1 to 3 μm.

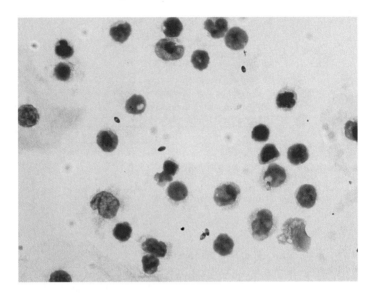

FIG. 10.7. Leishmania lymphadenitis (Diff-Quik stain, high magnification). Several bullet-shaped extracellular amastigotes can be seen scattered among lymphocytes and histiocytes.

The nucleus and bar-shaped kinetoplast (paranucleus) may not be visible in all organisms.

- Leishman-Donovan bodies are more commonly found in cases with more acute inflammation, and less often in cases with granulomas or numerous plasma cells.

Differential Diagnosis

- Granulomatous lymphadenitis.
- Histoplasma lymphadenitis: yeast forms that mimic amastigotes can be distinguished using a GMS stain which will not stain *Leishmania* organisms.

Ancillary Studies

- Parasites stain with Giemsa stains, but are negative with PAS and silver stains (GMS)
- Immunostain if available

- Serology
- Culture in appropriate media
- Animal inoculation

Herpes Simplex Virus Lymphadenitis

- Lymph node infection and enlargement due to infection by Herpes simplex virus (HSV) is rare, but has been reported in inguinal lymph nodes, particularly in patients with hematological malignancies.
- HSV infection manifests as a necrotizing lymphadenitis in lymph nodes.

Cytomorphologic Features

- Cytology samples have abundant necrotic debris with scattered neutrophils and a mixed lymphoplasmacytic infiltrate, but lack granulomas.
- Characteristic HSV viral inclusions such as multinucleation, margination of chromatin, and molding have been reported to occur in stromal cells, but not lymphoid cells.

Differential Diagnosis

- Acute suppurative lymphadenitis
- Cat scratch disease without granulomatous inflammation
- Other viral lymphadenitides (e.g., Epstein-Barr virus [EBV], measles)
- Lymph node infarction
- Malignancy, particularly hematologic malignancy given that most patients will have a history of a hematologic malignancy

Ancillary Studies

- Immunohistochemical or in situ hybridization stain for HSV1/2 ("cocktail")
- Viral culture
- Molecular methods to prove whether infection is due to HSV1 or HSV2

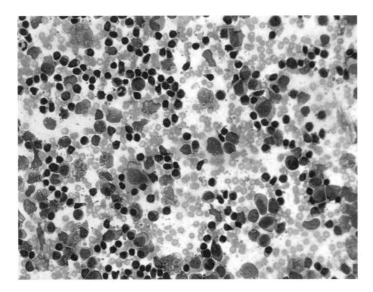

Fig. 10.8. Infectious mononucleosis (Diff-Quik stain, high magnification). This FNA is from a lymph node in an 8-year old boy with positive EBV serology. The lymphoid cells in this aspirate are polymorphous and include a prominent immunoblastic population and plasmacytoid cells. Flow cytometry confirmed the absence of a monoclonal population.

Infectious Mononucleosis Lymphadenitis (EBV Related Lymphadenopathy)

- Young children and toddlers typically have an asymptomatic self-limiting infection with EBV, whereas teenagers may have a more serious and contagious illness presenting with fatigue, fever, pharyngitis, lymphadenopathy, splenomegaly and sometimes hepatomegaly.
- Patients classically have tender cervical lymphadenopathy with a lymphocytosis containing atypical lymphocytes (Downey cells) reported in their peripheral blood smear (Fig. 10.8).

Cytomorphologic Features

- In a lymph node FNA a prominent immunoblast population is seen within a polymorphous lymphoid background admixed with tingible body macrophages and plasmacytoid lymphocytes.

- Occasionally, more pleomorphic atypical immunoblasts with binucleation, mimicking Reed-Sternberg (RS) cells, will be seen. Mitoses may be encountered in these cells.
- The key features that help to distinguish this reactive lymphadenopathy from non-Hodgkin lymphoma are the range (polymorphous appearance) of lymphoid cells present and the absence of clonality.

Differential Diagnosis

- Viral lymphadenitis with an infectious mononucleosis-like syndrome (HIV, Cytomegaloviral [CMV], HSV, HHV6)
- Toxoplasma lymphadenitis
- Autoimmune disease (SLE, rheumatoid arthritis)
- Lymphadenitis associated with drugs (e.g., phenytoin)
- Vaccination associated lymphadenitis
- Non-Hodgkin lymphoma
- Hodgkin lymphoma

Ancillary Studies

- Heterophil antibody testing (Paul-Bunnell test), MonoSpot test (more sensitive assay), and EBV-specific serology studies can be performed when infection is clinically suspected. The incubation of the virus is 40–60 days, so serology is usually positive at presentation.
- Immunostains: Unlike classical Hodgkin lymphoma, the RS-like cells in cases of infectious mononucleosis are positive for pan-B cell markers (CD20) and negative for CD15 and CD30.
- Flow cytometry should be performed particularly in those cases with an exuberant immunoblastic reaction that mimics a non-Hodgkin lymphoma (lymphocytes in reactive EBV lymphadenopathy are polyclonal). Flow cytometry will not exclude a Hodgkin lymphoma.

Cytomegaloviral (CMV) Lymphadenitis

- CMV is a rare cause of lymph node enlargement, which may present as an asymptomatic infection or with an infectious mononucleosis-like illness. CMV lymphadenitis can occur at any age and in immunocompetent or immunosuppressed patients.

- Involved lymph nodes usually have both reactive follicular and paracortical hyperplasia. The cells infected by CMV are histiocytes and occasionally endothelial cells, rather than lymphocytes.

Cytomorphologic Features

- Polymorphous lymphocytes, as seen in reactive lymphoid hyperplasia, are seen with an increase of monocytoid B-cells.
- Infected cells are often sparse and have characteristic CMV intranuclear inclusions and sometimes multiple small cytoplasmic inclusions.

Differential Diagnosis

- Reactive lymphoid hyperplasia
- Conditions with monocytoid B-cell hyperplasia (Table 10.3)
- Toxoplasma lymphadenitis
- Lymphoma: In classical Hodgkin lymphoma there is membranous CD15 staining, as opposed to cytoplasmic immunoreactivity seen in CMV infected cells.

Ancillary Studies

- Immunostains, including CMV immunostains. Cells containing CMV inclusions express CD15, with a Golgi reaction or diffuse cytoplasmic pattern.

HIV-Associated Lymphadenopathy

- Lymph node enlargement occurring in a patient with HIV infection may be due to HIV infection itself and/or secondary to co-infection (e.g., tuberculosis), an inflammatory process (e.g., Castleman disease or immune reconstitution inflammatory syndrome), or malignancy (e.g., lymphoma, Kaposi sarcoma, metastases).
- An infectious mononucleosis-like syndrome may occur in acute HIV infection that manifests with lymphadenopathy, pharyngitis, a rash, and malaise. Chronic HIV-related lymphadenopathy (progressive generalized lymphadenopathy) tends to present

with generalized lymphadenopathy, with nodes typically under 1 cm in size.

- Lymph node architecture changes with HIV infection chronicity and declining immunodeficiency (diminishing CD4 cell count). Nodal architecture progresses from hyperplastic geographic reactive follicles (pattern A), to follicle regression (pattern B), and ultimately presents with a "burnt out" fibrotic lymph node (pattern C). Late phase (pattern C) lymphadenopathy today is uncommon as individuals may be on highly active antiretroviral therapy (HAART).
- The formation of multinucleated giant cells may be seen in lymphoid tissue from HIV positive patients. These cells are produced by the syncytial aggregate of HIV-infected CD4 cells.

Cytomorphologic Features

- The architectural patterns of HIV lymphadenitis may not be easy to recognize by FNA alone. Patterns A (early HIV infection) and B (chronic HIV infection) will both show the cytomorphologic findings of reactive lymphoid hyperplasia, usually with admixed plasma cells and monocytoid B-cells. Lymphocyte depletion with follicular dendritic cells is seen in late stage HIV lymphadenopathy.
- Polykaryocytes or giant cells resembling Warthin-Finkeldey giant cells with hyperchromatic overlapping nuclei and scant cytoplasm may rarely be seen.

Differential Diagnosis

- Reactive lymphoid hyperplasia
- Castleman disease
- Lymphoma

Ancillary Studies

- HIV status and peripheral blood CD4 cell count
- p24 immunostain can be performed, with positive staining best localized to dendritic cells
- Special stains for mycobacteria and fungal infection as coexistent pathology should always be excluded

Spleen Infections

Bacilliary Peliosis

- This is a vascular proliferation caused by infection with *B. henselae*, occurring mainly in immunocompromised or AIDS patients.
- The spleen is rarely affected. More common sites of disease include the skin (bacillary angiomatosis), lymph nodes, bone, and liver.
- Vascular proliferation resembling granulation tissue associated with both neutrophils and mononuclear inflammatory cells is the morphologic hallmark.

Cytomorphologic Features

- Cytology samples show blood vessels with plump endothelial cells present in a background of neutrophils, debris, and granular material.
- Granular material containing bacteria may be seen.

Differential Diagnosis

- Carrion's Disease (Oroya fever) caused by *Bartonella bacilliformis*
- Granulation tissue
- Kaposi sarcoma
- Castleman disease
- Vascular tumors like hemangioma, littoral cell angioma, and angiosarcoma

Ancillary Studies

- Special stains: Gram stain can be used to demonstrate Gram-negative bacilli. A Warthin-Starry stain will highlight clusters of the Gram-negative bacilli
- Immunostain for Bartonella if available
- Electron microscopy in difficult cases
- Serology
- Culture of aspirated material
- Blood culture

Splenitis and Splenic Abscess

- Acute splenitis (also known as acute splenic tumor or septic spleen) is the result of a massive neutrophilic infiltrate and congestion within the red pulp accompanied by splenomegaly. This condition may be associated with sepsis or typhoid fever.
- Splenic abscess contains pus in a walled off area of the spleen. This usually occurs in the setting of bacterial endocarditis, immunosuppression, intravenous drug use, or splenic trauma. Bacteria like *Staphylococcus* or *Streptococcus* are the most common pathogens.

Cytomorphologic Features

- Aspirates contain abundant neutrophils that may be associated with inflammatory debris.
- Bacteria may be identified.

Differential Diagnosis

- Blood contamination with neutrophilia.

Ancillary Studies

- Gram stain
- Tissue culture
- Blood culture

Mycobacterial Infection

- Patients infected with mycobacteria can present with diffuse splenomegaly (e.g., multiple granulomas in miliary tuberculosis) or focal lesions in the spleen (e.g., solid spindle cell nodule in HIV+ patients).

Cytomorphologic Features

- Aspirates procured from granulomas show granulomatous inflammation with or without necrosis.
- In cases with atypical mycobacterial infection (e.g., MAI), specimens usually contain numerous histiocytes with foamy or granular cytoplasm.

- FNA of a solid spindle cell nodule will exhibit a predominant spindle cell population with abundant cytoplasm.
- Mycobacteria may be seen as a negative image with Diff-Quik stain.

Differential Diagnosis

- Fungal infection
- Noninfectious granulomatous disease (e.g., sarcoidosis, chronic granulomatous disease)
- Peliosis
- Felty syndrome (rheumatoid arthritis) where there is expansion of red pulp cords and sinuses with macrophages
- Proliferation of foamy macrophages due to other causes such as ingestion of exogenous mineral oil, immune thrombocytopenic purpura, metabolic storage disorders (Gaucher disease, Niemann-Pick disease, Tay-Sachs disease), thalassemia, and hyperlipidemia
- For splenic spindle cell lesion the differential includes inflammatory myofibroblastic tumor, vascular neoplasms like littoral cell angioma, and sarcoma.

Ancillary Studies

- Special stains for mycobacteria will be positive for organisms, which are usually abundant in cases of MAI. In spindle cell nodules the spindle cells contain mycobacteria.
- Immunostains to characterize spindle cells and exclude a vascular or other spindle cell tumor. These histiocytic spindle cells are positive for macrophage markers (e.g., CD68) and negative for keratin, actin, S-100, ALK, and endothelial antibodies.
- Tissue culture
- Blood culture

Infectious Mononucleosis

- Splenomegaly in infectious mononucleosis due to EBV infection may lead to splenic rupture and death.
- EBV infection results in white pulp hyperplasia without prominent germinal centers, and expansion of the red pulp sinusoids by immunoblasts.
- EBV infection may also be associated with hemophagocytic syndrome in the spleen.

Cytomorphologic Features

- Cytology material will show increased immunoblasts which have prominent nucleoli.
- Hemophagocytosis may be evident.

Differential Diagnosis

- Hodgkin and non-Hodgkin lymphoma
- Hemophagocytic syndrome due to other etiologies

Ancillary Studies

- Serology for evidence of EBV infection
- Immunostains such as EBV latent membrane protein (LMP) for staining EBV infected cells, and lymphoid cell markers to illustrate a reactive lymphoid process
- EBV in situ hybridization (EBER)
- Flow cytometry to exclude leukemia/lymphoma

Hydatid Cyst

- Hydatid cysts due to *Echinococcus granulosus* infection (cystic echinococcosis) can rarely occur in the spleen.

Cytomorphologic Features

- FNA of the cyst wall will show scattered fragments of an acellular, laminated membrane.
- Aspiration of fluid (hydatid sand) may yield numerous invaginated protoscoleces that bear hooklets as well as individual scattered hooklets (18–35 μm in length). Hooklets are usually present for longer because they resist degeneration.

Differential Diagnosis

- Noninfectious splenic cysts (epithelial, mesothelial)
- Pseudocyst
- Lymphangioma

Ancillary Studies

- Serology to confirm exposure to the parasite.

Suggested Reading

Caponetti G, Pantanowitz L. HIV-associated lymphadenopathy. Ear Nose Throat J. 2008;87:374–5.

Gaffey MJ, Ben-Ezra JM, Weiss LM. Herpes simplex lymphadenitis. Am J Clin Pathol. 1991;95:709–14.

Gupta SK, Kumar B, Kaur S. Aspiration cytology of lymph nodes in leprosy. Int J Lepr Other Mycobact Dis. 1981;49:9–15.

Hadfield TL, Lamy Y, Wear DJ. Demonstration of *Chlamydia trachomatis* in inguinal lymphadenitis of lymphogranuloma venereum: a light microscopy, electron microscopy and polymerase chain reaction study. Mod Pathol. 1995;8:924–9.

Monaco SE, Schuchert MJ, Khalbuss WE. Diagnostic difficulties and pitfalls in rapid on-site evaluation of endobronchial ultrasound guided fine needle aspiration. Cytojournal. 2010;7:9.

Shimizu K, Ito I, Sasaki H, Takada E, Sunagawa M, Masawa N. Fine-needle aspiration of Toxoplasmic lymphadenitis in an intramammary lymph node: a case report. Acta Cytol. 2001;45:259–62.

Silverman JF. Fine needle aspiration cytology of cat scratch disease. Acta Cytol. 1985;29:542–7.

Solis OG, Belmonte AH, Ramaswamy G, Tchertkoff V. Pseudogaucher cells in *Mycobacterium avium* intracellulare infections in acquired immune deficiency syndrome (AIDS). Am J Clin Pathol. 1986;85:233–5.

Stanley MW, Steeper TA, Horwitz CA, Burton LG, Strickler JG, Borken S. Fine-needle aspiration of lymph nodes in patients with acute infectious mononucleosis. Diagn Cytopathol. 1990;6:323–9.

Tallada N, Raventós A, Martinez S, Compañó C, Almirante B. Leishmania lymphadenitis diagnosed by fine-needle aspiration biopsy. Diagn Cytopathol. 1993;9:673–6.

11
Breast, Skin,
and Musculoskeletal Infections

Pam Michelow[1], Walid E. Khalbuss[2],
and Liron Pantanowitz[2]
[1]Cytology Unit, Department of Anatomical Pathology,
University of the Witwatersrand and National Health Laboratory Service,
Johannesburg, Gauteng, South Africa

[2]Department of Pathology, University of Pittsburgh Medical Center,
5150 Centre Avenue, Suite 201, Pittsburgh, PA 15232, USA

A plethora of infections may involve the skin, soft tissue, and musculoskeletal system. Almost all of these infections are amenable to being diagnosed by cytology using scrapings, split-skin smears, and fine needle aspiration. This chapter covers the cytopathology of infectious diseases in the breast, skin, subcutaneous tissue, deep soft tissue, bone and joints.

Breast Infections

- Breast cytology including FNA and infrequently nipple discharge evaluation may be useful in the management of breast infections.
- Most inflammatory lesions of the breast are benign in nature (Table 11.1).
- The most common microorganisms are bacteria, especially *Staphylococcus aureus*, including methicillin-resistant *Staphylococcus aureus* (MRSA).
- Unusual pathogens reported to involve the breast include cat scratch disease, mycobacteria (tuberculosis and atypical mycobacteria), actinomycosis, fungi (e.g., *Cryptococcus, Aspergillus,*

L. Pantanowitz et al., *Cytopathology of Infectious Diseases*,
Essentials in Cytopathology 17, DOI 10.1007/978-1-4614-0242-8_11,
© Springer Science+Business Media, LLC 2011

TABLE 11.1.   Inflammatory lesions of the breast.

Infectious
  Acute mastitis
  Puerperal mastitis
  Breast abscess
  Subareolar abscess
  Mycobacterial infection
  Fungal infections
  Cat scratch disease
  Actinomycosis
  Herpes simplex virus
  Parasitic infections
  Typhoid mastitis
  Myiasis (maggot infestation)

Benign inflammatory (noninfectious)
  Duct ectasia (periductal mastitis)
  Granulomatous lobular mastitis (idiopathic)
  Plasma cell mastitis
  Fat necrosis
  Silicone mastitis
  Diabetic mastopathy
  Sarcoidosis
  Vasculitis
  Phlebitis (Mondor disease)
  Breast infarct
  Collagen vascular disease
  Amyloid tumor
  Mastitis factitia (self-inflicted mastitis)

Malignant inflammatory (noninfectious)
  Inflammatory breast carcinoma

dimorphic fungi, chromomycosis), parasites, and maggot infestation. A rare case with herpes simplex virus cells has been reported in a hemorrhagic nipple discharge.

- Chronic infections may mimic breast cancer clinically, on imaging studies, and microscopically. They may manifest as a breast mass, with calcifications, inflammatory skin changes, and axillary lymphadenopathy.
- Unusual infections have been reported to be the initial presentation of HIV infection.
- Foreign bodies (e.g., nipple piercing, breast implants) occasionally result in associated infection.

- Breast cancer, particularly malignancies causing skin ulceration, can become secondarily infected. In such cases, it is important that malignant cells are not overlooked when there is an associated intense inflammatory background.
- Lymphoma (e.g., marginal zone lymphoma) of the breast should not be mistaken for chronic inflammation, nor should myeloid sarcoma be mistaken for acute inflammation.

Acute Mastitis and Abscess

- Mastitis is defined as inflammation of the breast with/without infection. Mastitis with infection may be lactational (puerperal) or nonlactational (e.g., related to mammary duct ectasia).
- A breast abscess is a localized area of infection with a walled-off collection of pus. Breast abscess develops in 5–10% of women with mastitis. Approximately 50% of infants with neonatal mastitis will develop a breast abscess. Aspiration of purulent material should always be submitted for culture.
- Subareolar abscess (Zuska disease) is an abscess located in the periareolar area of the breast, associated with squamous metaplasia of the lactiferous ducts, keratin plugging, duct dilation, and rupture. The exact etiology is unknown, but there may be an infective component.
- Mastitis due to infection is usually caused by bacteria. Most infections are due to *S. aureus*, followed by coagulase-negative staphylococci.
- Many cases, particularly abscesses, may be polymicrobial due to aerobes and anaerobes (Fig. 11.1).

Clinical Features

- Acute breast infections typically affects women 15–45 years of age (especially those lactating), infants under 2 months of age, and adolescent girls. Breast infection in men is rare, and may signify an underlying immune deficiency.
- Patients usually present with a tender breast mass. They may also have a purulent nipple discharge, drainage of pus from a mammary fistula, and tender ipsilateral axillary lymphadenopathy.
- Atypical presentations include bilateral breast mastitis and/or breast abscesses, multiple breast abscesses, nipple inversion and/or retraction, and septicemia and/or toxic shock syndrome.

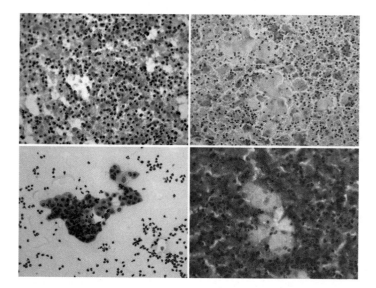

FIG. 11.1.   Acute mastitis. (*Top left*) Numerous neutrophils are shown from a breast aspirate consistent with a breast abscess (Pap stain, high magnification). (*Bottom left*) A group of reactive ductal epithelial cells is present in a background of neutrophils from a case of acute mastitis (Diff-Quik stain, high magnification). (*Right*) Anucleated squamous cells are shown in a background of acute inflammation obtained from a subareolar abscess caused by duct ectasia (*top image* is a Pap stain of intermediate magnification; *bottom image* is a Diff-Quik stain at higher magnification).

Cytomorphologic Features

- Numerous neutrophils are the hallmark of an acute infection. Frank pus may be obtained on aspiration.
- Background necrosis and admixed inflammatory cells (eosinophils, lymphocytes, plasma cells, and histiocytes) may be noted.
- Occasionally the causative pathogen or foreign material may be noted.
- Reactive ductal epithelial cells may be observed including cell enlargement and prominent nucleoli. These cells are cohesive and have associated myoepithelial cells compared with duct carcinoma.

- The presence of numerous anucleate and nucleated squamous cells with keratin debris associated with inflammatory cells, including foreign-body type giant cells, is indicative of duct ectasia.

Ancillary Studies

- Special stains (e.g., Gram stain, acid-fast stain)
- Microbiology culture

Chronic and Granulomatous Mastitis

- Chronic granulomatous inflammation of the breast may be related to infection (e.g., mycobacteria, fungi), a noninfectious etiology (e.g., sarcoidosis, Wegener's granulomatosis, foreign material including leakage from silicone implants), or an idiopathic condition (referred to as granulomatous lobular mastitis).
- Tuberculous (TB) mastitis is rare, even in tuberculosis-endemic countries, with a reported incidence of under 3%.
- Idiopathic granulomatous mastitis is an exceedingly rare breast condition.

Clinical Features

- Chronic breast infections may mimic breast cancer.
- TB mastitis can present as a painless mass (nodular, diffuse, or sclerosing type), breast edema, tender abscess, or with draining sinuses.

Cytomorphologic Features

- The hallmark feature is the finding of epithelioid macrophages lying singly or present in clusters.
- Varying quantities of multinucleated giant cells, lymphocytes, plasma cells, neutrophils, necrosis and ductal epithelial cells, with or without reactive atypia, may be seen.
- Rarely the causative agent (e.g., fungal elements) may be seen.

Ancillary Studies

- Polarization for foreign material
- Special stains (Gram, Ziehl-Neelsen, PAS and/or GMS)

- Microbiology culture including mycobacterial and fungal cultures
- Immunocytochemistry (e.g., CD68 for macrophages)
- Molecular studies (e.g., PCR for mycobacteria)

Parasitic Breast Infections

- Parasite infections typically present as a hard breast mass, and sometimes as an abscess. Persistent infections with old worms and/or embedded ova may present as calcifications on mammography.
- Mammary filariasis seen in tropical regions (India, China, South America) is mainly caused by *Wuchereria bancrofti*. FNA can detect microfilariae and adult worms. Eosinophils in these aspirates are a common finding.
- Other parasitic infections reported to occur in the breast include schistosomiasis, mammary cysticercosis, hydatid cyst, sparagnosis, and *Trichinella* infections.

Skin and Soft Tissue Infections

- Skin infections can be diagnosed by Tzanck preparations, slit-skin smears, and FNA of palpable lesions, vesicles, and/or cysts (Figs. 11.2–11.6).
  - *Tzanck preparation.* Scrapings taken from a vesicle or pustule (ideally taken from the base of the lesion) may show herpes simplex and varicella zoster cytopathic effect. In addition, the waxy cytoplasmic inclusions (molluscum bodies) of *Molluscum contagiosum* can be seen (Fig. 11.2).
  - *Slit-skin smear.* These smears are to be performed by making an incision involving an active lesion approximately 5 mm long and 3 mm deep. Pinching the skin decreases bleeding. The tissue is then scraped and slides prepared looking for microorganisms such as *Mycobacterium leprae in leprosy* or leishmaniasis.
- A wide variety of infections may involve the skin and underlying soft tissue (Table 11.2). Deep soft tissue infections that may be encountered include cellulitis, abscesses, necrotizing

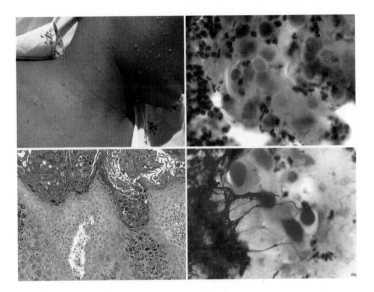

Fɪɢ. 11.2. *Molluscum contagiosum.* (*Top left*) An AIDS patient is shown with widely disseminated molluscum skin lesions. Some of the papules have a dimple in their center. (*Bottom left*) Skin biopsy shows keratinocytes containing large intracytoplasmic inclusions compressing the nucleus to the edge of the cell forming so-called molluscum bodies (H&E stain, intermediate magnification). (*Right*) Molluscum bodies are shown in a cytology sample present among inflammatory cells (*top image* with Pap stain and *lower image* with MGG stain, both at high magnification) (the *right images* are courtesy of Dr. Pawel Schubert, University of Stellenbosch, Cape Town, South Africa).

fasciitis, gangrene (e.g., Clostridial gas gangrene), cryptococcoma (Fig. 11.3), protothecosis and pyomyositis (suppurative myositis).

- Skin abscesses are mostly due to *Staphylococcus* spp., but many bacteria including *Streptococci* spp., *Clostridium* spp., and actinmycoses can cause them. Purulent material comprised of numerous neutrophils is noted.
- Granulomatous inflammation can be attributed to infections (e.g., mycobacteria) or noninfectious causes (e.g., sarcoidosis, foreign body reaction to a ruptured epidermal inclusion cyst).

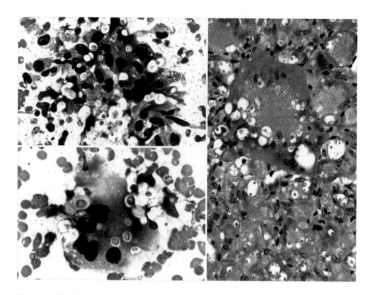

FIG. 11.3. Cryptococcosis. (*Left*) The images shown are from an HIV positive patient that presented with a large neck mass (cryptococcoma) suspected to be an extranodal soft tissue lymphoma based on radiological studies. There was no cervical lymphadenopathy seen. The specimen shows granulomatous inflammation associated with extra- and intracellular fungal organisms surrounded by a clear halo due to the cryptococcal capsules (Diff-Quik stain, high magnification). (*Right*) Histopathologic image showing yeasts in macrophages and giant cells (H&E stain, high magnification).

- Tuberculosis of the skin is traditionally classified into (1) primary infection, (2) secondary disease or reinfection (which includes lupus vulgaris, tuberculosis verrucosa, scrofuloderma, orificial, and disseminated cutaneous tuberculosis), and (3) cutaneous reactions (tuberculids) to a distant tuberculous infection. Scrofuloderma is involvement of the skin due to direct extension from underlying lymphadenitis, usually due to atypical mycobacteria. Atypical mycobacteria may also result in uncommon infections such as Buruli ulcer (*Mycobacterium ulcerans*) and swimming pool granuloma (*Mycobacterium marinum*). Mycobacterial specimens usually show granulomatous inflammation with/without necrosis associated with acid-fast bacilli.

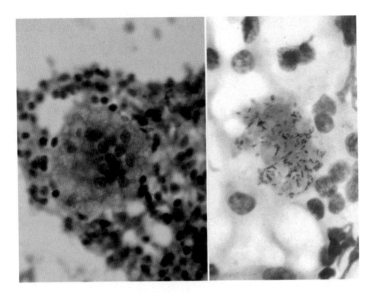

FIG. 11.4. Leprosy. (*Left*) A large foamy multinucleated macrophage is shown with vacuoles of various sizes (lepra cell) in an inflamed background (Pap stain, high magnification). (*Right*) Numerous bacteria can be seen within a lepra cell (Fite stain, high magnification) (images courtesy of Dr. Pawel Schubert, Stellenbosch University, Cape Town).

- Occasionally cytology samples may contain arthropods and related structures. Follicle mites (*Demodex*), measuring approximately 0.4 mm in length, are often located around the face, upper neck, and chest. *Demodex folliculorum* is found within hair follicles and *Demodex brevis* in sebaceous glands. These mites may cause folliculitis and possibly perifollicular inflammation (demodicosis). Cytologic findings in skin scrapings include mites that may be associated with squamous epithelial cells, and in cases of *Demodex* folliculitis with acute inflammation and hair follicle components. Mites still attached to hairs may be seen. They need to be differentiated from scabies (*Sarcoptes scabei*) which can also measure up to 0.4 mm in length. Jellyfish nematocysts (cylindrical hyaline structures) have been reported in skin scrapings. Myiasis is an infestation of the skin

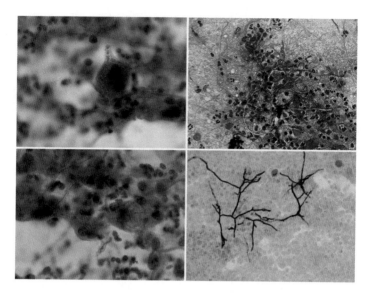

Fig. 11.5. Dermatophytosis. FNA in this case was obtained from multiple purulent neck masses caused by infection due to *Trichophyton violaceum*. (*Left*) *Pink* staining fungal elements are shown at high magnification with a Pap stain that can also be appreciated as negative images on the Diff-Quik stain (*top right*). Branching fungal hyphae are readily visible with a methenamine silver stain (*bottom right*, high magnification) (images courtesy of Dr. Pawel Schubert, Stellenbosch University, Cape Town).

by developing larvae (maggots) of a variety of fly species (e.g., botfly and tumbu fly). The diagnosis in cytologic material has been reported.

Leprosy

- Leprosy is a slowly progressive infection due to *M. leprae*. This organism is an intracellular Gram-positive bacterium that is also acid-fast, although less so than *Mycobacterium tuberculosis*.
- Cytology has been utilized in the diagnosis and classification of leprosy, as well as the evaluation of bacteriologic (bacterial index [BI]) and morphologic indices (MI) (Fig. 11.4).

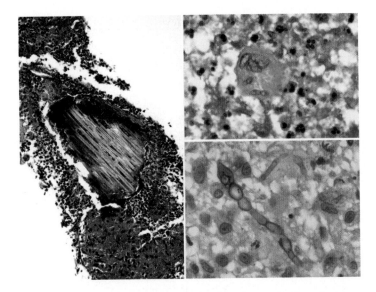

Fig. 11.6.   Dematiaceous fungi. (*Left*) Portion of a wood splinter is shown among inflammatory cells in this cell block identified in an elbow subcutaneous mass FNA (H&E stain, intermediate magnification). (*Top right*) A multinucleated giant cell is shown containing several round stacked brown (naturally pigmented) sclerotic bodies. These vegetative fungal cells resemble "copper pennies." Note the marked background inflammatory debris (H&E stain, high magnification). (*Bottom right*) Polymorphous hyphae with odd intercalated swellings are shown in a granulomatous background of this phaeomycotic cyst (PAS stain, high magnification).

Clinical Features

- Leprosy involves mainly the skin, nasal mucosa, and peripheral nerves.
- There are five different categories depending on the host response (Ridley-Jopling scale). These include tuberculous, borderline tuberculoid, mid-borderline, and borderline lepromatous and lepromatous leprosy.
- The WHO recommends classifying leprosy according to the number of lesions and presence of bacilli on a skin smear. The

TABLE 11.2.   Spectrum of skin infections.

Viral
  Poxviridae (e.g., molluscum contagiosum)
  Herpesviridae (e.g., HSV, varicella, Kaposi sarcoma)
  Papoviridae (e.g., verruca vulgaris, warts, condyloma acuminatum)
    Other viral diseases (e.g., HIV, HTLV-1)

Bacterial
  Superficial pyogenic infections (e.g., impetigo, ecthyma)
  Deep pyogenic infections (e.g., cellulitis, erysipelas, necrotizing fasciitis)
  Corynebacterial infections (e.g., erythrasma, trichomycosis)
  Neisserial infections
  Mycobacterial infections (tuberculosis, atypical mycobacteria, leprosy)
  Miscellaneous infections (e.g., cat scratch disease, chancroid, tularemia)
  Bacillary angiomatosis

Spirochetal
  Treponematoses (syphilis, bejel, yaws, pinta)
  Borrelioses

Mycoses
  Superficial filamentous infections (dermatophytoses, dermatomycoses)
  Yeast infections (e.g., candidasis, cryptococcosis)
  Systemic mycoses (e.g., blastomycoses, histoplasmosis, zygomycoses)
  Dematiaceous fungi (chromomycosis, phaeohyphomycosis, sporotrichosis)
  Hyalohyphomycoses
  Mycetoma
  Botryomycosis

Parasitic
  Protozoal (e.g., acanthamebiasis, leishmaniasis, toxoplasmosis)
  Helminths (e.g., cysticercosis, onchocerciasis, dirofilariasis)

Algal
  Prototheocosis

Infestations and animal injuries
  Arthropods (e.g., demodex, scabies, pediculosis, myiasis)
  Miscellaneous (e.g., marine injuries from jellyfish)

two categories are paucibacillary leprosy (five or less lesions with an absence of organisms on smear) and multibacillary leprosy (six or more lesions with possible visualization of bacilli on smear).

• The organism cannot be grown in vitro, and requires animal inoculation in mice or armadillos.

Cytomorphologic Features

- The cytomorphology of lepromatous and borderline lepromatous leprosy include large numbers of neutrophils and foamy macrophages (lepra cells).
- Lepra cells may be multinucleated with round to oval nuclei, finely granular chromatin, and inconspicuous nucleoli. The cells have abundant cytoplasm containing vacuoles of various sizes. Necrosis associated with a fatty background and epithelioid histiocytes may be seen.
- In tuberculoid and borderline tuberculoid leprosy, noncaseating granulomas comprised of epithelioid histiocytes, Langhans-type giant cells, and lymphocytes are seen.
- Negative images of mycobacteria may be encountered on Romanowsky-stained slides.
- With acid-fast stains, the bacilli are visible both intra- and extracellularly, 3–7 μm in length and may be beaded, straight, or curved.
- Bacilli are readily found in lepromatous and borderline lesions, but are scanty in borderline tuberculoid and not usually found in tuberculoid leprosy.
- Acid-fast stained smears can be used to determine a BI and Morphological Index (MI). The BI is an index of the bacillary load in the patient (density of bacteria is based on counting AFB per high power fields). The MI is an index of bacilli viability. Solid bacilli are judged to be viable while fragmented or granular bacilli are interpreted to be nonviable. At least 200 discrete bacilli should be evaluated.

Differential Diagnosis

- Other granulomatous infections (e.g., leishmaniasis, toxoplasmosis, histoplasmosis, mycobacteria)
- Noninfectious granulomatous reactions (e.g., foreign body)
- Sarcoidosis
- Sinus histiocytosis
- Whipple's disease
- Lipid granuloma
- Histiocytic disorders (e.g., Gauchers and Niemann-pick disease)

Ancillary Studies

- Special stains (e.g., Fite)
- Immunocytochemisry (*M. lepra* PGL-1 antibody test)
- Molecular studies (PCR)
- Lepromin skin test and lymphocyte transformation test (both usually positive in tuberculoid and borderline tuberculoid leprosy)

Cutaneous Mycoses

- A large proportion of infectious skin diseases are caused by fungi. These include dermatophytoses (ringworm), yeasts (e.g., *Candida*, *Cryptococcus*, dimorphic fungi), and the dematiaceous fungi.
- *Dermatophytosis* is a common fungal infection of the skin (tinea), hair (e.g., kerion), and nails (onychomycosis). The many keratinophilic fungal species belong to the genera *Microsporum*, *Trichophyton*, and *Epidermophyton*. Infections are generally made using skin scrapings examined microscopically with 10% potassium hydroxide, by biopsy or culture. Deep infections (pseudomycetoma) are uncommon, but when they occur these fungi cause a mixed suppurative and granulomatous reaction (Fig. 11.5).
- *Sporotrichosis* is caused by infection with the dimorphic fungus *Sporothrix schenckii*, usually following percutaneous implantation from infected vegetable matter (e.g., splinter, rose thorn). A single nodule at the trauma site may develop and subsequently spread as multiple nodules along local lymphatics. These nodules can ulcerate. Visceral involvement may rarely occur in immunosuppressed patients. Specimens demonstrate granulomas with or without abscesses and sometimes the presence of PAS positive hyaline material due to increased immune deposits. Sporothrix organisms may appear as yeast-like forms (2–8 μm), elongated cells (so-called cigar bodies) that measure 2–4×4–10 μm, or rarely true hyphae. These fungal elements stain with PAS, GMS, and anti-Sporothrix antibodies. They need to be differentiated from the septate hyphae and spores of alternariosis caused by *Alternaria* spp.
- *Dematiaceous* (*pigmented*) *fungi* are divided into two clinicopathological groups (Fig. 11.6):
  - *Chromomycosis* (*chromoblastomycosis*). This chronic fungal infection mainly affects the legs. It is caused by many fungi

(*Fonsecaea pedrosi*, *Phialophora carrionii*, *Aureobasidium pullulans*, *Rhinocladiella aquaspersa*). Lesions are characterized by granulomas with or without suppuration. Fungal forms are round, thick walled, golden brown due to their pigment, septate cells (called sclerotic bodies, muriform cells, or medlar bodies) that measure 5–12 μm. They may be free or within giant cells. PAS and GMS stains may obscure their natural pigment leading to a misdiagnosis.

    ○ *Phaeohyphomycosis* (*phaeochromomycosis*) includes a heterogeneous group of superficial, subcutaneous, and visceral infections. Common organisms include *Exophiala* spp., *Wangiella dermatidis*, *Curvularia pallescens*, *Phoma* spp., *Cladophialophora bantiana*, *Cladosporium* spp., and *Phialophora richardsiae*. Patients with systemic infections are usually immunosuppressed. Infection usually results in the formation of a circumscribed cyst or abscess, associated with granulomatous inflammation. Foreign material like a wood splinter is often found together with brown filamentous hyphae and yeast-like structures in a background of inflammatory debris.

- *Mycetoma* is a chronic infection of the skin and subcutaneous tissue that presents with draining sinuses that discharge colored (black, red, yellow, or pale) grains (aggregates of organisms). These lesions can extend deep into underlying bone. There are two etiologic types: actinomycetic mycetoma (caused by *Actinomycetes* or *Nocardia* spp.) and eumycotic (maduromycotic) mycetomas (caused by true fungi).
- *Botryomycosis* (bacterial pseudomycosis) is a chronic bacterial infection of the skin associated with suppuration and sinuses that drain small white granules composed of causal bacteria (e.g., *S. aureus*).

Cutaneous Parasites

- Parasitic infections that may involve the skin include ameba, flagellates (e.g., trypanosomes, leishmaniasis), trematodes (e.g., schistosomiasis), cestodes (e.g., cysticercosis, echinococcocis), and nematodes (e.g., onchocerciasis, dirofilariasis, larva migrans).
- *Leishmaniasis.* Infection due to Leishmania may manifest with cutaneous (oriental), mucocutaneous (American) and visceral

(kala-azar) disease (see also Chap. 4). Cutaneous ("dry" and "wet") leishmaniasis is a self-limited granulomatous condition of the skin with acute, chronic, recidivous (lupoid) and disseminated forms. Acute lesions contain massive amounts of chronic inflammatory cells, including parasitized macrophages. Chronic skin lesions contain fewer infected macrophages. A CD68 stain may help accentuate parasitophorous vacuoles containing organisms. Parasites may rarely be found in spindled fibroblasts. The parasites (amastigote phase) are round to oval and contain an eccentrically located kinetoplast. The kinetoplast may be lost with hydropic degeneration (swelling) of parasites, which is often the case when there is an associated marked acute inflammatory reaction. These organisms (Leishman-Donovan bodies) are best seen with a Giemsa stain. PCR can be used to confirm the diagnosis, even on old or dried material.

- *Cysticercosis.* Human cysticercosis caused by infection with the larval stage of *Taenia solium* (pork tapeworm) commonly manifests as subcutaneous and intramuscular nodules. Common sites of involvement include brain, muscle, eye, and heart. The larvae also have a predilection for subcutaneous tissue of the trunk, thighs, and upper arms. Nodular lesions, that may clinically resemble a lipoma or neurofibroma, are amenable to FNA. The nodules are composed of a cyst (usually 1 cm) filled with clear or milky white fluid and an ovoid larva (called a cysticercus cellulosae) that measures $3-10 \times 4-5$ mm attached at one end. The scolex has a rostellum, four suckers, and 22–32 hooklets in two rows. The cyst (bladder) wall is multilayered (100–200 μm thick), may be encased in fibrotic tissue and associated with eosinophils, chronic inflammatory cells, and foreign body giant cells. Cysticerci only cause an inflammatory response when they degenerate, not when they are viable. A cytological diagnosis can be easily made in cases where the actual parasite structure (scolex of the cysticercus larva) is identified in smears. However, in cases where the only finding is inflammatory cells (eosinophils, histiocytes) or granulomas present in a dirty granular background, these features should alert the pathologist to this possibility. When the cytological diagnosis of a parasitic cyst is suggested an excision biopsy should be recommended. Positive serology may be helpful.

Bone and Joint Infections

- Osteomyelitis may be caused by infection (viral, bacterial, myco-bacterial, and fungal including mycetoma) and noninfectious causes (e.g., acute fracture, sarcoidosis, histiocytic proliferation).
- *Bacterial osteomyelitis* may result from hematogenous spread (typically when bacteria are implicated), contiguous spread (e.g., diabetic foot, chronic leg ulcers) or direct inoculation (e.g., open fracture, introduction of orthopedic hardware). Bacterial osteo-myelitis is most often due to *S. aureus* infection, typically acute, occurs mainly in the long bones of children, and elicits a suppu-rative inflammatory response that includes osteonecrosis. Osteo-myelitis of the jaw may involve *Actinomyces*. Bacteria that may cause a granulomatous reaction include *Salmonella*, *Brucella*, *Bartonella*, *Coxiella burnetii* (causes Q fever), and *Burkholde-ria pseudomallei* (causes melioidosis) (Fig. 11.7).
- *Mycobacterial osteomyelitis* may be due to *M. tuberculosis*, atypical mycobacteria and leprosy. Tuberculous bone infections may be localized (e.g., Pott's disease of the spine). However, immunosuppressed patients such as those with AIDS frequently have multifocal bone involvement. Typically these specimens show necrotizing granulomatous inflammation.
- *Fungal osteomyelitis* may be attributed to almost all fungi. Bone involvement may occur from an isolated multisystem infection. Fungi that commonly demonstrate hematogenous spread to bone are *Candida* spp., *Cryptococcus,* and most of the dimorphic fungi. Radiology images may indicate significant bone destruc-tion, often with accompanying soft tissue infection.
- *Parasitic osteomyelitis* is mainly due to infection with *Echinoc-occus* (hydatid disease).
- *Arthritis* may be caused by infection of the joints (septic arthri-tis). Bacteria are the most common cause of synovial infec-tion, including septic bursitis. Typical bacterial culprits include *Staphylococcus*, *Streptococci*, *Gonococcus*, *Meningococcus*, polymicrobial infections including ancrobes, Lyme disease, and mycobacteria. A wide variety of viral infections (e.g., Parvovi-rus B19, Hepatitis B and C, HIV, Alphavirus) can lead to joint inflammation (rheumatic syndrome). Although less common, fungal causes of arthritis may be due to *Candida*, *Cryptococcus*,

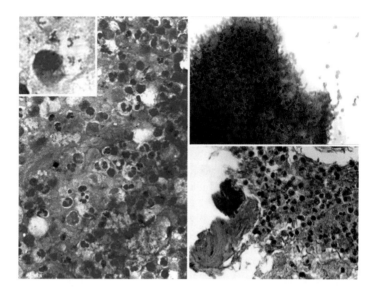

FIG. 11.7.   Acute osteomyelitis. (*Left*) FNA of bone showing acute inflammatory cells and debris that included groups of bacterial cocci (*upper left inset*) (Diff-Quik stain, high magnification). (*Right*) The images shown are from a 49-year-old female who presented with a thoracic vertebral lesion radiologically significant for osteomyelitis. (*Top right*) Most of the specimen shows marked cellular debris and acute inflammatory cells (Pap stain, high magnification). (*Bottom right*) The cell block in this latter case shows similar marked acute inflammation associated with osteonecrotic bone fragments (H&E stain, high magnification). A Gram stain on cell block material was positive for Gram-positive cocci.

Aspergillus, dimorphic fungi, and nearby mycetoma. Infection will need to be differentiated from noninfectious causes such as acute rheumatic fever and poststreptococcal arthritis. Synovial fluid characteristics as well as culture results may be helpful in this regard (Table 11.3).

Bacillary Angiomatosis

- Bacillary angiomatosis is an unusual vascular proliferation caused by infection with *Bartonella henselae*.
- It is seen predominantly in patients with AIDS, and may resemble Kaposi sarcoma clinically. However, cases in immunocompetent

TABLE 11.3. Synovial fluid characteristics in septic arthritis.

Condition	Appearance	Color	Consistency	Cellularity	Other elements
Normal	Clear	Yellow	Viscous	No or rare (<25%) neutrophils	No clots, crystals or organisms
Viral	Cloudy	Yellow	Low viscosity	Lymphocytes and some neutrophils (>50%)	May clot
Bacterial	Cloudy	Gray–green	Low viscosity	Abundant neutrophils (>75%)	Often clots, culture positive
Fungal	Variable	Variable	Low viscosity	Lymphocytes and some neutrophils (>50%)	None
Crystals	Cloudy	White	Low viscosity	Many neutrophils (<90%)	Crystals

persons and after organ transplantation have been described. If not treated, it may be life-threatening.

- Bone and soft tissue lesions may present with or without accompanying skin lesions. Skin lesions resemble pyogenic-like granulomatous inflammation.
- Histologically, lesions are characterized by a lobular proliferation of blood vessels lined by plump endothelial cells with an epithelioid appearance. The vessels are surrounded by a dense, neutrophilic infiltrate, and clusters of bacilli that can be highlighted with a Warthin-Starry silver stain.

Cytomorphologic Features

- The cytologic features are largely nonspecific including a specimen that contains blood and acute inflammatory cells.
- The diagnosis is best made on cell block material and with ancillary studies. The cell block will show a proliferation of small blood vessels, including some that are ectatic and filled with fibrin, erythrocytes, neutrophils, and leukocytoclastic debris.
- Blood vessels are lined by plump endothelial cells protruding into the vascular lumen. These endothelial cells have round or oval nuclei with moderate atypia, vesicular chromatin, and nuclear membrane folding. Their cytoplasm is finely vacuolated.

Ancillary Studies

- Special stain (the organisms can be detected with a Warthin-Starry silver stain).
- Immuncytochemistry (*Bartonella* antibodies are now available).
- Electron microscopy (these studies will show an extracellular aggregation of bacilli that have trilaminar walls including two electron-dense layers separated by a less electron-dense layer).

Suggested Reading

Dabiri S, Hayes MM, Meymandi SS, Basiri M, Soleimani F, Mousavi MR. Cytologic features of "dry-type" cutaneous leishmaniasis. Diagn Cytopathol. 1998;19:182–5.

EL Hag IA, Fahal AH, Gasim ET. Fine needle aspiration cytology of mycetoma. Acta Cytol. 1996;40:461–4.

Gupta RK, Naran S, Lallu S, Fauck R. Cytologic diagnosis of molluscum contagiosum in scrape samples from facial lesions. Diagn Cytopathol. 2003;29:84.

Handa U, Garg S, Mohan H, Garg SK. Role of fine-needle aspiration cytology in tuberculosis of bone. Diagn Cytopathol. 2010;38:1–4.

Kapila K, Verma K. Diagnosis of parasites in fine needle breast aspirates. Acta Cytol. 1996;40:653–6.

Malik A, Bhatia A, Singh N, Bhattacharya SN, Arora VK. Fine needle aspiration cytology of reactions in leprosy. Acta Cytol. 1999;43:771–6.

Nemenqani D, Yaqoob N, Hafiz M. Fine needle aspiration cytology of granulomatous mastitis with special emphasis on microbiologic correlation. Acta Cytol. 2009;53:667–71.

Rao RN, Krishnani N, Malhotra K, Suresh B, Mehrotra R. Dilemmas in cytodiagnosis of subcutaneous swellings: mimics and look-alikes of cysticercosis. J Clin Pathol. 2010;63:926–9.

Silverman J, Lannin D, Unverferth M, Norris H. Fine needle aspiration cytology of subareolar abscess of the breast. Spectrum of cytomorphologic findings and potential diagnostic pitfalls. Acta Cytol. 1986;30:413–9.

Thompson KS, Donzelli J, Jensen J, Pachucki C, Eng AM, Reyes CV. Breast and cutaneous mycobacteriosis: diagnosis by fine-needle aspiration biopsy. Diagn Cytopathol. 1997;17:45–9.

12
Head and Neck Infections

Pam Michelow[1], Walid E. Khalbuss[2],
and Liron Pantanowitz[2]
[1]Cytology Unit, Department of Anatomical Pathology,
University of the Witwatersrand and National Health Laboratory Service,
Johannesburg, Gauteng, South Africa

[2]Department of Pathology, University of Pittsburgh Medical Center,
5150 Centre Avenue, Suite 201, Pittsburgh, PA 15232, USA

Many patients present with lesions of the head and neck. These may be congenital, infectious, cystic, reactive, inflammatory, or neoplastic in nature. Clinical examination and radiologic imaging may not be sufficient to render an accurate diagnosis. Cytologic evaluation in the form of smears and fine needle aspiration (FNA) in this anatomical region is a rapid and accurate diagnostic modality with good sensitivity and specificity for infectious diseases. This chapter covers several key infections likely to be encountered in this site. Infections involving cervical lymph nodes are addressed in Chap. 10.

Salivary Gland Infections

- Bacteria, viruses, and fungi may all cause acute or chronic sialadenitis.
- The most common bacterium associated with infection of the salivary glands is *Staphylococcus aureus*. Other bacteria include *Hemophilus influenza*, *Klebsiella pneumonia*, *Salmonella* spp., *Pseudomonas aeruginosa*, *Prevotella*, and *Porphyromonas* spp., *Fusobacterium*, *Peptostreptococcus* spp., mycobacterium, cat scratch bacillus, *Treponema pallidum*, actinomyces, and *Burkholderia pseudomallei* (melioidosis).

L. Pantanowitz et al., *Cytopathology of Infectious Diseases*,
Essentials in Cytopathology 17, DOI 10.1007/978-1-4614-0242-8_12,
© Springer Science+Business Media, LLC 2011

- The most common cause of viral parotitis is paramyxovirus (mumps). Other viruses including *influenza*, *parainfluenza*, Coxsackie viruses A and B, ECHO virus, and cytomegalovirus have been cultured from salivary fluid in acute sialadenitis.
- Fungal infections of the salivary gland, mainly *Candida* and *Cryptococcus* have been reported.
- Rare parasitic infections described in the salivary glands include toxoplasmosis, cysticercosis, *Enterobius*, and hydatid disease.

Acute Sialadenitis

- Acute infection can involve any salivary gland, but is more common in the major glands (especially the parotid).
- Factors that increase the risk of infection are salivary stasis, salivary duct stenosis, dehydration, diabetes mellitus, anorexia, bulimia, hypothyroidism, malnutrition, HIV/AIDS, Sjögren's syndrome, and certain medications.
- Acute sialadenitis may result in an abscess. Patients present with tender, indurated, enlarged, ill-defined swelling of their salivary glands. Pus may discharge via the salivary duct orifice into the oral cavity.
- A neutrophilic infiltrate may be associated with destruction of ductal epithelium and loss of acini, especially with abscess formation (Fig. 12.1).

Cytomorphologic Features

- A marked inflammatory infiltrate that consists mainly of neutrophils with associated fibrin and debris is common.
- Occasional duct cells, sometimes with marked reactive changes, can be noted. Reactive atypia may mimic a neoplasm. Restricted numbers and limited atypia of epithelial cells in the presence of acute inflammation suggest sialadenitis rather than a neoplasm.
- Stone fragments may be seen if there is an associated sialolithiasis.
- Nontyrosine (amylase type) crystalloids (5–200 μm) may be identified. They are nonbirefringent, geometric in shape (rectangular, rhomboid), and typically fragment in aspirated material. They stain orange with Pap stain and pink in H&E stained cell blocks.
- Granulation tissue may be present.

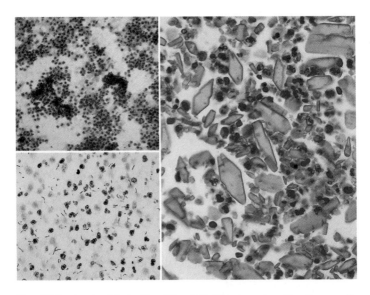

Fig. 12.1. Acute sialadenitis. (*Top left*) Direct smear of a fine needle aspiration (FNA) from a parotid gland showing numerous neutrophils and debris consistent with acute sialadenitis. Culture revealed *Staphylococcus aureus* (Pap stain, intermediate magnification). (*Bottom left*) Gram stain from a salivary gland FNA showing scattered Gram-positive bacteria (high magnification). (*Right*) Nontyrosine crystalloids admixed with acute inflammatory cells in a case of acute sialadenitis (H&E stain, cell block, high magnification).

Ancillary Studies

- Special stains (Gram stain, silver stain)
- Microbiology culture

Chronic Sialadenitis

- Chronic sialadenitis due to infection may present as a distinct mass, usually in the parotid gland. Noninfectious causes (e.g., Küttner's tumor) can have similar changes (Table 12.1).
- Chronic inflammation causes loss of acini, fibrosis, and duct dilatation.

TABLE 12.1.   Differential diagnosis of chronic sialadenitis.

Condition	Cytomorphology	Comment
Reactive lymphaden-opathy	Polymorphous lymphocytes	Within or adjacent to glands
	Tingible body macrophages	Contaminating epithe-lium can be present
	Lymphohistiocytic aggregates	
Benign lymphoepithe-lial cyst	Polymorphous lymphocytes	History of HIV or Sjögren syndrome
	Epithelial cells	
	Proteinaceous background	
Diffuse lymphocytosis syndrome	Increased CD8+ lymphocytes	History of HIV
Wharthin tumor	Polymorphous lymphocytes	Resembles oncocytic metaplasia
	Oncocytes	
	Cystic background	
Branchial cleft cyst	Benign squamous cells	Located outside salivary gland
	Reactive lymphocytes	
	Granular debris	
Mucoepidermoid carcinoma	Malignant cells (mucinous and/or squamous)	Cellular aspirate
	Background debris	
	Possible mucin	
Non-Hodgkin lymphoma	Monomorphic (atypical) lymphocytes	Ancillary studies required

Cytomorphologic Features

- Salivary epithelial cells are scant, especially acinar cells which are reduced in both size and number. Ductal cells may undergo squamous, mucinous, goblet, or oncocytic metaplasia.
- The background may contain blood, mucus, debris, varying numbers of mononuclear inflammatory cells, and fibrous tissue fragments.
- Microorganisms are rarely identified.

Ancillary Studies

- Special stains (e.g., Gram, GMS, PAS, acid-fast stains)
- Serology (for Sjögren's syndrome)
- Immunophenotyping (e.g., flow cytometry) to exclude a non-Hodgkin lymphoma
- Microbiology culture

Granulomatous Sialadenitis

- There are infectious and several noninfectious causes (e.g., sarcoidosis, Wegener's granulomatosis).
- Infections include mycobacteria, histoplasmosis, toxoplasmosis, cat scratch disease, and rhinosporidiosis. Infection of the salivary gland may be the primary site of presentation.
- Patients usually present with a firm, unilateral, or bilateral swelling with or without pain. Occasional cases may produce draining sinuses and facial nerve palsy, mimicking cancer.

Cytomorphologic Features

- Epithelioid and possible multinucleated histiocytes are present with a variable background of acute and chronic inflammatory cells with/without necrosis.
- Inflammation with foamy macrophages and associated reactive epithelial atypia can be mistaken for mucoepidermoid carcinoma.
- The causative organism (e.g., mycobacteria, fungi) may be seen.

Ancillary Studies

- Special stains for mycobacteria (AFB) and fungi (GMS, PAS)
- Immunocytochemistry (macrophages are CD68 positive)
- Serology (e.g., toxoplasmosis, autoimmune disease)
- Microbiology culture
- PCR for microorganisms

Thyroid Gland Infections

- Infective thyroiditis is an infrequent occurrence (Table 12.2). This is because the thyroid gland is relatively resistant to infection due largely to iodine concentration. Cultures may reveal a single agent or polymicrobial infection (approximately 30% of cases).
- In children, infection usually occurs when the thyroid is joined directly to the oropharynx (e.g., congenital pyriform sinus fistula). Thus, the causative agents are those that spread contiguously from the oral cavity to the thyroid.

TABLE 12.2 Causes of infective thyroiditis.

Viral

  Measles, influenza, EBV, CMV, enterovirus, adenovirus, echovirus, mumps,
    St. Louis encephalitis viruses

Bacterial

  (Common) *Streptococcus, Staphylococcus, Peptostreptococcus* spp.,
    Gram-negative bacilli
  (Uncommon) *Klebsiella* spp., *Haemophilus influenza, Salmonella* spp., Entero-
    bacteriaceae, *Eikenella corrodens*, mycobacteria, actinomycosis, *Bartonella,
    Treponema pallidum*

Fungal

  Coccidiomycosis, Aspergillosis, Cryptococcosis, Histoplasmosis, Candidiasis,
    Pneumocystis jirovecii

Parasitic

  Hydatid disease, *Strongyloides stercoralis,* cysticercosis, malaria

- In adults, infection may be from hematogenous spread, a thyroglossal duct remnant, underlying neoplasia (e.g., infected fistula), or direct extension from a nearby site (e.g., esophagus, neck abscess). Patients with immunosuppression (e.g., HIV positive) are at increased risk.
- There have been occasional case reports where FNA resulted in the development of acute suppurative thyroiditis, emphasizing the need to maintain sterility when performing an FNA.
- The presentation may be acute or insidious with a painful, swollen thyroid. Dysphagia, dystonia, fever, and erythema of the skin overlying the thyroid may be noted. De Quervain thyroiditis clinically may mimic acute thyroiditis. Thyroid function tests are usually normal.
- Bacteria tend to cause acute suppurative thyroiditis (acute inflammatory cells), whereas viral infections present mainly with subacute thyroiditis.
- On FNA, a marked inflammatory infiltrate with numerous neutrophils, macrophages, and debris is seen. Follicular cells, with or without reactive atypia, may be encountered. Occasionally the causative organism is noted.
- The presence of associated fluid and/or foamy macrophages with follicular cells favors the diagnosis of an infected thyroid cyst.
- In the absence of native thyroid epithelium, it may not be possible to distinguish acute thyroiditis from an abscess in a lymph node. Radiologic imaging may help determine the site.

- In anaplastic carcinoma, scant malignant cells may be masked by an intense inflammatory infiltrate. If the patient does not respond to antimicrobial agents, an alternative diagnosis should be considered.
- The causative organism may not always be seen in cytologic material. Therefore material should be stained (Gram, AFB, GMS, PAS) and aspirates submitted for microbiology culture (aerobic and anerobic bacteria, mycobacteria, fungi).
- Granulomatous (De Quervain) thyroiditis often presents with a tender thyroid that mimics acute thyroiditis clinically. Multinucleated giant cells are a prominent feature in addition to granulomatous inflammation and occasional degenerated follicular cells.
- Autoimmune (Hashimoto's thyroiditis) presents with a diffusely enlarged thyroid that, on occasion, may be painful. FNA yields a heterogeneous population of lymphocytes, plasma cells, macrophages, and lymphohistiocytic aggregates in addition to Hürthle cells.

Oropharyngeal Infections

- Normal oropharyngeal flora do not usually cause disease. Altered local factors, systemic disease, and unusual organisms may overcome the defensive mechanism of this flora to cause infection.
- Many viral infections can involve the oropharynx such as herpes viruses, HIV, HPV, EBV, rubeola (measles), rubella, mumps, and *Molluscum contagiosum.*
- HPV transmission can be sexual or vertical. The latter route of infection may be related to juvenile onset laryngeal papillomatosis. Oral verruca are due to HPV 2 and 4, focal epithelial hyperplasia due to HPV 13, benign condyloma and papillomatosis due to HPV 6 and 11, and squamous cell carcinoma related to HPV types 16, 18, 31, 33, and 35. HPV related lesions in this location do not exfoliate easily and their diagnosis is based primarily on histology, not cytology.
- Peritonsillar abscess (quinsy) is the most common deep infection in the head and neck. FNA will show abscess material. It is usually the result of a polymicrobial infection.

- Although a wide variety of fungal infections may affect the oral mucosa, candidiasis is the most common yeast infection of the oropharynx.
- Parasites that involve the oropharynx include cysticercosis (tapeworm), echinococcosis (hydatid disease), trichinosis (round worm), and mucocutaneous leishmaniasis (also known as espundia).

Herpes Simplex Virus (HSV)

- Herpes simplex virus (HSV) is a DNA virus. HSV-1 is transmitted through infected saliva or active perioral lesions while HSV-2 is spread by sexual contact. Both types may cause oral lesions. Clinical lesions associated with both types are indistinguishable.
- Primary HSV oral lesions occur predominantly in small children and are associated with fever, malaise, and neck lymphadenopathy. Painful oral lesions may extend from the mouth to the lips, coalesce, and ulcerate.
- Latent infection residing in ganglia may re-activate (e.g., following stress or immunosuppression) causing a secondary herpetic lesion (cold sore or fever blister), often on the lips.
- A Tzanck preparation or smear (vesicle-based scraping submitted for microscopic examination) is often done to diagnose HSV infection (Fig. 12.2).

Cytomorphologic Features

- Herpetic viral changes of Cowdry type A and B are evident, which includes nuclear enlargement and molding, multinucleation, peripheral condensation of chromatin, and eosinophilic intranuclear inclusions.
- Acute and chronic inflammatory cells and debris are seen in the background.
- The cytomorphology resembles varicella zoster virus infection, but the clinical picture differs.

Ancillary Studies

- Immunocytochemistry for HSV
- Direct fluorescent assay

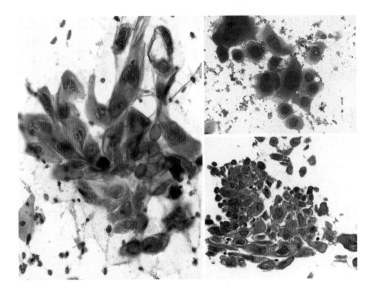

FIG. 12.2. Oral herpes simplex virus (HSV) infection showing characteristic viral cytopathic changes with (*left image*) Pap stain, (*top right*) Diff-Quik stain, and (*bottom right*) in H&E stained cell block material (high magnification).

- PCR for viral DNA
- Serology
- Viral isolation from tissue culture

Cervicofacial Actinomycosis

- *Actinomyces* are filamentous, branching, Gram-positive anaerobic bacteria. The most common isolate is *Actinomyces israelii*. Almost all species are commensals of the mouth.
- Cervicofacial infection often involves the jaw ("lumpy jaw") leading to multiple abscesses, extensive fibrosis, and sinuses from which pus with sulfur granules (bacterial colonies) may drain.
- Trauma (like tooth extraction) or immunosuppression, are predisposing factors for actinomycosis (Figs. 12.3 and 12.4).

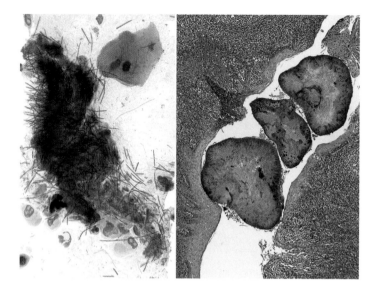

FIG. 12.3. Oral actinomyces flora. (*Left image*) Filamentous bacteria are shown without associated acute inflammatory cells (Pap stain, high magnification). Actinomyces granules without inflammation are shown in this tonsillectomy specimen, which are frequently embedded within tonsillar crypts (H&E stain, intermediate magnification).

Cytomorphologic Features

- Cytologic specimens contain long, thin, and sometimes branched filamentous bacteria that may radiate from a central area within a sulfur granule.
- True infection is usually associated with numerous neutrophils, unlike contamination from oral flora.

Ancillary Studies

- Special stains (e.g., Gram, Ziehl-Neelsen, Fite). *Actinomyces* needs to be distinguished from *Nocardia* as *actinomyces* responds to penicillin while Nocardia is treated with sulfa drugs. Unlike *actinomyces*, *Nocardia* often stains with acid-fast stains. *Actinomyces* also tends to stain well with GMS.
- Microbiology culture.

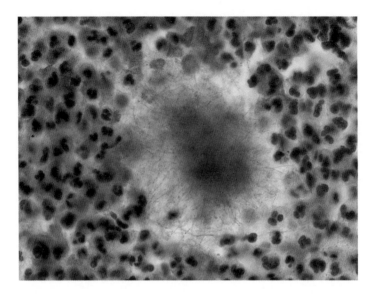

Fig. 12.4. Actinomycosis. This image shows a cluster of *Actinomyces* filamentous bacteria surrounded by acute inflammatory cells in an FNA obtained from an infected cervical lymph node in an HIV positive patient (Pap stain, high magnification) (image courtesy of Dr. Pawel Schubert, Stellenbosch University, South Africa).

Oral Candidiasis

- Candida normally colonizes the oral cavity. Clinical evidence of infection (candidiasis or candidosis) depends on the immune status of the host, mucosal environment, and strain of *Candida* spp.
- *Candida albicans* is most frequently associated with oral candidiasis.
- Clinical presentations include pseudomembranous candidiasis (thrush), central papillary atrophy, cheilitis, as well as erythematous, hyperplastic, and mucocutaneous lesions.
- Oral Candida may be the presenting feature of HIV infection or other cause of immunosuppression (Fig. 12.5).

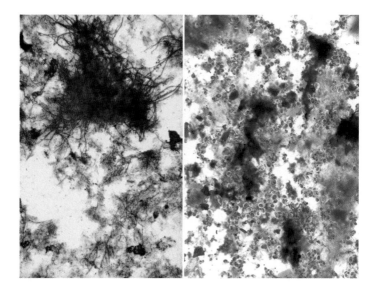

Fɪɢ. 12.5. Oral candidiasis. (*Left image*) Oral smear showing abundant pseudohyphae and yeasts of *Candida albicans* (PAS stain, intermediate magnification) (photo courtesy of Dr. Shabnum Meer, University of the Witwatersrand, South Africa). (*Right image*) Many spores can be seen associated with debris in this case where *Candida* contaminated a herpetic oral ulcer (Diff-Quik stain, high magnification).

Cytomorphologic Features

- Pseudohyphae and/or yeasts are seen. Pseudohyphae are elongated and constricted along their length. Yeasts are round to oval in shape and 2–4 µm in size.
- *Candida glabrata* exists only in a yeast form, with no pseudohyphae.
- If yeasts are prominent, the differential includes histoplasmosis, cryptococcosis, and blastomycosis.
- If pseudohyphae predominate, they need to be distinguished from Aspergillus (septate and branches at 45°) and mucromycosis (aseptate and branches at 90°), both of which do not form budding yeasts.

- Reactive squamous epithelial and inflammatory cells are present in the background.
- There may be associated bacteria and pathology related to another underlying entity (e.g., herpes, carcinoma).

Ancillary Studies

- Wet mount (saline and 10% potassium hydroxide) prepared from fresh material.
- Special stains (PAS with diastase, GMS, others). *Candida* is also Gram positive.
- Microbiology culture

Sinonasal Infections

- Infections of the nasal cavity and sinuses are common.
- Typical viral infections are due to rhinovirus, adenovirus, parainfluenza, and influenza viruses.
- *Staphylococcus aureus*, *Streptococci* spp., *Peptostreptococci* spp., and *Pseudomonas aeruginosa* are common bacteria associated with sinusitis. Bacterial rhinosinusitis, however, is an uncommon complication of acute viral rhinosinusitis.
- Sinonasal fungal infections may be:
  - ○ Noninvasive. This includes a fungal ball (also called mycetoma or if appropriate, aspergilloma), allergic fungal rhinosinusitis, and saprophytic infection. Nasal discharge cytology has been used to diagnose allergic fungal sinusitis, looking for fungal hyphae of *Aspergillus*, as well as thick allergic-type mucin, eosinophils, and Charcot-Leyden crystals.
  - ○ Invasive. Such mycotic infections may be due to mucormycosis (zygomycosis), aspergillosis, and *Fusarium*. Mucormycosis is most commonly due to infection with the class Zygomycetes (e.g., *Mucor*, *Rhizopus*, *Absidia* spp.). The ribbon-like fungal hyphae of such zygomycetes are nonseptate or pauciseptate, branch at right angles, and usually associated with necrosis (Fig. 12.6).
- Several infectious diseases of the nose and paranasal sinuses can present with granulomatous inflammation. These include not only invasive fungal rhinosinusitis, but also rhinoscleroma,

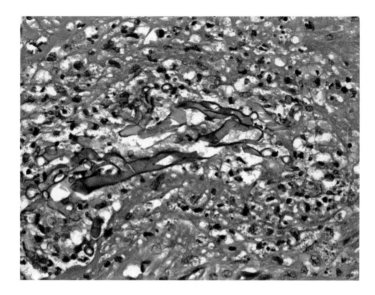

FIG. 12.6. Mucormycosis (phycomycosis). The image shows broad nonseptate hyphae within fibrinopurulent material identified in a 70-year male patient with fungal sinusitis (H&E stain, high magnification). Culture grew out *Rhizomucor* spp. in this case (image courtesy of Dr. Raja Seethala, University of Pittsburgh Medical Center, USA).

rhinosporidiosis, tuberculosis, and leprosy. The differential diagnosis also includes noninfectious causes like sarcoidosis and Wegner's granulomatosis.

- Parasites such as fly larvae may be identified in the nasal cavity.

Rhinoscleroma

- Rhinoscleroma (or just scleroma) is associated with the bacterium (coccobacillus) *Klebsiella rhinoscleromatis*, acquired by direct inhalation of infected material.
- Specimens show a mixed inflammatory infiltrate of plasma cells, lymphocytes, and foamy macrophages (called Mikulicz cells) that contain bacteria.
- Bacteria stain with silver stains like the Warthin-Starry stain.

Rhinosporidiosis

- Rhinosporidiosis is due to chronic infection with *Rhinosporidium seeberi*, believed to be an aquatic protistan parasite rather than a fungus. Contact with stagnant water is a risk factor. This infection is endemic in India and Sri Lanka.
- In addition to infecting the upper airways (causing polypoid mucosal lesions), the conjunctiva and skin may be involved.
- Specimens show sporangia and endospores present in a background of mixed inflammatory cells (plasma cells, lymphocytes, histiocytes, neutrophils, and possible giant cells) and metaplastic columnar cells. Neutrophils tend to form rosettes around the spores.
- The sporangia are large (100–300 μm), thick walled, and contain hundreds to thousands of small round endospores (6–12 μm).
- Sporangia and spores both stain with PAS, GMS, and mucicarmine.
- The differential diagnosis includes *Coccidioides immitis,* which produces spherules (30–60 μm), and *Mucorales,* which produces sporangia (30–70 μm). Myospherulosis may also mimic rhinosporidiosis (see Chap. 15).

Infected Embryologic Cysts

- Embryologic cysts in the head and neck region (e.g., branchial cleft cyst, thyroglossal duct cyst, cystic hygroma) may become infected.
- These cysts are often asymptomatic until they become infected.
- Infected cysts on FNA yield purulent material containing numerous neutrophils and debris.
- Inflamed cysts can show reactive changes that may mimic squamous cell carcinoma.
- Repeated infections can cause fibrosis and the lining epithelium to become denuded and replaced by granulation tissue (Figs. 12.7 and 12.8).

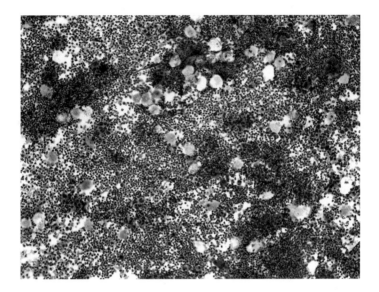

Fig. 12.7. FNA of an infected branchial cleft cyst in a 39-year old male shows abundant neutrophils mixed with benign squamous cells (Pap stain, low magnification).

Eye Infections

- All structures of the eye can become infected.
- Specimens from the eye suitable for cytologic evaluation include conjunctival and corneal scrapings and aspirates of the anterior chamber, vitreous cavity, and lacrimal glands.
- Impression cytology of the ocular surface utilizes a collection device, usually filter paper, applied to the conjunctiva or cornea and then removed. This provides well-preserved cells and is suitable for microscopic evaluation as well as PCR, flow cytometry, immunocytochemistry, and culture. HSV, *Acanthameba*, varicella-zoster virus, adenovirus, and rabies have been diagnosed using impression cytology in combination with various ancillary techniques.
- *Pththirus pubis* (crab louse) may infect eye lashes and could therefore be present as a contaminant on specimens procured from the eye.

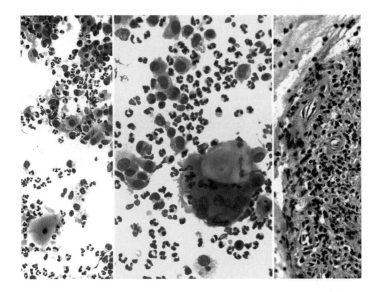

Fig. 12.8. Infected branchial cleft cyst. The aspirate contains mucinous and metaplastic epithelium present with acute inflammatory cells (Diff-Quik stain, *left* intermediate magnification, *middle image* high magnification). The cell block contains fragments of granulation tissue (H&E stain, *right image*, intermediate magnification).

Viral Ophthalmic Infections

- Viruses can infect the eyelids (e.g., herpes simplex), lacrimal apparatus (e.g., Epstein Barr virus), conjunctivae (e.g., adenovirus), intraocular structures (e.g., cytomegalovirus), and the cornea (keratitis).
- Herpes simplex keratitis is one of the most important causes of viral keratitis and is associated with significant morbidity and mortality. Viral inclusions are rarely identified with corneal scraping and ancillary investigations such as PCR, ISH, and electron microscopy may be required. Immunoreactivity for HSV in these samples may be predominantly present in the cytoplasm rather than the nucleus.

Chlamydial Eye Infection

- Trachoma, caused by *Chlamydia trachomatis*, is an important cause of blindness. Infection may lead to inversion of the upper eyelids, misdirected eyelashes, corneal scarring, and visual loss.
- Cytologic evaluation of conjunctival scrapings, swabs, and ocular impression cytology is useful for making the diagnosis, although diagnostic ancillary studies such as direct fluorescent antibody tests and culture are being used more frequently.
- Cytomorphology of Romanowsky-stained smears shows lymphocytes, neutrophils, and conjuctival cells with basophilic intracytoplasmic inclusions.

Bacterial Eye Infection

- Infection of the lacrimal gland is usually bacterial in nature. *Staphylococcus aureus* is the most common pathogen but other pathogens include streptococci, gonococci, mycobacteria, and syphilis.
- Bacterial conjunctivitis usually presents with a purulent discharge that may be examined microscopically. Infection may be due to a variety of bacteria such as *Neisseria gonorrhea*, *Neisseria meningitides*, and *Staphylococcus*.
- Drying of the cornea or hypoxia predispose to infection with *Staphylococci*, *Streptococci*, and *Pseudomonas*.
- Intraocular bacterial infection may be due to surgery, trauma, and hematogenous spread. The best source of material for microscopic evaluation and culture is vitreous fluid, in which neutrophils are present. A Gram stain in such samples is necessary.

Fungal Eye Infection

- The cornea is by far the most common site of ocular fungal infection. Trauma is an important predisposing factor as is topical steroid use.
- Corneal scrapings are suitable for microscopic evaluation, special stains, and culture.
- Conjuctival specimens may reveal *Candida*, *Sporothrix schenckii*, and *Rhinosporidium seeberi*.

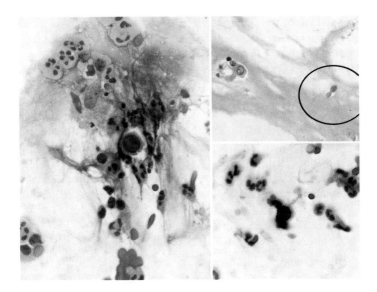

FIG. 12.9. Ocular cryptococcosis. FNA of the vitreous fluid in this patient revealed (*left image*) encapsulated Cryptococcal yeasts (Pap stain, high magnification) with narrow-based budding (*top right image*) (H&E stain, cell block, high magnification). (*Bottom right image*) Yeasts stain positively with mucicarmine stain (high magnification).

- Fungal keratitis is often due to filamentous species (e.g., *Fusarium*, *Candida*, and *Aspergillus*).
- In the vitreous, the presence of macrophages and multinucleated giant cells indicates a granulomatous process, suggestive of mycobacterial infection (Fig. 12.9).

Parasitic Eye Infection

- Conjunctival scrapings are useful to diagnose fly larvae, nematodes, and trematodes.
- Acanthameba keratitis can occur after trauma to the cornea, and has been reported following the use of unsterile saline contact lens solution. Corneal scrapings are examined for characteristic trophozoites and cysts (round to oval, 12–18 μm, double-walled) on Romanowsky, calcofluor white, and trichrome stains, in addition to fluorescent microscopy and culture. The background contains reactive epithelium.

- Aspirates from the anterior chamber can be used to diagnose *Entameba histolytica* and nematodes. Parasites can be the cause of neutrophils in vitreous samples.

Ear Infections

- While otic smears for cytologic evaluation are a useful technique used in veterinary practice, they are not utilized much in human medicine.
- Otitis externa (swimmer's ear) is caused by excessive moisture remaining in the ear canal, or disruption of the ear canal mucosa by trauma.
- The most common bacteria responsible for outer ear infections are *Staphylococcus aureus* and *Pseudomonas aeruginosa*. Other bacteria are less common. In a minority of cases (less than 10%), a fungus is the cause of swimmer's ear.
- Confirmation of infection can be achieved by culture, rather than cytologic examination of smears.

Suggested Reading

Braz-Silva PH, Magalhães MH, Hofman V, Ortega KL, Ilie MI, Odin G, et al. Usefulness of oral cytopathology in the diagnosis of infectious diseases. Cytopathology. 2010;21:285–99.

Deshpande AH, Munshi MM. Rhinocerebral mucormycosis diagnosis by aspiration cytology. Diagn Cytopathol. 2000;23:97–100.

Gori S, Scasso A. Cytologic and differential diagnosis of rhinosporidiosis. Acta Cytol. 1994;38:361–6.

McQuone S. Acute viral and bacterial infections of the salivary glands. Otolaryngol Clin North Am. 1999;32:1–17.

Rivasi F, Longanesi L, Casolari C, Croppo GP, Pierini G, Zunarelli E, et al. Cytologic diagnosis of Acanthamoeba keratitis. Report of a case with correlative study with indirect immunofluorescence and scanning electron microscopy. Acta Cytol. 1995;39:821–6.

Sah SP, Mishra A, Rani S, Ramachandran VG. Cervicofacial actinomycosis: diagnosis by fine needle aspiration cytology. Acta Cytol. 2001;45:665–7.

Schnadig VJ, Rassekh CH, Gourley WK. Allergic fungal sinusitis. A report of two cases with diagnosis by intraoperative aspiration cytology. Acta Cytol. 1999;43:268–72.

13
Immunosuppressed Host

**Pam Michelow[1], Sara E. Monaco[2],
and Liron Pantanowitz[2]**
[1]Cytology Unit, Department of Anatomical Pathology,
University of the Witwatersrand and National Health Laboratory Service,
Johannesburg, Gauteng, South Africa

[2]Department of Pathology, University of Pittsburgh Medical Center,
5150 Centre Avenue, Suite 201, Pittsburgh, PA 15232, USA

Immunosuppression is the result of reduced activity or efficiency of the host immune system to fight infection. An individual may be immunosuppressed due to a congenital condition (e.g., severe combined immunodeficiency or SCID), an acquired condition (e.g., human immunodeficiency virus [HIV] infection, autoimmune disease), or an iatrogenic cause (e.g., transplantation, splenectomy, chemotherapy, or immunosuppression drugs such as corticosteroids or cyclosporine). A weakened immune system for other reasons is said to be immunocompromised. Potential etiologies in these patients are diverse, including common community-acquired infections to uncommon opportunistic infections (Fig. 13.1). While the inflammatory response associated with many microbial infections in this setting is often impaired, unusual cases may result in pseudotumor formation following infection simulating malignancy. Moreover, the quantity and morphology of several microorganisms is likely to be altered because of prophylactic therapy and/or antimicrobial resistance. The risk of infection in such patients is usually dependent upon their epidemiologic exposure (e.g., latent infection with reactivation, nosocomial infection), degree of immunosuppression (e.g., lowered CD4 count in an HIV positive patient), and comorbid conditions (e.g., indwelling catheter). An overview of specific infections and conditions in the immunosuppressed patient is reviewed in this chapter.

L. Pantanowitz et al., *Cytopathology of Infectious Diseases*,
Essentials in Cytopathology 17, DOI 10.1007/978-1-4614-0242-8_13,
© Springer Science+Business Media, LLC 2011

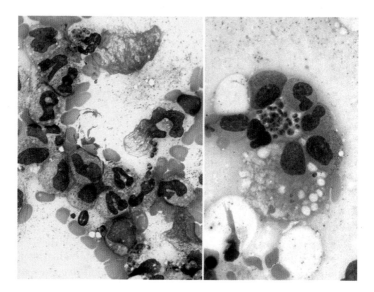

FIG. 13.1. *Penicillium marneffei* infection in AIDS. This dimorphic fungus is an opportunistic pathogen which has emerged to become an AIDS-defining illness in the endemic areas of Southeast Asia. Cytology specimens used to make the diagnosis include FNA of lymph nodes, sputum cytology, and touch smears of skin. The images show several yeasts associated with white blood cells in (*left*) peripheral blood and (*right*) marrow (May-Grünwald Giemsa stain, high magnification) (images courtesy of Kit-Fai Wong, Queen Elizabeth Hospital, Hong Kong).

Transplantation

- Posttransplant infections (Table 13.1) may occur early after transplantation (first month), after an intermediate period (1–6 months), or after 6 months.
  - *Early period*: Infection may be derived from the donor or recipient (e.g., CMV, *Toxoplasma gondii*), surgical complications (line sepsis, aspiration pneumonia), or hospitalization.
  - *Intermediate period*: Patients are at greatest risk for developing an opportunistic infection due to exogenous immunosuppression. This includes *Pneumocystis* pneumonia,

TABLE 13.1. Transplant-related opportunistic infections.

Viral
  Cytomegalovirus (CMV)
  Herpes simplex virus (HSV)
  Varicella zoster virus (VZV)
  Epstein–Barr virus (EBV)
  Adenovirus
  Merkel cell polyomavirus (MCPyV)
  BK polyomavirus
  Human papillomavirus (HPV)

Bacterial
  Listeria monocytogenes
  Nocardia
  Legionella
  Mycobacterium tuberculosis
  Atypical mycobacteria (*M. avium intracellulare or MAI*)

Fungal
  Candida
  Aspergillus
  Cryptococcus neoformans
  Pneumocystis jirovecii
  Trichosporon beigelii
  Fusarium
  Zygomycetes
  Histoplasma capsulatum
  Coccidioides immitis

Parasitic
  Toxoplasma gondii

BK polyomavirus, respiratory viruses, mycobacteria, and gastrointestinal parasites.

○ *Late period*: These transplant recipients are at stable and often reduced levels of immunosuppression. They are at risk for developing common infections (e.g., community-acquired pneumonia) and/or more rare infections (e.g., disseminated histoplasmosis).

• In the transplant patient, viral coinfection may cause direct effects (clinical infection with symptoms such as esophagitis or diarrhea) and indirect consequences such as oncogenesis (e.g., EBV-related posttransplant lymphoproliferative disorder or PTLD, human herpesvirus-8 [HHV8] associated Kaposi sarcoma).

Human Immunodeficiency Virus (HIV) Infection

- The hallmark of HIV infection is characterized by this retrovirus leading to selective depletion of CD4 T-lymphocytes. This acquired immune deficiency allows for the development of opportunistic infections and neoplasia.
- The stages of HIV infection include (1) primary infection (so-called acute seroconversion syndrome), (2) seroconversion (development of detectable antibodies), (3) clinical latent period (with or without persistent generalized lymphadenopathy or PGL), (4) early symptomatic infection (previously called acquired immunodeficiency syndrome [AIDS]-related complex or ARC), (5) AIDS, and (6) advanced HIV disease (CD4 count <50/mm^3).
- Normal CD4+ T-cell blood count measurements are ≥500 cells/mm^3. CD4+ below 200 cells/mm^3 is indicative of AIDS. Other conditions that may also define an AIDS diagnosis are shown in Table 13.2.
- HIV may induce a direct viral cytopathic effect on host cells, mainly lymphoid and histiocytic cells, by causing the formation of multinucleated giant cells. These p24-positive Warthin-Finkeldey-type giant cells may be observed rarely in lymph node specimens and in abundance in fine needle aspirates of salivary gland lymphoepithelial lesions.
- Mortality and morbidity associated with HIV infection has declined since the advent of combination antiretroviral therapy (ART), also called highly active antiretroviral therapy (HAART).
- Immune reconstitution inflammatory syndrome (IRIS) occurs in some HIV-infected patients after commencing ART leading to a paradoxical worsening of symptoms. Microorganisms frequently associated with IRIS include *Cryptococcus*, mycobacteria, varicella zoster, herpes virus, and cytomegalovirus.

Human Papilloma Virus (HPV)-Related Disease

- Immunosuppressed individuals are at increased risk of HPV-associated malignancies including cervical, anal, penile, vulvar, vaginal, and oropharyngeal carcinoma.

TABLE 13.2. AIDS-defining conditions.

Infections
  Pneumocystis pneumonia
  Esophageal and airway candidiasis
  Disseminated atypical mycobacterial infection
  Tuberculosis
  Cytomegalovirus disease (including retinitis)
  Recurrent bacterial pneumonia
  Toxoplasmosis
  Chronic cryptosporidiosis
  Disseminated histoplasmosis
  Chronic herpes simplex
  Progressive multifocal leukoencephalopathy (JC virus)
  Chronic intestinal isosporiasis
  Chronic intestinal cryptosporidiosis
  Extrapulmonary cryptococcosis
  Disseminated or extrapulmonary coccidioidomycosis

Neoplasms
  Kaposi sarcoma
  Large B-cell non-Hodgkin lymphoma
  Invasive cervical cancer

Other
  Wasting
  HIV-associated dementia (and encephalopathy)
  Lymphoid interstitial pneumonia (in children under 13 years)

- While many HPV-related conditions associated with HIV have decreased with HAART, their incidence has remained unchanged.

Cervicovaginal Disease

- HIV-infected women harbor a wider range of HPV types, have more persistent HPV, higher rates of progressive squamous intraepithelial lesion (SIL), and present with invasive cervical cancer 10–15 years earlier than HIV-negative counterparts with more advanced disease.
- With HIV infection there is a tenfold increase in the rate of abnormal Pap tests compared to HIV-negative women, especially when the CD4 count falls below <200 cells/mm^3.

- Although there are currently no consensus guidelines, HIV-infected women should undergo more frequent Pap test screening and/or HPV testing.

Anal Disease

- Invasive squamous cell carcinoma of the anus, associated with high-risk HPV types, is higher among HIV-positive women and men, especially in men who have sex with men (MSM). The incidence continues to increase despite the widespread use of ART.
- Anal cytology (Anal Pap test) is covered in detail in Chap. 7. The sensitivity of anal cytology to identify anal squamous lesions ranges between 69 and 93%, but suffers from low reported specificity (32–59%).
- There are currently no consensus guidelines regarding anal screening.
- Unlike cervical cancer, HPV testing of anal cytology samples has shown poor positive predictive value for high grade anal intraepithelial neoplasia (AIN).

Lymphadenopathy

- HIV-related lymphadenopathy may occur at any stage of HIV disease and can be due to a wide variety of reactive, infectious, and neoplastic causes (Table 13.3). Most of these entities are discussed in detail in Chap. 10.
- The most common FNA diagnoses made from HIV-related lymph nodes are reactive lymphadenopathy followed by infection and then malignancy.
- Rare infectious causes of HIV lymphadenopathy may be encountered such as *Pneumocystis jirovecii* lymphadenitis.
- HIV-infected patients are at increased risk of developing multicentric Castleman disease (MCD), which is often associated with HHV8 infection. Although atypical follicular dendritic cells are thought to be diagnostic of Castleman disease, they are not consistently found on FNA of lymph nodes.

TABLE 13.3. Causes of HIV-related lymphadenopathy.

HIV-associated lymphadenopathy
Mycobacterial infection (tuberculous, atypical and BCG-related)
Suppurative lymphadenitis (bacterial infection including mycobacteria)
Fungal infection (e.g. *Cryptococcosis*, *histoplasmosis*)
Viral infection (e.g., EBV, CMV, HSV)
Castleman disease
Non-Hodgkin lymphoma
Hodgkin lymphoma
Kaposi sarcoma
Bacillary angiomatosis
Metastatic cancer

- On occasion, more than one disease may be encountered in the same lymph node (e.g., mycobacterial infection together with Kaposi sarcoma or lymphoma) (Fig. 13.2).

Oropharyngeal Disease

- Immunosuppressed patients, especially those with HIV infection, may manifest with diverse diseases of the oropharynx.
- *Oral candidiasis.* True infection should be suspected when fungal elements (yeasts, hyphae, and pseudohyphae) are intermingled with inflammatory cells and debris. The presence of thrush is a frequent source of *Candida* contamination in gastrointestinal and respiratory tract samples (e.g., bronchoalveolar lavage) in these patients.
- *Oral hairy leukoplakia* (OHL) (Fig. 13.3). This EBV-associated disease causes white patches on the side of the tongue, typically with a corrugated or hairy appearance, but can also be smooth and flat. Cytology specimens may show prominent nuclear beading (peripheral margination and clumping of chromatin), eosinophilic intranuclear inclusions, and ground glass nuclei. Detection of EBV DNA can be confirmed by PCR or in situ hybridization, as well as viral culture.
- *Herpes simplex virus.* The diagnosis can be confirmed using a Tzanck smear, immunohistochemical stains for HSV1/2, direct fluorescent assay, PCR for viral DNA, and viral culture.

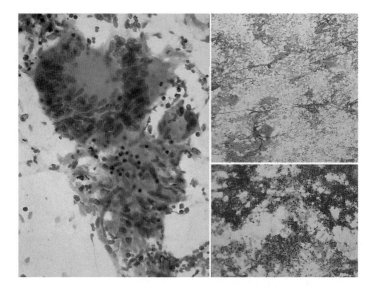

Fig. 13.2. Tuberculous lymphadenitis due to *Mycobacterium tuberculosis* infection. (*Left*) Lymph node FNA showing classic granulomatous inflammation morphology with a Langhans type giant cell and adjacent epithelioid histiocytes (Pap stain, high magnification). (*Top right*) Mycobacterial infection consisting predominantly of necrosis (Pap stain, low magnification). (*Bottom right*) Mycobacterial infection presenting as an abscess with numerous neutrophils in a necrotic background (Pap stain, intermediate magnification).

- Patients may also manifest with gingival disease (linear gingival erythema, necrotizing ulcerative gingivitis), periodontitis, and aphthous ulcers.
- Neoplasms likely to be encountered in this setting include HPV-related squamous cell carcinoma, Kaposi sarcoma, and lymphoma.

Salivary Gland Lesions

- Many HIV-infected patients may present with enlargement of their salivary glands, typically of the parotid, due to benign lymphoepithelial cysts (BLECs), intraparotid lymphadenopathy,

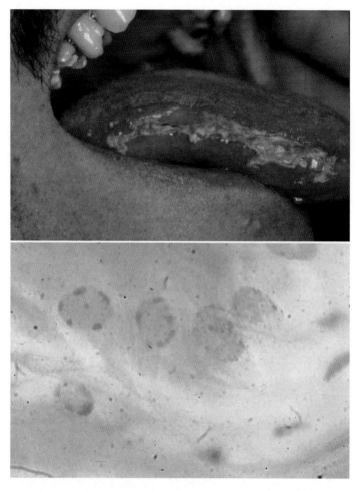

FIG. 13.3. Oral hairy leukoplakia. (*Top*) Patient with *white patches* shown on the side of the tongue. (*Bottom*) Oral smear showing EBV infected epithelial cells with prominent nuclear beading (Pap stain, high magnification) (photographs courtesy of Dr. Shabnum Meer, Division of Oral Pathology, University of the Witwatersrand, South Africa).

or less often infection (e.g., *Cryptococcus*, CMV sialadenitis, mycobacteria) and neoplasia.

- *BLEC* is bilateral in up to 20%. FNA yields straw-colored or turbid fluid with or without a residual mass after aspiration. Cyst aspiration is both diagnostic and therapeutic. On FNA, there is a triad of (1) polymorphous reactive lymphoid cells, (2) cyst contents with foamy histiocytes and proteinaceous background, and (3) occasional epithelial cells (squamous, metaplastic, or glandular including ciliated and mucinous types). The differential diagnosis includes branchial cleft cyst, Sjögren syndrome, Warthin tumor, and non-Hodgkin lymphoma.

- *Diffuse infiltrative lymphocytosis* (DILS) presents in HIV-infected patients with a Sjögren-like syndrome of dry eyes and mouth and salivary gland enlargement. The salivary glands and several other body sites (e.g., lacrimal glands, kidney, lung, gastrointestinal tract, and breast) are infiltrated by CD8+ T-lymphocytes. There is an increased risk of lymphoma and some authors recommend follow up by FNA.

Lymphoproliferative Disorders

Posttransplant Lymphoproliferative Disorder (PTLD)

- PTLD is a well-recognized complication of transplantation. Most cases are observed in the first year after transplantation. The greater the immunosuppression, the higher the incidence of PTLD and the earlier it occurs.

- In most cases, PTLD is associated with EBV infection of B-cells. Therefore, evaluation of tumor for the presence of EBV is very important, and can be accomplished by demonstrating the presence of EBV-encoded RNA (EBER) using in situ hybridization in tumor cells.

- EBV is uncommon with PTLD that presents in adults, late after transplantation, tumors that are monomorphic, and more resistant to treatment. PTLD of T-cell and NK-cell phenotypes is also usually not associated with EBV infection, and does not respond to immunosuppression dose reduction. Hence, it carries an unfavorable prognosis.

- The World Health Organization (WHO) classification for the pathological diagnosis of PTLD includes four categories: (1) early lesions (plasmacytic hyperplasia, infectious mononucleosis-like lesion), (2) polymorphic PTLD, (3) monomorphic PTLD (classified according to the B-cell or T-cell lymphoma that it resembles), and (4) classical Hodgkin lymphoma-type PTLD.

AIDS-Related Lymphomas (ARL)

- Lymphomas are an AIDS defining condition, except for low grade B-cell lymphomas and Hodgkin lymphoma. AIDS-related lymphomas (ARL) are divided by the WHO into three categories:
  - Lymphomas also occurring in immunocompetent patients: Burkitt lymphoma, diffuse large B-cell lymphoma, extranodal marginal zone B-cell lymphoma of mucosa-associated lymphoid tissue type, peripheral T-cell lymphoma, and Hodgkin lymphoma.
  - Lymphomas occurring more specifically in HIV-infected patients: Primary effusion lymphoma (PEL) and plasmablastic lymphoma.
  - Lymphomas also occurring in other immunodeficiency states: Polymorphic or PTLD-like B-cell lymphoma.

Plasmablastic Lymphoma

- This is an aggressive lymphoma that is EBV-associated (EBER-positive, LMP-negative).
- Tumors commonly present in the oral cavity, but have been described in many other sites. Two subtypes have been described: (1) oral mucosa type and (2) plasmablastic lymphoma with plasmacytic differentiation.
- Lymphoma cells (plasmablasts) are large, round to oval with abundant cytoplasm, a paranuclear hof, eccentrically situated nuclei, and single or multiple nucleoli. They often mimic other poorly differentiated neoplasms including carcinoma. There may be associated background apoptosis and tingible body macrophages.

- Tumor cells are positive for plasma cell markers (CD138, CD38, MUM1), CD79a, CD30, and EMA. They may be negative or weakly positive for CD45 (LCA), CD20, and PAX5.

Human Herpesvirus-8 (HHV8)-Associated Lymphomas

- These lymphomas include classic (body cavity based) PEL and the solid (extracavitary) variant of PEL. Classic PEL presents with effusions (pleural, peritoneal, pericardial, and rarely CSF or joint space) and no mass or nodal disease. Solid PEL may manifest with an effusion in addition to nodal or solid tissue lymphoma.
- The cytology of either PEL subtype is characterized by large atypical lymphoid cells ranging in appearance from immunoblastic to anaplastic phenotype (Fig. 13.4).
- In most cases, PEL cells lack B-cell and T-cell markers, but coexpress CD30, EMA, plasma cell antigens (CD38, CD138, MUM-1) and HHV8.
- PEL is associated not only with HHV8, but also sometimes with EBV infection. HHV8 immunoreactivity can be very helpful in diagnosing HIV-associated lymphomatous effusion (Fig. 13.5).

Hodgkin Lymphoma

- Hodgkin lymphoma is currently among the most common non-AIDS defining cancer (NADC) encountered, particularly the mixed cellularity and lymphocyte-depleted subtypes.
- Approximately 75–100% of these AIDS-associated cases have EBV coinfection.
- In HIV patients, Hodgkin lymphoma may be widely disseminated with frequent extranodal disease, but rare mediastinal involvement.

Central Nervous System Disease

- *Meningitis.* The etiology of meningitis in HIV-infected patients is multifactorial and includes infection, inflammatory conditions (e.g., IRIS), CNS lymphoma, and HIV itself.

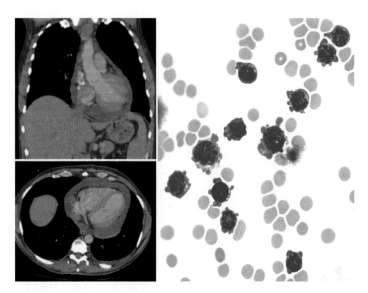

FIG. 13.4. Primary effusion lymphoma. (*Left*) CT scan images show a large pericardial effusion in a 44-year-old HIV+ man who presented with fever and cardiac tamponade. Over 1 L of fluid was drained. (*Right*) The pericardial fluid shows large anaplastic lymphoma cells (Wright-Giemsa stain, high magnification) that were immunoreactive with the LNA-1 antibody for HHV8. (Images reproduced with permission from Braza JM, Sullivan RJ, Bhargava P, Pantanowitz L, Dezube BJ. Images in HIV/AIDS. Pericardial primary effusion lymphoma. AIDS Read. 2007;17(5):250–2. Courtesy of UBM Medica).

- ○ Cryptococcal meningitis is the most common opportunistic infection causing meningitis in HIV-infected individuals. Other invasive fungal infections (*Aspergillus, Candida*) are also important pathogens, especially in HIV-negative persons with an immune deficiency.
- ○ Mycobacterial infection, coccidiomycosis, histoplasmosis, candidiasis, and syphilis produce meningitis more frequently in HIV-positive persons compared to HIV-negative patients.
- ○ Viral infections like CMV can cause meningoencephalitis.
- ○ Bacteria such as meningococci and pneumococcal meningitis carry a high risk of mortality in HIV-infected people.

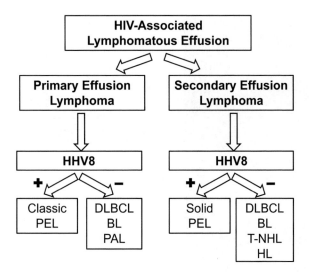

Fig. 13.5. Algorithmic approach to HIV-associated lymphomatous effusions. *BL* Burkitt lymphoma; *DLBCL* diffuse large B-cell lymphoma;
HHV8 human herpesvirus-8; *HL* Hodgkin lymphoma; *NHL* non-Hodgkin
lymphoma; *PAL* pyothorax-associated lymphoma; *PEL* primary effusion
lymphoma (reproduced with permission from Pantanowitz L, Dezube BJ.
HIV-related lymphomas. Int Pleural Newslett. 2009;7:18–9).

- *Mass lesions.* Space occupying lesions in the HIV positive patient
  may be due to infections such as toxoplasmosis, mycobacteria,
  and cryptococcus, as well as neoplasms such as primary CNS
  lymphoma (PCNSL) and metastases.
  - Toxoplasmosis is characterized radiologically by multiple
    enhancing brain lesions. The diagnosis is often misdiag-
    nosed in intraoperative cytology specimens because the par-
    asites are easily overlooked. They are typically seen within
    pseudocysts (bradyzoites). This should be kept in mind when
    there are nonspecific changes with an atypical lymphocytic
    infiltrate.
  - PCNSL is associated with EBV. The cytomorphology of this
    B-cell lymphoma is that of a diffuse large B-cell lymphoma.

- *Progressive multifocal leukoencephalopathy* (*PML*). This is a subacute demyelinating disorder due to JC virus, a polyomavirus that targets oligodendrocytes. JC virus reactivates in conditions of immune suppression.
  - Neuroimaging findings together with CSF analysis for JC viral antigen using PCR are usually diagnostic.
  - Routine cytologic CSF analysis is typically normal. FNA samples and brain smears may reveal foci of white matter demyelination, eosinophilic inclusions in oligodendrocytes, and abnormal giant astrocytes.
  - In equivocal cases, stereotactic brain biopsy provides a definitive diagnosis (Figs. 13.6 and 13.7).

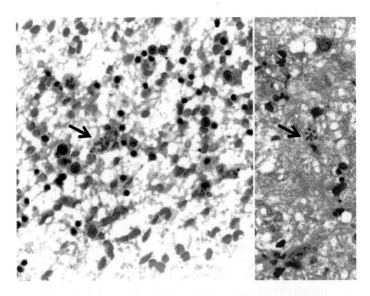

FIG. 13.6.   AIDS-associated brain toxoplasmosis. (*Left*) An intraoperative smear shows a "bag of parasites" (*arrow*) among scattered chronic inflammatory cells (H&E stain, high magnification) that (*right*) can also be seen in the brain surgical biopsy specimen (H&E stain, high magnification). Toxoplasma infection was confirmed using immunohistochemistry.

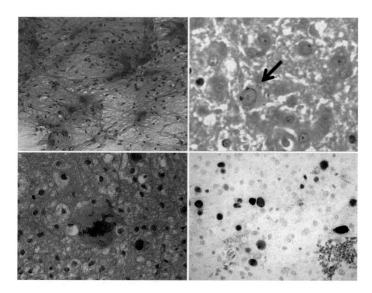

FIG. 13.7. Progressive multifocal leukoencephalopathy (PML). (*Top left*) Brain smear showing reactive gliosis and foam cells (H&E stain, intermediate magnification). (*Top right*) Oligodendrocyte (*arrow*) with a ground glass intranuclear inclusion (H&E stain, high magnification). (*Bottom left*) Enlarged astrocyte with a bizarre nucleus is shown among several background foamy macrophages (H&E stain, high magnification). (*Bottom right*) Infected cells show strong positive staining with a JC virus immunostain (high magnification) (image courtesy of Dr. Clayton A. Wiley, Neuropathology, University of Pittsburgh Medical Center, USA).

Pulmonary Disease

- *Infection.* Specific microorganisms likely to be encountered include conventional causes of bacterial pneumonia, mycobacterial infection, *P. jirovecii*, *Cryptococcus neoformans*, and various viral infections (e.g., CMV, HSV).
  - ○ A potential pulmonary pathogen may be identified in approximately 25% of HIV+ individuals with negative BAL cytology using other diagnostic modalities (e.g., culture, biopsy).
  - ○ Uncommon infections have been reported in AIDS patients such as microsporidiosis and malakoplakia associated with *Rhodococcus equi*.

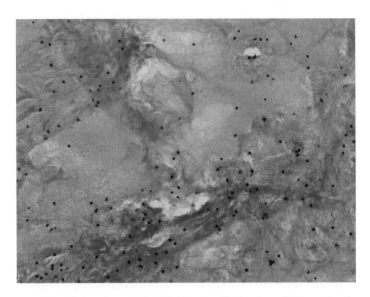

FIG. 13.8. Tuberculous (TB) effusion. An effusion in an HIV+ patient is shown with mature lymphocytes, serous material, and a dearth of mesothelial cells. Culture of the fluid revealed *Mycobacterium tuberculosis* (Pap stain, low magnification).

- *Neoplasia.* Lung tumors that may be seen in HIV+ patients include Kaposi sarcoma, lymphoma, and carcinoma.
  - Lung carcinoma in HIV+ patients is predominantly adenocarcinoma, which tends to present at a younger age and with more advanced stage than in HIV-negative people.
- *Effusions.* Pleural effusion in HIV-infected patients is common, with a prevalence of 14–27%.
  - The etiology may include infections (parapneumonic effusions, mycobacteria, empyema, CMV, *P. jirovecii*), neoplasia (mainly Kaposi sarcoma and lymphoma), and miscellaneous conditions (e.g., fluid overload, hypoalbuminemia, nephropathy, chronic liver disease, and pulmonary embolism).
  - Macroscopically, a mycobacterial effusion yields shiny green fluid that contains very few mesothelial cells (Fig. 13.8) and typically increased numbers of lymphocytes (often >50% lymphocytes). In HIV+ patients an AFB smear may be positive

in ~20% of cases, with pleural fluid culture positive in many more (40%) specimens. Pleural fluid adenosine deaminase (ADA) levels are often elevated.

○ Mesothelial cells in recurrent pleural effusions from patients with AIDS-associated Kaposi sarcoma and Castleman disease may be infected with HHV8.

Renal Disease

- BK polyomavirus infection in immunocompromised individuals can cause renal dysfunction and abnormal urine cytology (covered in Chap. 8).
- In some (1–10%) renal transplant recipients, BK virus may infect and replicate within the renal graft (called BK nephropathy). As a result, up to 80% of these patients may lose their renal grafts. Nephritis can arise soon (within days) after transplantation to as late as 5 years.
- In bone marrow transplant patients, BK virus is a frequent cause of hemorrhagic cystitis.

Spindle Cell Lesions

Specific spindle cell lesions that should be considered in the setting of immunosuppression include the following:

- *Mycobacterial spindle pseudotumor.* These lesions contain spindle-shaped macrophages (CD68+) that harbor numerous mycobacteria (AFB positive). They predominantly involve lymph nodes, but may affect the skin and bone marrow. They are most often associated with atypical mycobacteria like *Mycobacterium avium intracellulare* (MAI).
- *Kaposi sarcoma.* Aspirates procured from these lesions contain clusters and bland spindle cells (CD34+, CD31+, D2-40+) present in a bloody background. Nuclear immunostaining with LNA-1 for HHV8 (KSHV) is diagnostically helpful in these cases.
- *EBV-associated mesenchymal tumors.* Leiomyoma, leiomyosarcoma, and myopericytoma present with spindle cells that

are positive with smooth muscle markers and EBER by in situ hybridization. In HIV+ patients, these tumors usually occur in unusual sites and may be multifocal.

- *Follicular dendritic cell sarcoma.* These neoplasms can present in nodal and extranodal sites. An association with EBV has been shown in some cases. Neoplastic spindle to ovoid cells show morphologic and phenotypic features of follicular dendritic cells (positive for CD21, CD35, CD23, clusterin, and fascin) (Figs. 13.9 and 13.10).

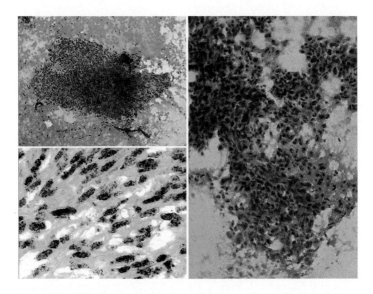

Fig. 13.9. HIV-associated spindle cell lesions. (*Top left*) FNA from a neck lymph node showing LNA-1 negative spindle cells arranged in a large cluster. Culture revealed *Mycobacterium tuberculosis* confirming the diagnosis of Mycobacterial spindle cell pseudotumor (Pap stain, intermediate magnification). (*Bottom left*) Kaposi sarcoma spindle cell nuclei stain positively with LNA-1 confirming HHV8 infection (immunostain, high magnification). (*Right*) Lung FNA from an HIV+ male showing loose aggregates of spindle cells with eosinophilic cytoplasm and nuclear atypia in a necrotic background. Ancillary investigations confirmed the presence of a leimyosarcoma (Pap stain, intermediate magnification).

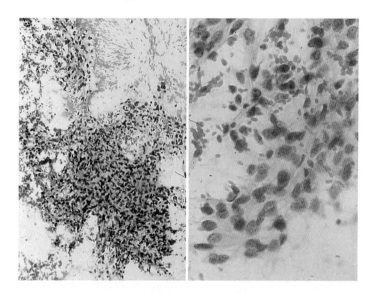

FIG. 13.10. Follicular dendritic cell sarcoma showing fascicles and sheets of atypical spindle cells with moderate amounts of cytoplasm, finely granular chromatin, and small nucleoli (Pap stain, *left* intermediate magnification, *right* high magnification).

Suggested Reading

Ellison E, Lapuerta P, Martin S. Fine needle aspiration (FNA) in HIV+ patients: results from a series of 655 aspirates. Cytopathology. 1998;9:222–9.

Gattuso P, Castelli MJ, Peng Y, Reddy VB. Posttransplant lymphoproliferative disorders: a fine-needle aspiration biopsy study. Diagn Cytopathol. 1997;16:392–5.

Hanks D, Bhargava V. Fine-needle aspiration diagnosis of HIV-related conditions. Pathology. 1996;4:221–52.

Kocjan G, Miller R. The cytology of HIV-induced immunosuppression. Changing pattern of disease in the era of highly active antiretroviral therapy. Cytopathology. 2001;12:281–96.

Lobenthal SW, Hajdu SI. The cytopathology of bone marrow transplantation. Acta Cytol. 1990;34:559–66.

Michelow P, Meyers T, Dubb M, Wright C. The utility of fine needle aspiration in HIV positive children. Cytopathology. 2008;19:86–93.

Naresh K. Lymphoproliferative disorders in the immunosuppressed. Diagn Histopathol. 2009;16:206–15.

Pantanowitz L, Dezube BJ. Evolving spectrum and incidence of non-AIDS-defining malignancies. Curr Opin HIV AIDS. 2009;4:27–34.

Pantanowitz L, Kuperman M, Goulart RA. Clinical history of HIV infection may be misleading in cytopathology. Cytojournal. 2010;7:7.

Pantanowitz L, Michelow P. Review of human immunodeficiency virus (HIV) and squamous lesions of the uterine cervix. Diagn Cytopathol. 2011;39:65–72.

Siddiqui MT, Reddy VB, Castelli MJ, Gattuso P. Role of fine-needle aspiration in clinical management of transplant patients. Diagn Cytopathol. 1997;17:429–35.

14
Ancillary Investigations

**Pam Michelow[1], Tanvier Omar[2],
and Liron Pantanowitz[3]**

[1]Cytology Unit, Department of Anatomical Pathology,
University of the Witwatersrand and National Health Laboratory Service,
Johannesburg, Gauteng, South Africa

[2]Division of Cytopathology, Department of Anatomical Pathology, School of
Pathology, National Health Laboratory Service, and University of
Witwatersrand, Johannesburg, Gauteng, South Africa

[3]Department of Pathology, University of Pittsburgh Medical Center,
5150 Centre Avenue, Suite 201, Pittsburgh, PA 15232, USA

Cytomorphology alone using routine stains such as the Papanicolaou
(Pap), Diff-Quik (DQ), and hematoxylin and eosin (H&E) stains
may be adequate to diagnose several infections in cytology material. However, the use of ancillary investigations improves cytologic diagnostic accuracy, may help subtype microorganisms, and
determine their antimicrobial sensitivity. Identification of infectious organisms by the laboratory relies primarily on microscopy,
special stains (histochemistry and immunocytochemistry), and
culture. With the well-established success of cell block technique,
many cytology samples can now be effectively stained using immunocytochemistry. A fresh specimen may not always be available
to submit for microbiology culture. In addition, culture may have
limited utility in some clinical cases due to the prolonged incubation required for the growth of fastidious pathogens and the inability to culture others. While microscopy and culture techniques
remain very useful, newer detection methods are being introduced
into routine clinical practice such as in situ hybridization (ISH),
flow cytometry, and molecular tests. One of the best examples in
cytopathology of new technologies being rapidly incorporated

L. Pantanowitz et al., *Cytopathology of Infectious Diseases*,
Essentials in Cytopathology 17, DOI 10.1007/978-1-4614-0242-8_14,
© Springer Science+Business Media, LLC 2011

into laboratory diagnostic tests is for the detection of human papillomaviruses (HPV). HPV testing technologies can be divided into four main types of methods: (1) direct probe methods (Southern, dot blot, and ISH), (2) signal amplification system (hybrid capture), (3) target amplification system (polymerase chain reaction [PCR], nuclei acid sequence-based amplification), and (4) emerging technologies (microarrays).

Routine Cytology Stains

Papanicolaou (Pap) Stain

- The Pap stain is the most widely used routine cytologic stain applied to alcohol-fixed material. Hematoxylin is used as a nuclear stain and Orange G-6 (OG-6) and eosin-azure (EA) as cytoplasmic counterstains. This stain is not entirely standardized and slight differences exist in dye composition and stain technique.
- The Pap stain provides good nuclear and cytoplasmic details of many organisms, in addition to the host's cellular changes like inflammation, repair, and neoplasia that may be induced by the infective process. Most viral changes including nuclear and cytoplasmic inclusions are best seen in Pap-stained smears.

Romanowsky Stains

- Romanowsky stains are applied to air-dried smears and blood smears. Several different types of Romanowsky stains exist (e.g., DQ, May-Grunwald and Giemsa [MGG]), but all are based on a combination of reduced eosin, methylene blue, and thiazine dyes.
- Romanowsky stains are used, for the most part, to stain cytoplasm, and extracellular substances. Bacteria, fungi, and parasites are often easier to detect on Romanowsky, as compared to Pap, stained smears. They also allow one to identify the negative image (unstained element) of certain microorganisms (e.g., mycobacteria) if present.

Hematoxylin and Eosin (H&E) Stain

- The H&E stain consists of hematoxylin and eosin. Most cytology laboratories reserve H&E for staining cell blocks. H&E stains are also occasionally used for intraoperative cytology preparations (e.g., touch or squash preparations).
- Like the Pap stain, the H&E stain provides good nuclear and cytoplasmic details of many organisms, in addition to the host's cellular changes stimulated by infection. OG-6 is not present in the H&E stain, limiting the detection of keratin in squamous cells.

Toluidine Blue

- Toluidine blue is a rapid stain for use on fresh specimens to assess specimen adequacy.
- Some organisms (e.g., *Pneumocystis jirovecii*) can be readily identified with Toluidine blue staining, allowing the specimen to be placed in the appropriate microbiologic medium for best culture results.

Cell Blocks

- Cell blocks are created by placing cytology material into a fixative, of which several are available such as 10% buffered formalin. The liquid specimen is centrifuged to create a cell pellet, which is embedded for sectioning as for biopsy material.
- Both conventional exfoliative and aspiration cytology have limited material available for ancillary investigations. The use of cell block technique allows for many sections to be made and hence multiple special stains and immunostains can be performed for infectious diseases. Large structures floating in liquid-based specimen vials may only be identified in cell block material.

Special Stains

- Most staining methods available for formalin-fixed tissues can be successfully adapted for cytology smear and cell block material.
- With the exception of acid-fast and Gram stain where air-dried material is preferred, the stains described below are better

performed on alcohol-fixed material. If only air-dried material is available, prior rapid fixation for 10 s in 95% alcohol is advised to ensure that material does not wash off during staining.

- Routinely stained slides can be used for special stains if needed, but require decolorization in acid alcohol for 2–10 minutes prior to the specific staining process.

- Positive controls should be run with each test. While it is preferable to use cytology specimens as controls, this is often not possible due to the limited number of available cytology slides. Formalin-fixed tissue sections are more easily available and serve as useful substitutes.

Wet Mount Preparation

- A saline (0.85% NaCl) wet prep may be used to detect the microscopic presence of various microorganisms in liquid specimens. The prep is observed using brightfield microscopy. Material must usually be examined within 30 min once obtained. It can be used on vaginal secretions to diagnose motile *Trichomonas vaginalis* trophozoites, clue cells, and yeast.

- A wet prep with 20% potassium hydroxide (KOH) lyses epithelial cells allowing for easier visualization of certain microorganisms (e.g., Candida). Placing a drop of KOH on a slide of the wet prep may cause a foul, fishy odor if there is anaerobic overgrowth or infection (known as the "whiff" test).

Bacterial Stains

Gram Stain

- The Gram stain differentially stains Gram positive and Gram negative bacteria. It is well suited for use with air-dried smears.

- The differential staining results from differences in the chemical (peptidoglycan) composition and thickness of the cell walls of Gram positive and Gram negative organisms.

- There are four basic steps of the Gram stain: (step 1) apply a primary stain (crystal violet or methylene violet); (step 2) add a trapping agent (Lugol's iodine); (step 3) rapid decolorization

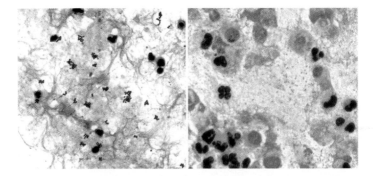

Fig. 14.1.   Gram stained bacteria (Gram stains, high magnification). (*Left*) Clusters of Gram positive *Staphylococcus aureus* cocci are shown in this specimen from an infected skin wound. (*Right*) Numerous Gram negative *Haemophilus* rods and coccobacilli are present in the background among neutrophils and bronchial cells in this bronchoalveolar lavage specimen.

with alcohol or acetone; and (step 4) counterstain with safranin (or neutral red).

- Gram negative bacteria stain red and Gram positive bacteria appear blue-black. The age of bacteria, antibiotic treatment, fragility of the cell wall, over-decolorization, and decalcification may cause Gram positive bacteria to appear Gram negative.
- Other microorganism may also stain. For example, fungi like *Candida albicans* and cryptococcus as well as intracellular microsporidia stain gram positively.
- Modified Gram stains like the Brown and Hopp's or Gram-Twort stains are better suited for use with formalin-fixed tissue sections. These methods should be employed when staining of cell block material is required.
- Caution: Crystal violet is toxic when swallowed and in vapor form causes ocular irritation. Iodine is a corrosive and can cause cutaneous burns (Fig. 14.1).

Stains for Helicobacter pylori

- In cytology laboratories where gastric washing cytology is regularly assessed, special staining for *H. pylori* may be necessary. Several staining methods can be employed:

- *Cresyl violet acetate*: This rapid, simple stain employs no counterstain. *H. pylori* organisms stain purple. The background stains in lighter hues of the same color. This will also stain *Pneumocystis* cysts.
- *Gimenez*: This stain is good for slow-growing and fastidious bacteria. The stain uses carbol fuchsin to stain the organisms a magenta color. The counterstain with 1% malachite green achieves a blue-green background. This staining process requires steps and care should be taken not to overstain the background. Gimenez can also be used to highlight *Legionella bacilli*.
- *Toluidine blue*: This reliable metachromatic stain uses a phosphate buffer at pH 6.8 to stain *H. pylori* dark blue. The background stains a lighter shade. Toluidine blue also stains *Pneumocystis* cysts.
- *Silver stains*: Other stains sometimes used include silver stains such as Warthin–Starry, Genta, or Steiner methods.
- Specific immunocytochemistry can also aid in bacterial detection. It is highly specific and has a higher sensitivity than bacteriological culture and other classical histological staining methods.

Warthin-Starry Stain

- This is a fastidious stain used for identifying spirochetes, *Bartonella henselae* and *Bartonella quintana*, Donovan bodies, and *H. pylori*. It is also capable of demonstrating *Klebsiella* and *Leptospira* bacteria as well as microsporidia, although this is rarely indicated.
- The stain employs a silver heat impregnation technique. Once silver salts deposit onto the organisms, they are reduced with hydroquinone to produce a silver metal.
- Microbes appear somewhat magnified and stain black in a golden brown background.
- Stains with necrotic material or cells with intracellular debris that show nonspecific staining are difficult to interpret. The incubation step of this stain is critical to provide a well-stained slide. Over- or underdeveloped sections are frustratingly difficult to interpret. Nonspecific precipitation can be removed by rapid rinsing in 2.5% iron alum.

- Dieterle stain is another silver impregnation stain that can be used to identify similar organisms as for the Warthin-Starry stain, and may also stain *Mycobacterium tuberculosis*.

Acid-Fast Stains for Mycobacteria (AFB)

- These stains are preferentially performed on air-dried material to prevent alcohol disruption of bacterial cell walls.
- The lipid capsule of mycobacteria is hydrophobic, rendering them resistant to Gram staining. However, these bacteria can be stained using concentrated dyes, particularly when the staining process is combined with heat. Once stained, these microorganisms resist a dilute acid and/or ethanol-based decolorization procedure. Hence, once stained, the mycobacterial capsule is acid, and variably alcohol-fast. This chemical property forms the basis of the various acid-fast stains (Table 14.1).
- It is advisable to use a fairly pale methylene blue counterstain to enhance visualization of bacilli, especially since some mycobacteria are often sparse.
- Mycobacteria may also stain with other stains. For example, *Mycobacterium* spp. are also Grocott methanamine silver (GMS) positive and *Mycobacterium avium-intracellulare complex* (MAC) stains with periodic acid-Schiff (PAS).
- Modified AFB stains can also stain *Nocardia*, *Rhodococcus*, *Legionella micdadei*, the spines on *Schistosoma* spp. ova, *Echinococcus* hooklets, and *Cryptosporidium* spores (Figs. 14.2 and 14.3).

Fungal Stains

- Fungi are usually visualized as spores and/or hyphae. Specific host responses together with the size, septation, budding, and branching characteristics of these fungal elements assist in fungal speciation.
- Factors that may influence the appearance of fungal elements include the age of the fungal lesion, effects of antifungal therapy, type of infectious tissue, and host immune response.
- Fungi possess polysaccharide-rich cell walls. The oxidation of these carbohydrate components to dialdehydes forms the

TABLE 14.1. Acid-fast stains for mycobacteria.

Stain	Action	Result
Auramine-rhodamine	Constituent fluorochromes bind to cell wall	Bacilli fluoresce orange-yellow in a black background under ultra-violet light
Ziehl-Neelsen	Phenol facilitates staining of cell walls with carbol fuchsin, resisting decolorization by strong acid alcohol. Heat is required	Mycobacteria stain red to purple and are slightly curved, rod shaped bacilli, and occasionally beaded
Kinyoun	Modification of the Ziehl-Neelsen stain. Heat is not required and the concentrations of carbol fuschin and phenol are higher	
Modified Fite	Staining principle similar to Ziehl-Neeslen. Peanut oil can be added to enhance acid-fastness. Acid alcohol is replaced by sulfuric acid. Xylene is avoided to protect delicate walls of atypical mycobacteria	Preferable for atypical mycobacteria, *M. leprae*, and *Nocardia*. Organisms stain red
Triff	Combination of carbol fuschin, Mayer's hematoxylin to stain nuclei, eosin yellow to stain cytoplasm, and alcohol saffron as a counterstain	Utilized for *M. leprae* which stains red

basis of PAS and GMS stains (Table 14.2). GMS is preferred for screening, because it gives better contrast and stains even degenerated and nonviable fungi. Overstaining with GMS prevents the internal structure (e.g., hyphal septae) to be visualized. Mucormycosis may be only weakly positive for GMS. *Histoplasma capsulatum* organisms are not adequately demonstrated by the PAS reaction.

- The cell wall or capsule of several fungi will stain with mucicarmine, including *Cryptococcus*, *Blastomyces*, and *Rhinosporidium*. In some cases, poorly encapsulated or capsule-deficient cryptococci may not stain positively with mucicarmine stain. Alcian blue can also demonstrate the mucoid capsule of *Cryptococcus neoformans*.

Fig. 14.2. A Ziehl-Neelsen stain demonstrating acid-fast bacilli (AFB) that on culture proved to be *Mycobacteria tuberculosis* (high magnification).

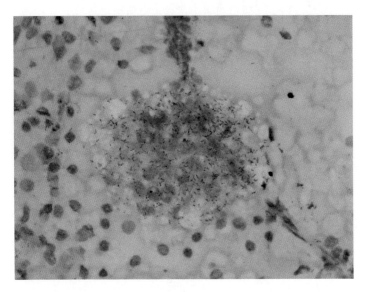

Fig. 14.3. Modified Fite stain demonstrating *Mycobacteria leprae* (high magnification) (image courtesy of Dr. Pawel Schubert, University of Stellenbosch, Cape Town, South Africa).

TABLE 14.2. Characteristics of routinely used fungal stains.

Stain	Action	Fungi	Comment
McManus periodic acid-Schiff (PAS)	Schiff's reagent stains glycogen and fungal cell walls oxidized by periodic acid magenta. Mayer's hematoxylin is used to stain nuclei. Light green may be used as a counterstain	Useful for a variety of fungi including *Candida, Cryptococcus, Histoplasma, Aspergillus, Mucormycosis,* and *Blastomycosis.* Also highlights rabies viral inclusions and mycobacteria when present in large numbers	Basic fuschin is carcinogenic and direct contact or inhalation is best avoided
Grocott methanamine silver (GMS)	Polysaccharide cell walls are oxidized in chromic acid to expose aldehydes prior to silver impregnation. Light green or H&E can be used as a counterstain	Highlights fungal cell walls and *Pneumocystis jirovecii* cysts. Some bacteria, actinomycetes and *Nocardia* stain brown-black. Useful in staining carbohydrate centers of dead mycobacteria where cell wall integrity is compromised. Also stains *E. histolytica,* encysted amoebas, CMV intracytoplasmic inclusions, echinococcal cyst wall and algae	Over-incubation and uneven temperatures result in distortion of internal fungal morphology

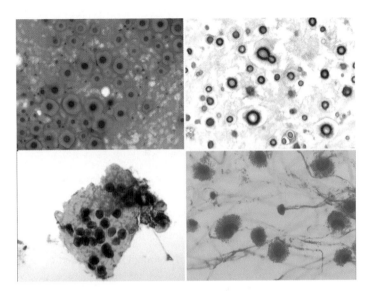

FIG. 14.4. Fungal stains (high magnification). (*Upper left*) PAS highlighting *Cryptococcus* in an FNA of a lymph node. (*Bottom left*) GMS demonstrates *Pneumocystis jirovecii* cysts in an alveolar cast from a bronchoalveolar lavage. (*Upper right*) Mucicarmine highlights several encapsulated *C. neoformans* yeast. Note the narrow-based budding of an organism in the upper center of the image. (*Bottom right*) Lactol-phenol cotton blue stain is used to illustrate *Aspergillus flavus* isolated from fungal culture.

- Fontana-Masson stain may demonstrate the cell wall of *C. neoformans* and also stains all dematiaceous (pigmented) fungi (e.g., *Phaeohyphomycosis*).
- Lactol-phenol cotton blue (LPCB) staining is used to examine fungal cultures in the mycology laboratory. It is also used to detect acid-fast parasites in stool and gastrointestinal aspirate specimens (Fig. 14.4).

Stains for Rickettsia

- Rickettsial infections are caused by small Gram negative obligate intracellular coccobacilli transmitted by ticks, fleas, lice, and mites. In humans, the organisms invade and multiply in vascular endothelium. Multi-organ involvement can occur. Diagnosis of an infection is usually made by complement fixation, immunofluorescence, or PCR of tissue or blood.

- While their visualization is rarely required in cytology, they can be seen with Romanowsky stains or by means of Macchiavello's stain.

Stains for Viruses

- Several viral infections often result in morphologically visible cytopathic effects that permit a diagnosis to be made in conventionally stained cytological preparations. Viral inclusions may be nuclear and/or intracellular. Table 14.3 lists several stains available for viral infections.
- The increasing availability of monoclonal antibodies and hybridization probes to detect viruses has made the use of special stains less popular (Fig. 14.5).

Stains for Parasites

- The diagnosis of protozoal infections has been simplified by the availability of new diagnostic modalities including serological agglutination tests, immunohistochemistry, immunofluorescence, and PCR. Moreover, in cytological material, protozoal morphology can usually be appreciated on routine staining.
- The preferred stain for blood parasites is a Giemsa stain.
- Tri-PAS is a useful stain to confirm the presence of amoeba in cytology smears. It extends the conventional PAS stain by adding a Mayer's hematoxylin counterstain and orange G to demonstrate erythrophagocytosis. Ameba are weakly hematoxyphilic and color pinkish orange. Engulfed red cells stain orange.
- Ova in schistosomiasis stain readily with H&E, Pap, GMS, and Ziehl-Neelsen stains. For echinococcosis (hydatid disease), the laminated membrane can be highlighted by PAS or GMS stains, and the refractile hooklets can be illustrated with a modified Fite stain.
- Fecal material for microbiology specimens is stained with Trichrome, iron hematoxylin, and/or modified acid-fast stains.

TABLE 14.3. Stains for viral infections.

Stain	Action	Positive result	Comment
Macchiavello	Basic fuchsin is differentiated with citric acid and counterstained with methylene blue	Viral inclusions (e.g., Negri bodies in rabies), rickettsia and chlamydia	Organisms stain red and tissue cells blue
Lendrum's phloxine-tartrazine	Trichrome stain that uses hematoxylin to stain nuclei blue, phloxine to stain viral inclusions bright red and tartrazine to serve as a differentiator	*Molluscum contagiosum* and measles	Russell bodies, keratin, Paneth cells are resistant to tartrazine differentiation and may be a source of false-positive interpretation
Shikata's Orcein	Potassium permanganate oxidizes sulfur containing proteins to form sulfonate residues which react with orcein. Rectified spirits are used to differentiate	Hepatitis B surface antigen is demonstrated in the cytoplasm of hepatocytes. Infected cells stain dark red or brown in a light brown background	Orcein should be freshly prepared each week
Feulgen	Acid hydrolysis with hydrochloric acid breaks down DNA bonds in nuclear material. The exposed nucleic acid components are stained using the PAS stain	Cytomegalovirus inclusions stain magenta	This is an uncommonly used stain for the demonstration of DNA
Tzanck smear	Smear of blister fluid in herpes virus infection stained with a Pap or H&E stain	Highlights herpes cytopathic effect (HSV I and II, VZV) and nonherpetic findings	Sensitivity is lower if the herpetic lesion has crusted

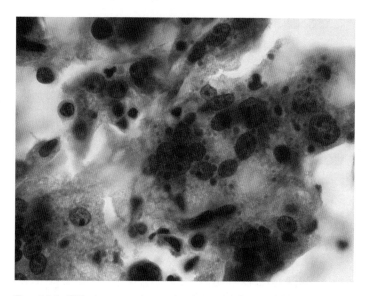

Fig. 14.5. Phloxine-tartrazine stain demonstrating multinucleated cells with viral nuclear and cytoplasmic inclusions staining red consistent with measles infection in this lung FNA (high magnification) (image courtesy of Dr. Pawel Schubert, University of Stellenbosch, Cape Town, South Africa).

Immunocytochemistry

- Immunocytochemistry uses antibodies to detect the presence of proteins or antigens in cells and tissues. The material to be tested can be smears, imprints, cytospin cell suspensions on glass slides, or cell blocks. Cell blocks are preferred for immunocytochemistry as they allow for optimal antigen retrieval. However, alcohol-fixed and air-dried material can be successfully used with some modifications.
- Where smears, imprints, and cytospins are being prepared specifically for immunocytochemistry, they should preferably be air-dried prior to fixation in acetone using charged/adhesive slides. Acetone is less destructive of tissue epitopes than alcohol, and will allow for superior antigen retrieval.
- All alcohol-fixed material should be decolorized in acid-alcohol before being postfixed in 10% buffered formalin for 30 seconds

followed by incubation in 0.25–0.5% Triton X-100 in PBS for 10 minutes to permeabilize cell membranes. This step can be omitted following acetone or methanol fixation. This is followed by routine staining as per the manufacturer's instructions.

- Immunocytochemistry is useful where microorganism speciation is needed and there is no fresh tissue for culture available, or culture will take too long for a diagnosis. It is also useful in cases with atypical morphology or unusual presentation of an infectious disease.
- Immunochemistry for diagnosing infectious diseases is expanding as the number of commercial antibodies available for use increases. Immunostains allow for the confirmation of morphological observations, especially where the cytological features are not definitive. It is particularly useful for rapid diagnoses in cases where culture is not available or too time consuming. To date, antibodies to a range of bacterial, mycobacterial, viral, fungal, and parasitic organisms have been developed (Table 14.4). These immunostains are often more sensitive and specific than their special stain counterparts (Figs. 14.6–14.8).

In Situ Hybridization

- ISH utilizes a complementary and known DNA or RNA strand (probe) to localize a specific DNA or RNA sequence. Several different methods are used to identify the hybridized probe-target complex including fluorescent tags (FISH), chromagens (CISH), and nonisotopic labeling systems (NISH). PCR can then be used to amplify the DNA or RNA sequences obtained using ISH.
- Fresh or destained archival material can be utilized for FISH, although destained archival material yields less consistent results. Air-dried and fixed smears including liquid-based preparations and paraffin-embedded cell blocks are suitable for ISH.
- The advantage of ISH over immunocytochemistry is that the actual gene product is identified rather than protein uptake or receptor-bound proteins, reducing false-positive, and false-negative results that may occur with immunocytochemistry. ISH allows staining to be correlated with cellular morphology.

TABLE 14.4. Useful commercially available immunocytochemistry antibodies for microbe identification.

Microorganism	Localization	Comment
Actinomycetes	Bacteria	Antibodies for Actinomyces genus, A. israelii and A. naeslundii
Adenovirus	Nuclear	Pan-adenovirus marker; monoclonal antibody is reactive with all 41 serotypes of adenovirus
Aspergillus	Fungal elements	Genus specific only. Stains fungus cell wall, septa, and cytoplasm
Bartonella henselae	Bacteria	Polyclonal antibody that does not differentiate between B. henselae and B. quintana. There is also a monoclonal antibody specific for B. henselae
BK virus	Nuclear	Specific for BK virus. The antibody is directed against the large T cell antigen of SV40 virus
Candida albicans	Fungal elements	Does cross-react with other yeasts
Cryptococcus	Fungal elements	Stains different Cryptococcus neoformans and serotypes
Cytomegalovirus	Nuclear and cytoplasmic	No cross-reaction with other herpes viruses or adenovirus
EBV latent membrane protein	Membranous and cytoplasmic	Monoclonal antibodies to LMP-1 or LMP-2
Epstein Barr virus	Nuclear	Acetone fixed tissue only; replicating and latent infection (EBNA2)
Giardia intestinalis	Extracellular	Stains protozoa on luminal surface of epithelia
Helicobacter pylori	Bacteria	Also cytoplasmic staining
Hepatitis B core Ag	Nuclear and cytoplasmic	Targets core antigen in infected cells
Hepatitis B surface Ag	Cytoplasmic	Targets surface antigen in infected cells (HBsAg)
Hepatitis C virus	Cytoplasmic	Sensitivity variable
Herpes simplex virus 1 and 2	Nuclear and cytoplasmic	Some cross-reactivity may be observed. Polyclonal antibody does not distinguish between HSV-1 and HSV-2
Human Herpesvirus 8	Nuclear	Targets latent nuclear antigen-1 (LNA-1); also called latent associated nuclear antigen-1 (LANA)
Human immunodeficiency virus	Granular staining close to infected cell	Targets P24 protein. Not suited to tissues that have had prolonged fixation in formalin

Human papilloma virus (HPV)	Nuclear	Major capsid protein antibody expressed in HPV type 6, 11, 16, 18, 31, 33, 42, 51, 52, 56 and 58
Merkel cell polyomavirus	Nuclear	Majority (not all) Merkel cell tumors are positive
Mycobacterium bovis	Cell wall of organism	Raised against BCG
Mycobacterium tuberculosis	Cell wall of organism	Species specific. With anti-BCG polyclonal antibody has shown better sensitivity than AFB staining, except in cases where there are very few bacilli. A polyclonal antibody against the *M. tuberculosis*-secreted antigen MPT64 is also useful
Parvovirus B19	Nuclear and cytoplasmic	Recognizes an epitope common to VP1 and VP2 proteins of human Parvovirus B19
Pneumocystis jiroveci	Cyst wall	Specific to *P. jiroveci* (formerly *P. carinii*). Stained rings correspond to individual cyst walls
Prion protein	Cytoplasmic	Also called prion protein PrP antibody
Respiratory syncytial virus	Cytoplasm and cell membrane	There are multiple types and subtypes of RSV that may not be covered by all clones
Toxoplasma gondii	Parasites	Stains bradyzoites and tachyzoites. Targets *Toxoplasma gondii* p30 surface antigen
Varicella Zoster virus	Cytoplasmic	Specific for varicella zoster; does not cross-react
Zygomycoses	Fungal elements	Genus specific only

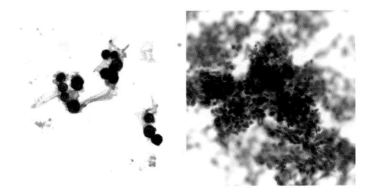

Fig. 14.6. Immunocytochemistry. (*Left*) A CSF specimen showing immunoreactive cryptococcal yeast (high magnification). (*Right*) Direct smear of a Merkel cell carcinoma showing positive staining of tumor cells with CM2B4, a monoclonal antibody to exon 2 peptides of the Merkel cell polyomavirus (MCPyV) T antigen (intermediate magnification).

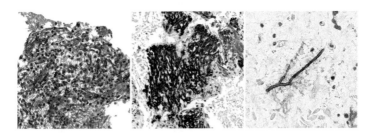

Fig. 14.7. Aspergillus immunocytochemistry. (*Left*) Multiple hyphae of *Aspergillus* spp. are present with inflammatory cells in this cell block from a bronchoalveolar lavage (PAS stain, intermediate magnification). (*Middle*) *Aspergillus* hyphae in this BAL case are immunoreactive in cell block material (intermediate magnification). (*Right*) Immunostains can help identify rare branching *Aspergillus* hyphae as depicted in this lung cytology specimen (high magnification). The commercially available monoclonal antibody for aspergillosis usually detect several *Aspergillus* spp. like *A. fumigatus*, *A. flavus*, and *A. niger*.

- ISH is useful for the detection of a wide range of organisms including viruses like human papillomavirus, cytomegalovirus, hepatitis viruses, herpes simplex viruses, and Epstein-Barr virus (EBV); bacteria such as *Helicobacter pylori*, legionella,

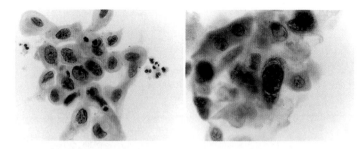

Fig. 14.8. Pap test immunocytochemistry. (*Left*) High grade squamous intraepithelial cells (HSIL) are shown on a ThinPrep Pap test (Pap stain, high magnification). (*Right*) These HSIL cells demonstrate p16 nuclear and cytoplasmic immunoreactivity, a surrogate marker indicative of HPV infection (high magnification). In dysplastic cells of the uterine cervix E7 protein of high-risk HPV inactivates retinoblastoma protein (pRB) which in turn leads to the overexpression of p16.

and tuberculosis; and fungi such as blastomyces, coccidioides, cryptococcus, histoplasmosis, sporothrix, and parasites including malaria, cryptosporidium, and amebae.

- For the detection of HPV, ISH allows for both the diagnosis of integrated HPV, and visualization of HPV within these infected cells. ISH is available for both low-risk and high-risk HPV types. Low-risk HPV-related lesions (e.g., papillomas) often contain low viral copy numbers, show only patchy staining, and may not be uniformly positive for HPV. High-risk HPV-positive lesions and tumors (e.g., HSIL) may show more diffuse positivity for HPV.
- EBV-encoded RNA (EBER1 and EBER2) is expressed in cells infected with EBV. ISH for EBER has been recommended as perhaps the best test for detecting and localizing latent EBV in tissue and cytology samples. False-positive EBER interpretations may occur as a result of confusion related to latent infection of background lymphocytes instead of lymphoma cells, nonspecific staining, or cross-reactivity with mucin, yeast, or plant materials. False-negative results may occur with RNA degradation.
- Before concluding that a slide for ISH to localize is negative, it is important to evaluate a control slide that was run in parallel, demonstrating that RNA or DNA is present and available for hybridization in the cells of interest (Fig. 14.9–14.11).

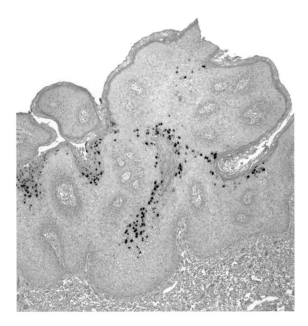

Fig. 14.9.   HPV-ISH of a cervix condyloma. Tissue biopsy of this condyloma shows patchy positive nuclear staining for low-risk HPV in surface koilocytes (low magnification).

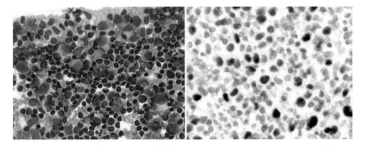

Fig. 14.10.   Infectious mononucleosis. (*Left*). FNA of a lymph node in an 8 year old boy with infectious mononucleosis shows several atypical lymphocytes (Diff-Quik stain, intermediate magnification). (*Right*) In situ hybridization (ISH) for EBER in this specimen shows nuclear positivity in several of the larger lymphocytes (intermediate magnification) (courtesy of Dr. Sara Monaco, Department of Pathology, University of Pittsburgh Medical Center, USA).

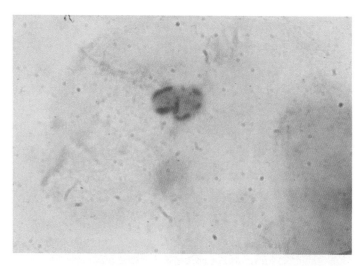

FIG. 14.11. ISH demonstrating Epstein-Barr virus in an oral smear from a patient with hairy leukoplakia (high magnification) (courtesy of Dr. Shabnum Meer, Division of Oral Pathology, University of the Witwatersrand, Johannesburg).

Fluorescent Stains

- Certain organisms when combined with fluorescent molecules will fluoresce when viewed with a fluorescent light microscope. This is based on the ability of some organisms to produce fluorescent light after absorption of ultraviolet light. Fluorescent molecules are called fluorophores or fluorochromes and include green fluorescent protein and fluorescein. Several fluorescent stains may be used simultaneously permitting information on multiple parameters to be collected concurrently.

- This technique is useful to rapidly identify various bacteria and fungi that cause identical clinical conditions. Both *P. jirovecii* and mycobacteria fluoresce when stained with a Papanicolaou stain and viewed under a fluorescent microscope autofluoresce. *P. jirovecii* cysts appear greenish yellow with irregular shapes while mycobacteria appear as brilliant green bacilli.

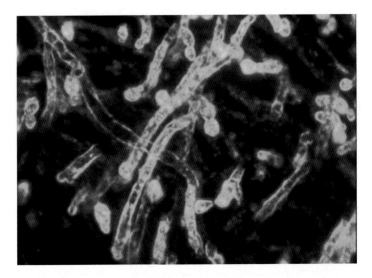

FIG. 14.12. Fluorescence of Candida from an oral smear (high magnification) (courtesy of Dr. Shabnum Meer, Division of Oral Pathology, University of the Witwatersrand, Johannesburg).

- Fluorescent stains available for clinical use include the acridine-orange stain, auramine-rhodamine stain, and Calcofluor stains. The acridine-orange stain is used to detect thin bacteria (e.g., *Helicobacter*) and fungi. The auramine-rhodamine stain is used to detect acid-fast and partially acid-fast bacteria. Calcofluor white stains yeast (e.g., *Pneumocystis*), fungi and some parasitic organisms (e.g., *Microsporidium*, *Acanthamoeba*, *Naegleria*, and *Balamuthia* spp.). Contaminants (e.g., cotton fibers) may fluoresce strongly and must therefore be separated from fungal hyphae.
- The direct fluorescence monoclonal antibody stain (DFA) for *Pneumocystis* appears to have higher diagnostic sensitivity than silver stains like GMS (Figs. 14.12 and 14.13).

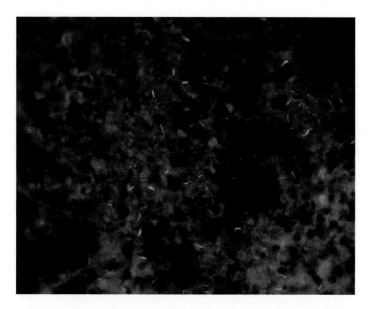

FIG. 14.13. Autofluorescence of *Mycobacterium tuberculosis* in a lymph node when viewed under a fluorescent microscope (Pap stain, high magnification) (courtesy of Prof. Colleen Wright, Stellenbosch University, Cape Town).

Flow Cytometry

- Particles in a liquid sample are passed individually in front of an intense light source. Light scatter and fluorescence of different wave lengths are measured. Multiple parameters can be measured simultaneously. A single cell suspension is required for flow cytometry, which makes cytologic specimens ideal.
- Flow cytometry has numerous applications including lymphoma and leukemia diagnosis, identifying and counting microbes (such as bacteria, viruses, fungi, parasites), and evaluating the host response to infection.
- Flow cytometry is useful in managing HIV-infected patients by measuring CD4 T-cell counts and CD4/CD8 ratios.

Serology

- In terms of infectious disease, serology involves the use of blood tests to detect the presence of antibodies against a microorganism. Some microorganisms (antigens) stimulate their human host to produce antibodies. There are several serology techniques that can be used depending on the antibodies being studied including enzyme-linked immunosorbent serologic assay (ELISA), agglutination, precipitation, complement fixation, and fluorescent antibodies.
- Serology provides an indirect marker for current or past infection. IgM is useful as a measure of acute phase infection. A fourfold or greater rise in antibody titer is indicative of acute infection. IgG indicates past infection and determines if protective antibodies are present.
- Serology is very useful in diagnosing atypical pneumonia, syphilis, brucellosis, and many viral infections such as hepatitis, HIV, and EBV if infectious mononucleosis is suspected.

Signal Amplification Assay

- The nucleic acid hybridization assay is used to detect and quantify RNA or DNA targets. The assay does not require preamplification of the nucleic acid to be detected. Enzymes are used to indicate the extent of hybridization, but unlike PCR are not used to manipulate the nucleic acids. This technology facilitates high throughput assays that can be used on a large number of samples (e.g., HPV testing).
- The Digene Hybrid Capture II (HC II) assay is a nucleic acid hybridization microplate assay. It is an FDA-approved test used to detect HPV DNA from both low- and high-risk HPV types. There are several steps involved in the HC II assay (Fig. 14.14).

Polymerase Chain Reaction (PCR)

- PCR is the amplification of a specific DNA or RNA sequence whereby thousands or several millions of copies of that sequence are generated. PCR is performed using cycles of repeated heating and cooling. At lower temperatures, double-stranded DNA

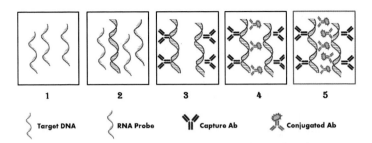

FIG. 14.14. Hybrid Capture II assay steps. (*1*) Target DNA is denatured. (*2*) RNA-probes hybridize with target DNA. (*3*) The RNA-DNA hybrids are captured onto the microplate well surface. (*4*) Amplification of hybrids with multiple antibodies conjugated to an enzyme (alkaline phosphatase). (*5*) The enzyme cleaves a chemiluminescent substrate, emitting light that gets measured.

separates into two single-stranded DNA pieces. At medium temperatures, short DNA fragments (primers) containing sequences complementary to the target region pair up (anneal) with the single-stranded DNA together with a DNA polymerase that starts to copy the template. The template is then coupled to the primer, producing a double-stranded DNA molecule. As the process is repeated, more and more copies are exponentially produced. The copies are referred to as amplicons. Very small quantities can be amplified and analyzed, making cytology an appropriate medium for PCR.

- In the past, traditional PCR was time consuming. Today, rapid cycle or real-time PCR methods are quicker and easier to perform. These are carried out in a closed system in which both amplification and detection occur, reducing the potential for contamination and false-positive results. Monoplex assays for the detection of a single organism and multiplex assays, whereby several organisms can be simultaneously detected are available.

- PCR is useful for the diagnosis of organisms that are slow growing, fastidious or cannot be easily cultured (e.g., *M. tuberculosis*, *Legionella pneumophila*, or *P. jirovecii*). PCR also permits quantification of these organisms.

- Problems related to PCR include false-positive (e.g., due to contamination) and false-negative (e.g., technical failure) results.

- Postamplification analysis consists of several different techniques to obtain additional information that cannot be acquired from the amplification technique alone and include melt curve analysis, reverse hybridization, DNA sequencing, and microarray technology.

- *Melt curve analysis*. This assesses variants in DNA sequences including mutations and single nucleotide polymorphisms. The melting profile or temperature-dependent separation between two DNA strands of a PCR product depends on its guanine-cytosine content, length, sequence, and heterozygosity. This can be measured with saturating dyes that fluoresce in the presence of double-stranded DNA. This technique has been used to genotype various organisms (e.g., hepatitis viruses, mycobacteria, salmonella species) and to investigate antimicrobial resistance.

- *Reverse hybridization*. This technique is able to detect a variety of pathogens. The amplicon (PCR product) is labeled and applied to a nitrocellulose membrane strip containing the relevant probes. The amplicon will then hybridize to the complementary species-specific probe, forming a banding pattern on the nitrocellulose strip. Multiple species can be detected in a single strip. This technique has been used to detect various subtypes of mycobacteria, HIV, hepatitis C, and fungi.

- *DNA sequencing*. This establishes the nucleic acid sequence of the amplicon through Sanger sequencing (enzymatic procedure to synthesize DNA chains of varying length to determine the order of nucleotide bases) or pyrosequencing (determining the sequence of nucleotide bases based on the incorporation of each nucleotide as the strand of DNA is being synthesized). Once the DNA sequence has been ascertained, it is compared to an existing database to find a match. This technique has proved very useful in identifying mycobacterial species, Nocardia, and other actinomycetes, in addition to detecting antimicrobial resistance.

- *Microarray technology*. This technique permits one to study the expression of thousands of genes simultaneously using hybridization of RNA or DNA that is placed in a specific order on a solid surface and analyzed with the aid of a computer. This can be used to rapidly identify pathogens, investigate antimicrobial resistance, and determine host response to infection (Fig. 14.15).

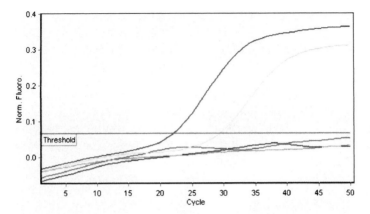

Fig. 14.15. Real-time PCR amplification curve for HHV-8 over 50 cycles. The colored lines indicate different patients. Patients indicated with *blue* and *yellow lines* are positive for HHV-8 DNA, while the samples from patients indicated by *red*, *purple* and *pink lines* do not have HHV-8 DNA (courtesy of Sharlene Naidoo, Department of Anatomical Pathology, University of the Witwatersrand, Johannesburg).

Electron Microscopy (EM)

- The role of electron microscopy (EM) has been greatly diminished in recent times with the development of new techniques described above. This holds true for the diagnosis of infectious diseases. However, the ultrastructural features of many pathogens have been well described and EM can certainly serve as a useful adjuvant diagnostic modality when others are unavailable or unsuccessful.

Culture and Sensitivity

- Samples can be sent for culture and antimicrobial susceptibility when an infectious process is suspected. Enriched media (e.g., blood agar, chocolate agar) are designed to support the growth of most microorganisms. Selective media (e.g., MacConkey agar) are designed to support the growth of only certain microorganisms and suppress the growth of others. Some organisms

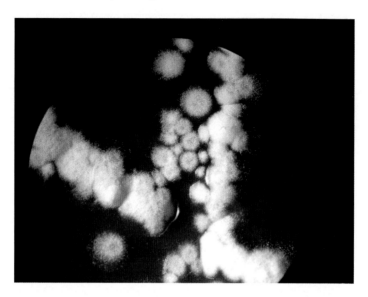

Fig. 14.16. Culture plate of *Nocardia* spp. This photograph was taken through a dissecting microscope and shows waxy and bumpy colonies on culture (courtesy of Dr. Warren Lowman, Department of Microbiology, University of the Witwatersrand, Johannesburg).

have very specific growth requirements (e.g., *Legionella*) and will require more specialized media. Others may grow slowly and thus may require an extended incubation (e.g., *Bartonella*). Therefore, it is important to clearly communicate with the microbiology laboratory the source of the specimen and suspected pathogens.

- Cytological findings at the time of specimen procurement (i.e., immediate evaluation) are able to help direct specific adjuvant investigations (e.g., bacterial, fungal, or mycobacterial culture). Material should be expelled into appropriate containers and/or culture media. Alternatively, it can be washed into a sterile container with saline to prevent desiccation of material. Aspiration of pus may be related to an infection and hence such material should be sent for culture. A dedicated pass often yields the best results, but if unfeasible, needle rinses in culture media after smears are made may be employed (Fig. 14.16).

Acknowledgements Thanks to Carina Aitken, Head of the Special Stains Section, Department of Anatomical Pathology, School of Pathology, University of Witwatersrand, Johannesburg, SA, for invaluable advice on special staining procedures and pitfalls.

Suggested Reading

Armbruster C, Pokieser L, Hassl A. Diagnosis of Pneumocystis carinii pneumonia by bronchoalveolar lavage in AIDS patients. Comparison of Diff-Quik, fungifluor stain, direct immunofluorescence test and polymerase chain reaction. Acta Cytol. 1995;39:1089–93.

Atkins KA, Powers CN. The cytopathology of infectious diseases. Adv Anat Pathol. 2002;9:52–64.

Bancroft J, Gamble M. Theory and practice of histological techniques. 6th ed. London: Churchill Livingstone; 2008.

Bravo L, Procop G. Recent advances in diagnostic microbiology. Semin Hematol. 2009;46:248–58.

Eyzaguirre E, Haque AK. Application of immunohistochemistry to infections. Arch Pathol Lab Med. 2008;132:424–31.

Hubbard RA. Human papillomavirus testing methods. Arch Pathol Lab Med. 2003;127:940–5.

Lott RL. Fungi. In: Brown RW, editor. Histologic preparations: common problems and their solutions. Chicago: CAP Press; 2009. p. 85–94.

Nuovo GJ. The surgical and cytopathology of viral infections: utility of immunohistochemistry, in situ hybridization, and in situ polymerase chain reaction amplification. Ann Diagn Pathol. 2006;10:117–31.

Oliveira A, French C. Application of fluorescence in situ hybridization in cytopathology. A review. Acta Cytol. 2005;49:587–94.

Woods GL, Walker DH. Detection of infection or infectious agents by use of cytologic and histologic stains. Clin Microbiol Rev. 1996;9:382–404.

15
Mimics and Contaminants

**Liron Pantanowitz[1], Robert A. Goulart[2],
and Rafael Martínez-Girón[3]**

[1]Department of Pathology, University of Pittsburgh Medical Center,
5150 Centre Avenue, Suite 201, Pittsburgh, PA 15232, USA

[2]New England Pathology Associates, Mercy Medical Center, Sisters
of Providence Health System/Catholic Health East, 299 Carew Street,
Springfield, MA 01104, USA

[3]CF Anatomía Patológica y Citología, Instituto de Piedras Blancas,
Piedras Blancas, Asturias 33450, Spain

Many potential artifacts and contaminants may be encountered
when examining cytology slides that could mimic true microorganisms or cytopathic changes secondary to infection and thereby
lead to an erroneous diagnosis. An artifact is an undesired alteration or artificial change in cytological material introduced by a
technique and/or technology, or unexpected material, e.g., talc.
Such modifications may occur at the time the sample is collected
or they may occur during or after laboratory processing of the
sample. The observation of bacteria in cytology specimens is a
common finding in certain specimen types, such as sputa, vaginal
smears, and voided urine. In most instances, they should not be
interpreted as a true infection, but rather as a contamination by the
saprophyte flora.

When artifacts and contaminants are encountered, their significance and ways to avoid them should be determined. Critical issues
to resolve include whether the finding is an isolated (or random)
event, or if it signifies a more widespread (or systematic) problem
with specimen collection and/or processing. Both artifacts and contaminants may lead to problems with interpretation, creating confusion with other structures of major relevance. The clinical context
of the patient (age, immune status, comorbid conditions, travel

L. Pantanowitz et al., *Cytopathology of Infectious Diseases*,   351
Essentials in Cytopathology 17, DOI 10.1007/978-1-4614-0242-8_15,
© Springer Science+Business Media, LLC 2011

history, and immigration) is extremely important in these cases. Intracellular organisms represent true infection, whereas generally the lack of an intimately associated inflammatory response, necrosis, or cellular reactive changes in an immunocompetent host favors a contaminant. Additional helpful indicators favoring the presence of contamination rather than true infection include (1) the presence of the structure on either the Pap or Romanowsky stain but not both, (2) the structure lies on a different focal plane than the inherent cellular material suggesting they were deposited there at a different time, and (3) the structure is at the edge of the glass slide.

In certain settings, these contaminants can be introduced by patients into cytology samples, such as oral food particulate material contaminating a respiratory specimen or fibers from a vaginal pessary or sanitary pad seen in a cervicovaginal Pap test. An interpretation of contamination should not be reported to avoid subjecting the patient to unnecessary therapy, undue follow-up, and perhaps further tests, whereas true infection should be diagnosed and requires careful study of the patient's immune status, prompt investigation, and appropriate therapy.

There are a host of endogenous and exogenous structures (Table 15.1) that may be mistaken for microorganisms (so-called pseudomicrobes). These structures continue to pose diagnostic problems for many cytologists due to a lack of familiarity or experience with them. This chapter covers several cytology artifacts and contaminants that are likely to be seen in practice.

Mimics of Viral Infection

- Koilocytes are squamous epithelial cells that exhibit structural changes following HPV infection. These cellular changes include nuclear enlargement and irregularity, hyperchromasia, and a perinuclear halo. When intracytoplasmic glycogen gets dissolved, leaving a large clear space around the nucleus, these cells in a Pap test may mimic koilocytes (Fig. 15.1). However, such koilocyte-like cells lack all other morphological features of dysplasia. Nonspecific perinuclear halos within superficial and intermediate squamous cells in Pap tests may be associated with

TABLE 15.1. Endogenous and exogenous structures that mimic micro-organisms.

Endogenous structure	Potential mimic
Blood	Pneumocystis cast, Cryptococcus yeast
Platelets	Extracellular parasites
Calcification	Parasite ova and fungi
Psammoma body	Parasite ova
Mucus	Worms
Ciliocytophthoria	Ciliated parasite and flagellated protozoa
Leisegang rings	Parasitic ova and fungal yeast
Myospherulosis	Endosporulating fungi
Tissue fiber (skeletal, elastic)	Worms
Exogenous structure	
Pollen	Parasite ova
Dirt	Bacteria
Vegetable matter	Viral change and worms
Synthetic fibers and thread	Worms
Dust and powder	Parasite ova
Lubricant	Pneumocystis cast

inflammatory conditions (e.g., *Trichomonas* infection), but can also be an artifact due to slide preparation. These halos differ from true koilocytes by their small size, indistinct edge, and the symmetry of the halo about the nucleus.

- Vegetable parenchymal cells may also resemble koilocytes. In Pap tests, certain gels and pessaries containing excipient vegetable material are thought to be the source of such contaminants. Additionally, a number of unusual contaminants may be detected in Pap tests due to women using environmental products, sometimes under the guidance of traditional healers. Laboratory personnel should be aware of the local practices of their communities and ethnic groups in order to be able to identify these contaminants.
- Cellular degeneration can be mistaken for viral changes including Herpesvirus and Adenovirus, as well as the commonly seen Polyomavirus effect in degenerated urothelial cells. Retroplasia, characterized by the retraction of nuclear material, is a degenerative phenomenon that may be interpreted as viral infection, especially CMV (Fig. 15.2) and Herpes virus infection.

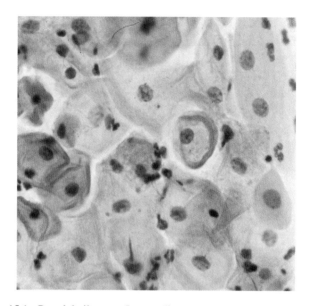

Fig. 15.1. Pseudokoilocytes. Intermediate squamous cells from this Pap test resemble koilocytes due to the loss of perinuclear intracytoplasmic glycogen. Note that their nuclei do not have dysplastic features character-istic of true koilocytes, but resemble those of nearby intermediate squa-mous cells (Pap stain, high magnification).

- Reactive-atypical endocervical cells may resemble the cytologic changes associated with Herpes Simplex Virus (HSV) infection (Fig. 15.3). This is a known potential pitfall in endocervical brush specimens. Despite the presence of multinucleation and nuclear molding in reactive endocervical cells, the chromatin pattern, presence of macronucleoli, and absence of intranuclear inclusions are important to establish the appropriate differential diagnosis.

Ancillary Studies

- Immunocytochemistry for specific viruses.

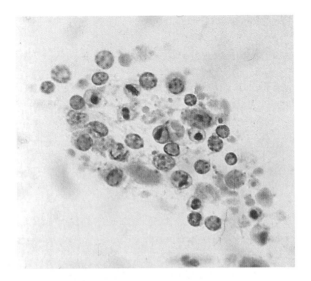

Fig. 15.2. Retroplasia. These bronchial epithelial cells on a sputum smear show degenerative changes. Note the chromatin condensation (retroplasia) mimicking intranuclear inclusions similar to CMV (Pap stain, high magnification).

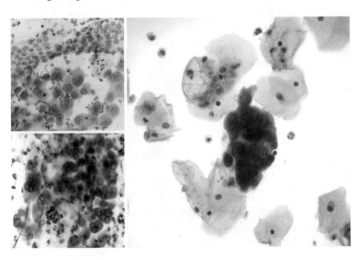

Fig. 15.3. Pseudo-herpes on a Pap test. Reactive endocervical cells, often with multinucleation, are shown mimicking herpetic infection on a conventional smear (*left*) and a ThinPrep (*right*) Pap test. Note the sheet of normal endocervical cells present in the top of the *upper left image* (Pap stains, *left* intermediate magnification, *right* high magnification).

Mimics of Bacterial Infection

- Normal bacterial flora is a common finding in vaginal specimens (lactobacilli), oropharyngeal contamination in sputa, and voided urine. These should not be interpreted as a true infection, but rather as a contamination by the saprophyte flora (Fig. 15.4).
- If a fluid is placed in an unsterile container, has a long time delay in reaching the laboratory, or is not refrigerated, overgrowth of contaminating bacteria may be marked.

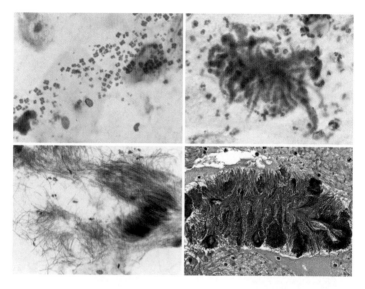

Fig. 15.4. Normal oral flora. (*Upper left*, high magnification) Sarcina forms on a sputum smear, illustrating their characteristic appearance in tetrads (buckets of eight elements). This type of bacteria is frequently observed as a commensal flora in the mouth (Pap stain). (*Bottom left*, high magnification) *Leptotrichia buccalis* present as a contaminant on a sputum smear (Pap stain). (*Upper right*, high magnification) Actinomyces-like organisms contained within a sputum smear. Their presence indicates oral contamination and not a true infection (Pap stain). (*Bottom right*, intermediate magnification) Oropharyngeal contamination composed of anucleate squames and filamentous bacteria present within the cell block of a bronchoalveolar lavage specimen (H&E stain).

- Bacteria may be introduced onto slides by bacterial growth contaminating stain solutions.
- Dirt, granular debris, precipitate material, pencil graphite, and silver nitrate crystal contamination in Pap tests may resemble clumps of bacteria. If these contaminants are not part of the specimen, they will be slightly out of the plane of focus with the routine cellular material.
- In vitreous fluid, small fusiform melanosomes released from degenerating choroid tissue may resemble bacteria. These rods may also be phagocytosed by macrophages.

Ancillary Studies

- Gram stain
- Bacterial culture

Mimics of Fungal Infection

- Various fungi (e.g., *Alternaria*, *Aspergillus*, *Cladosporium*, *Fusarium*, *Penicillium* spp., etc.) are ubiquitous in the environment (Table 15.2) and thus may easily be introduced into cytology samples or make their way onto glass slides (Figs. 15.5 and 15.6) from contamination of collection materials (e.g., spatulas), laboratory equipment (e.g., stain solutions and dishes), and cell blocks. One may find the entire conidiophore (fruiting body composed of specialized fungal hyphae that produce conidia) or other fungal elements such as a swollen vesicle, phialides (dilated portion of the conidiophore), and/or isolated conidia (spores). Any of these fungi, however, may become opportunistic pathogens in the immunosuppressed host. Numerous spores arranged in chains, sometimes characteristic of *Aspergillus* and *Penicillium*, can resemble coccoid bacteria or erythrocytes.
- In respiratory cytology samples, *Candida* spp. elements obtained from the mouth frequently represent a "contaminant" of the respiratory specimen. This is often the case in immunosuppressed patients, such as individuals with AIDS who have oral thrush.

TABLE 15.2. Comparison of different airborne fungal contaminants.

Fungus	Fungal elements
Alternaria	Club-shaped septate conidia
Aspergillus	Fruiting body and septate hyphae
Cladosporium	Dark conidia with branching chains
Fusarium	Sickle-shaped septate conidia
Penicillium	Fruiting structures and septate hyphae

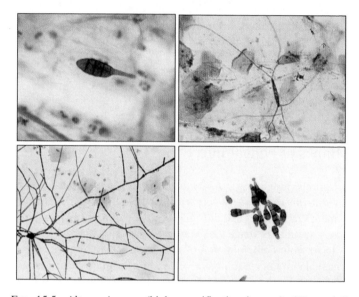

FIG. 15.5. *Alternaria* spp. (high magnification images). (*Upper left*) Sputum smear containing a "racket-shaped" macroconidia (Pap stain). (*Bottom left*) Alternaria tenuissima in a cervicovaginal smear. Several branching hyphae are originating from a macroconidia placed at the left of the image (Pap stain). (*Upper right*) Sputum smear showing macroconidia with four attached septated hyphae (Pap stain). (*Bottom right*) Brown club-shaped septate macroconidia seen in fungal culture (Lactol Phenol Cotton Blue stain).

- Erythrocytes, particularly degenerating and "ghost" red blood cells, may mimic yeast (Fig. 15.7). Table 15.3 illustrates a number of the morphological features that can be used to differentiate red blood cells from true yeast. Foamy alveolar

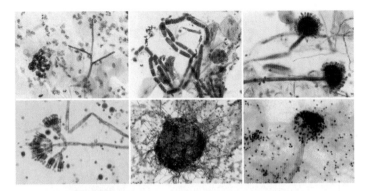

FIG. 15.6. Fungal contaminants. (*Upper left*) *Cladosporium* spp. found on a cervicovaginal smear. At the *left* of the image, we can observe the typical spores (ovoid in shape and forming short chains), and at the *right*, septate and branched hyphae (Pap stain, high magnification). (*Bottom left*) *Penicillium* spp. present within a sputum smear. These species, the most abundant genus of fungi in soils and food, are recognized by their brush-like spore-bearing structures. Branching is an important feature for identifying *Penicillium* spp. (Pap stain, high magnification). (*Upper middle*) *Geotrichum* present within a sputum smear. This fungus appears as long segmented hyphae and rectangular arthroconidia with squared ends. *Geotrichum* is a ubiquitous saprophyte found in soil, decomposing organic matter, and contaminated food. It is also a transient commensal of the oropharynx, being frequently isolated from sputum and stool samples of normal persons (Pap stain, high magnification). (*Bottom middle*) Cervicovaginal smear with the presence of a dense *Chaetomium* spp. fungal mass-like ball surrounded by numerous filaments corresponding to long hyphae (Pap stain, intermediate magnification). (*Upper right*) Fruiting bodies of *Aspergillus* spp. These structures have swollen vesicles at the end of a conidiophore. Hyphal segments are also observed (Pap stain, high magnification). (*Bottom right*) Aspergillus-like artifact. This is really a cotton fiber with a cannonball of leukocytes that resembles a fruiting body in a Pap smear (Pap stain, high magnification).

casts seen with Pneumocystis infection in the lung are better circumscribed than lysed red blood cells. True Pneumocystis casts may also be mimicked by debris, lubricant, amyloid, and alveolar proteinosis.

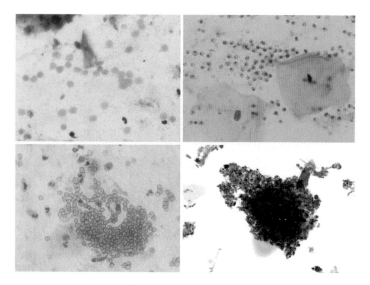

FIG. 15.7.   Red blood cell fungal mimics. (*Upper left*) Acetic acid effect is shown on erythrocytes in a Pap smear. Due to their decoloration, these red blood cells may be misinterpreted as fungal yeast. Their size, relatively uniform morphology, and absence of both budding and clear halos are important keys to the differential diagnosis (Pap stain, high magnification). (*Bottom left*) Erythrocytes contained within a bronchoalveolar lavage (BAL) smear mimic *Pneumocystis* microorganisms. Red blood cells have irregularities and thickenings in their outlines and condensation of content in the center (Pap stain, high magnification). (*Upper right*) Degenerated erythrocytes on a cervicovaginal smear, likely due to ethanol. Because of their appearance, they could be confused with fungal yeasts (Pap stain, high magnification). (*Bottom right*) Granular bloody cast seen in a BAL specimen resembling an alveolar cast of *Pneumocystis* infection. Unlike a true cast, this blood aggregate has irregular edges (Pap stain, intermediate magnification).

- Spermatozoa may mimic yeast, particularly when only their head is visible in stained material.
- Many vegetable or synthetic fibers as well as contaminating threads on cytology slides can resemble portions of fungal hyphae, especially when these are highlighted with a GMS stain (Fig. 15.8).

TABLE 15.3. Cytomorphological features comparing common yeast to erythrocytes.

Structure	Yeast	Erythrocyte
Size (μm)	3–6	5–7
Shape	Round-ovoid	Round
Color	Variable	Red-orange
Budding	Yes	No
Clear halos	Yes	No
Appendages	No	No

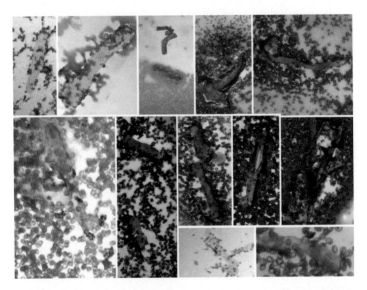

FIG. 15.8. Fungal mimics. Multiple structures are shown that resemble fungal hyphae, as seen within several direct smear preparations (Pap and Diff-Quik stains, high magnification).

- Macrophages containing phagocytosed material within intra-cytoplasmic vacuoles may be mistaken for organisms such as *Histoplasma capsulatum*.
- Talc granules from talcum powder can mimic fungal yeast (Fig. 15.9). Talc is a mineral composed of hydrated magnesium silicate. The granules form crystalloid, transparent, and polygonal

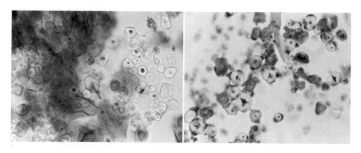

FIG. 15.9. Talc. (*Left*) Talc crystals on a cervicovaginal smear appear as crystalloid, transparent, and polygonal structures with a dark striation in the middle (Pap stain, high magnification). (*Right*) Talc crystals within a sputum smear (Pap stain, high magnification).

structures with a dark striation in the middle. Using polarized light, the typical "Maltese cross" image will appear.

- Pollen grains may mimic parasite ova (Fig. 15.10). They can be differentiated by their larger size, thick cell wall, and refractile appearance. Sporangia are plant, fungal, or structures from algae containing spores that may be encountered in respiratory cytopathology. Some sporangium-like spherules may mimic *Coccidiodes immitis* sporangia containing endospores.
- Calcification may resemble fungal yeast when it is fragmented or hyphae when it is linear and branching (Fig. 15.11).
- Myospherulosis is the alteration of red blood cells, following exposure to fats or fat products (e.g., petrolatum, lanolin, human fat), into many 4–7 μm smooth, refractile or oily, spherules that are typically enclosed in a sac-like structure (parent body). The spherules can also be dispersed singly. This can occur after hemostatic packing (e.g., of the nasal cavity or paranasal sinuses with petrolatum-based ointment and gauze), via intramuscular injection with ointments, or from endogenous lipid breakdown (postsurgical or blunt trauma). Myospherulosis is not an uncommon finding in FNA of fat-containing sites like the breast and subcutaneous tissue, and may be seen accompanying fat necrosis. Altered red blood cells do not appear to be lysed following exposure to hemolytic solutions. These structures are readily

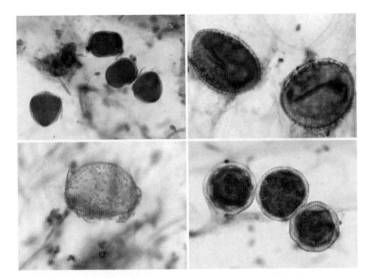

FIG. 15.10. Pollen grains (high magnification images). (*Upper left*) Pollen grains belonging to the *Betulaceae* family seen within a sputum smear. In these structures, a refractile capsule and three surface apertures (pores) are observed (Pap stain). (*Bottom left*) Pollen grain belonging to the *Pinaceae* family present within a sputum smear. Because their airborne sacs are broken, the undulations on the wrinkled surface may mimic an *Ascaris lumbricoides* egg (Pap stain). (*Upper right*) Pollen grains belonging to the *Liliaceae* family detected on a sputum smear. The grains are large (about 300×150 µm), ovoid in shape, with refractile capsules and notable folds on the surface (Pap stain). (*Bottom right*) Pollen grains belonging to the *Caryophyllaceae* family present within a sputum smear. Due to their round shape (approximately 70 µm in diameter) and evident capsule, these structures may be mistaken for *Toxocara* eggs (Pap stain).

seen with a Pap stain, but fail to stain with GMS and PAS stains. They may resemble endosporulating fungi like coccidiomycosis and rhinosporidiosis, as well as other sporangia.

Ancillary Studies

- Special stains (GMS, PAS) for fungi
- Fungal culture

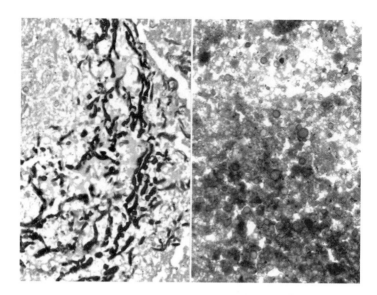

Fig. 15.11. Calcification mimicking fungal (*left*) hyphae and (*right*) yeast (H&E stain, intermediate magnification).

Mimics of Parasitic Infection

- Parasite worms can be mimicked (Fig. 15.12) by human tissue fibers (e.g., skeletal muscle or elastic fibers), suture material, strands of mucus (e.g., Curschmann spirals), vegetable matter (e.g., plant hairs) as well as contaminating exogenous synthetic fibers and plant threads (cotton, cellulose, rayon, etc.) or ferruginous bodies (seen mainly in patients with pneumoconiosis). The presence of unusual shapes (e.g., sharp kinks) and lack of both external (e.g., mouth, hooks, etc.) and internal (e.g., digestive or reproductive tract) recognizable anatomical structures are often essential to differentiate artifacts from real worms. Curschmann spirals are formed from inspissated mucus and can be found in cervical Pap tests, respiratory tract specimens, and even fluids which contain mucus. Skeletal muscle fibers typically have nuclei distributed longitudinally along the periphery and have cross striations. Their presence in respiratory specimens may be derived from food contamination or aspiration.

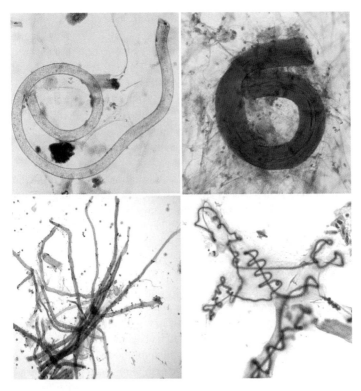

Fig. 15.12. Worm mimics. (*Upper left*) Synthetic fiber observed on a sputum smear. In spite of the characteristic spiral arrangement mimicking a filariform larva of *Strongyloides stercoralis*, the presence of numerous fine dots covering the entire surface and the two ends terminating abruptly are very characteristic. Moreover, note the absence of internal anatomical structures (Pap stain, high magnification). (*Bottom left*) Multiple synthetic fibers present in a CSF liquid based slide (Pap stain, intermediate magnification). (*Upper right*) Striated skeletal muscle fiber in a sputum smear. In spite of its spiral arrangement, the right end is interrupted sharply, there is an absence of internal structure, and the large diameter (about 60–100 μm in width) is an important key to not confuse this with a true parasite (Pap stain, high magnification). (*Bottom right*) Curschmann spiral embedded in mucus in a respiratory sample (Pap stain, high magnification).

Synthetic fibers covered in dots are indicative of rayon, whereas those with a series of lines forming a fringe along the entire length are characteristic of cotton. Because several of these artifacts are refractile and may be birefringent, the utilization of polarized light is a useful ancillary technique to recognize them. Sutures or retained foreign material (e.g., fibers from retained surgical gauze or sponges) are typically accompanied by either acute inflammation (if recently introduced into the patient) or foreign-body type granulomatous inflammation (if the surgical procedure was performed in the patient's remote past).

- Parasite ova can be mimicked by psammoma bodies, crystals in urine sediment, corpora amylacea, bile microspheroliths, pollen, vegetable cells, dust, and even certain powders contaminating slides. In urine, the presence of a lateral spine, miracidium inside eggs, and background eosinophilia can help differentiate urine crystals (especially "lemon-like" uric acid crystals) from true *Schistosoma haematobium* eggs.

- Cellular degeneration may mimic certain parasites (Fig. 15.13). In cervicovaginal Pap tests, the presence of bare nuclei among cellular inflammatory debris in cases with atrophic change and cytolysis could be misinterpreted as trichomoniasis. Degenerative changes in leukocytes may also mimic the presence of trichomonas on a cervicovaginal smear. Compared to bare nuclei of parabasal cells and degenerated cells, trophozoites of *Trichomonas vaginalis* are pyriform in shape, measure 7–30 μm in length × 6–15 μm in width, have four anteriorly directed flagella and one directed posteriorly, a nucleus situated in the anterior portion of the organism, and cytoplasmic granules. Flagella may be hard to visualize.

- Ciliocytophthoria are degenerated anucleate, apical remnants of ciliated epithelial cells (Fig. 15.14) that may be mistaken for the oval ciliated parasite *Balantidium coli* or multi-flagellated protozoa (Hypermastigida). Detached ciliary tufts may be seen in respiratory specimens associated with viral infection (particularly adenovirus), Pap tests, or peritoneal fluid specimens where they are associated with physiologic shedding from the female genital tract, and as contaminants in amniotic fluid during amniocentesis. Motile forms may be observed in fresh (wet) nasopharyngeal and peritoneal specimens. In fresh specimens, cellular tufts may retain cilial motility for several hours.

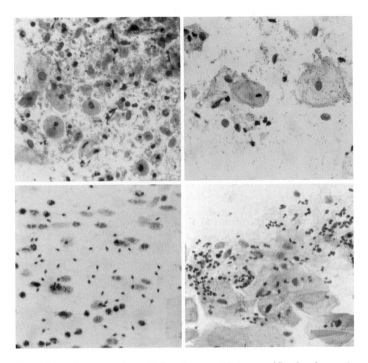

FIG. 15.13. Degenerative cellular changes (high magnification images). (*Upper left*) Atrophic changes in a conventional cervicovaginal smear. Due to the background with abundant cellular debris, bare nuclei, and cellular necrosis, this pattern could be misinterpreted as trichomoniasis (Pap stain). (*Bottom left*) Degenerative changes in leukocytes, mimicking the presence of *Trichomonas* on a conventional cervicovaginal smear. Numerous spermatozoa are also observed (Pap stain). (*Upper right*) Cytolytic changes are shown on a conventional cervicovaginal smear. This pattern, with the presence of bare nuclei and cellular debris, could also be misinterpreted as trichomoniasis. Numerous lactobacilli are also seen (Pap stain). (*Bottom right*) Neutrophils with fragmented nuclei are present within a conventional cervicovaginal smear. These elements may be mistaken for microorganisms, such as fungal yeast (Pap stain).

Infections due to *B. coli* are rare and mainly involve the large intestine. *B. coli* are much larger (40–100 μm) than ciliocytophthoria (10–12 μm). Ciliocytophthoria usually demonstrate cilia resting on a terminal bar predominantly along one edge whereas *B. coli* are uniformly covered with cilia. Also, ciliocytophthoria

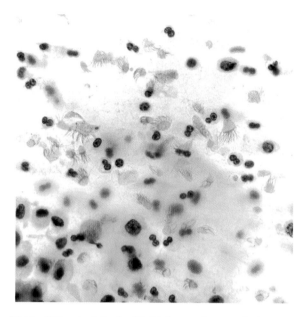

FIG. 15.14. Ciliocytophthoria. Multiple anucleate, apical remnants of ciliated epithelial cells are shown scattered among a few inflammatory cells in this Pap test slide (Pap stain, high magnification).

are anucleate compared to *B. coli* which contain a macronucleus. Multi-flagellated protozoa show irregular insertion of flagella, absence of a terminal bar, and prominent nuclear halos. One may also find detached single cilia in brochoalveolar lavage specimens that mimic bacilliform structures.

- Leisegang rings (or bodies) are nonpolarizable laminated ring-like structures (Fig. 15.15) occasionally found in benign cysts and abscesses. They are of variable size (3–800 μm), usually have a double-layer outer wall, faint radial striations, and an amorphous central core. They may be confused with parasites (especially eggs), but also with algae and psammoma bodies. Unlike ova, they lack flattening on one side or at the poles and show marked variation in size. They are easily observed with Pap (green color), H&E (pink), Diff-Quik (purple) stains, and a few other (Masson's trichrome, acid-fast, Gram) stains which accentuate their concentrically laminated morphology. They do not stain with GMS, PAS, or von Kossa stains.

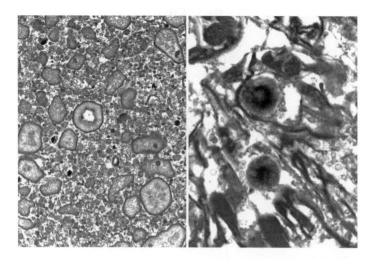

FIG. 15.15. Leisegang rings. These cell block specimens prepared from fine needle aspirates of hemorrhagic cysts show laminated ring-like structures. (*Left*) The bodies present are of variable size and shape. Some rings contain a distinct double-layer outer wall (H&E stain, intermediate magnification). (*Right*) In these two darker colored Leisegang rings, one can see faint radial striations and an amorphous central nidus (H&E stain, high magnification).

Ancillary Studies

- Light polarization or specialized illumination (e.g., Nomarski technique) used to enhance the contrast in unstained, transparent samples.
- Serology for parasite exposure and eosinophilia
- Von Kossa stain for calcification

Plant Contaminants and Mimics

- Slides may contain plant tissue cells (sclerenchyma) including fibers and sclereids (Fig. 15.16). Each has hard cell walls. Fibers are generally long and slender whereas sclereids are shorter and more variable in shape. An asterosclereid is a type of sclereid cell that tends to be radially branched. Plant cells have been

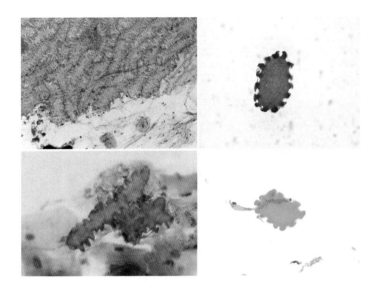

FIG. 15.16. Asterosclereids. (*Upper left*) A fragment of epidermal plant tissue is contained within a sputum smear. Note at the *bottom* of the image the presence of two squamous cells (Pap stain, intermediate magnification). (*Bottom left*) Plant epidermal cells present in a cervicovaginal smear. They have characteristic undulating thick walls (Pap stain, high magnification). (*Right*) Single asterosclereid cells are shown with Diff-Quik (*Upper right*, high magnification) and Pap (*Bottom right*, high magnification) stains.

reported to resemble koilocytes and tumor cells in cytology specimens.

- Trichomes (meaning "growth of hair") are the fine appendages (e.g., hairs) found on some plants (Fig. 15.17). These plant hairs may have blunt or tapering ends and an internal refractile core.
- Pollen grains come in a wide variety of shapes (most often spherical), sizes (6–100 μm), and surface markings characteristic of their plant species (Fig. 15.10). A mature pollen grain has a double wall that includes a thin delicate inner wall (called the intine) and a tough outer cuticle (called the exine). Unlike parasite ova, an internal structure is not visualized. They usually do not show birefringence under polarized light compared to crystals. Pollen can mimic yeast, parasitic ova, and psammomatous calcification.

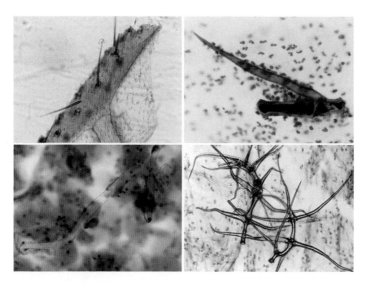

Fig. 15.17. Trichomes. (*Upper left*) Epidermal plant tissue observed on a sputum smear showing numerous hairs (trichomes) and pores (stomata) (Pap stain, intermediate magnification). (*Bottom left*) Single trichome is shown in a Pap test specimen mimicking an *Enterobius vermicularis* worm (Pap stain, high magnification). (*Upper right*) Trichome seen on a cervicovaginal smear. Note the thorny appearance and thick walls (Pap stain, high magnification). (*Bottom right*) Trichomes shown on a sputum smear. In spite of its branching appearance, the presence of thick walls, no budding, and lack of septae are important features that help to differentiate these structures from true fungal hyphae (Pap stain, high magnification).

- Sporangia are plant, fungal, or algal structures containing spores. Sporangium-like structures may be encountered that mimic true sporangia. The absence of free endospores around these structures and absence of a well-defined cell wall favor an artifact mimicking sporangia.
- Algae are plant-like organisms (autotrophic protists) that grow in water. Their presence on cytology slides as single structures or as colonies (Fig. 15.18) is mainly due to tap water contamination from using aqueous solutions or washing slides in water. They can be unicellular or multicellular and may assume different and peculiar morphologies (e.g., filamentous, spheroid, crystalloid, etc.). They include diatoms (phytoplankton) and

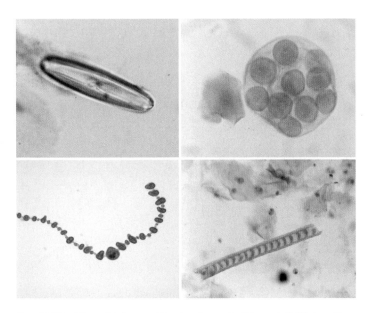

Fᴵɢ. 15.18.   Algae (high magnification images). (*Upper left*) Diatom frus-
tule (*Navicula* spp.) present within a sputum smear. Note the characteristic thick silicified cell wall, elongate shape, and presence of transversal
striations in this diatom (Pap stain). (*Bottom left*) The freshwater red algae
belonging to Rhodophyta was identified in this Pap smear. The round
forms are arranged as beads on a necklace (Pap stain). (*Upper right*) Sputum smear in which a sphere-like structure containing numerous round
cells was identified, compatible with *Eudorina* spp. (Pap stain). This
could be mistaken for adenocarcinoma. (*Bottom right*) In this cervicovaginal smear, there is an unbranched filament (*Ulothrix* spp.) with identical
C-shaped chloroplasts and thick cellular walls (Pap stain).

dinoflagellates (flagellated plankton). Diatoms range in size
from 2 to 200 μm and are contained within a unique hard
silicate crystalloid cell wall (shell). Their morphology varies.
While most diatoms are circular in shape, some may be elliptical, triangular, or even square. Some of these plant cells consist of filaments (e.g., *Ulothrix*). Certain filamentous organisms
enclosed in a gelatinous sheath (e.g., *Oscillatoria* spp.) may
mimic parasite worms. Most dinoflagellates are unicellular forms
with two flagella. These flagellated structures may be confused

with pathogens (e.g., fungi, parasites) or other elements such as fibers, pollen grains, crystals, fecal contamination, and even malignant cells. *Volvocales* algae (also called Chlamydomonadales) can form spherical (moruliform) colonies embedded in a clear matrix that may resemble adenocarcinoma. Freshwater red algae (Rhodophyta) characteristically form round elements arranged as beads on a necklace (Fig. 15.18). These "strings of pearls" have been interpreted by some authors to represent blue bobs in postmenopausal atrophy on Pap tests. In forensic pathology, the presence of diatoms in certain organs (e.g., lung, bone marrow, etc.) provides complementary evidence in the diagnosis of death by drowning.

Ancillary Studies

- Expert consultation (e.g., microbiologist, botanist)

Animal Contaminants and Mimics

- Entire insects or parts (head, thorax, wing, jointed leg, antennae) of an insect may sometimes be trapped under a coverslip of a glass slide (Fig. 15.19).
- Carpet beetle hairs are infrequent contaminants (Fig. 15.20). Carpet beetles are one of the most common insects found in homes. Adult carpet beetles are oval and approximately 1/8 in. long. Their larvae are covered with short hairs or bristles.
- Dust mites occasionally can be found in cytology specimens (Fig. 15.21). The average dust mite measures 0.4 mm in length by 0.25 mm in width. Their body is somewhat rectangular shape and like all acari they have eight legs.
- Several small invertebrates (zooplankton) including aquatic crustaceans (water fleas), rotifers (commonly called wheel animals), and ciliates (e.g., *Vorticella*) may be identified as contaminants. Daphnia (freshwater water fleas) is the most commonly known genus. Their body is covered by a carapace and they have 5 or 6 pairs of legs and prominent antennae. They may have elaborate appendages and filaments (Fig. 15.22) that facilitate their flotation and food capture. Rotifers are approximately 0.1–0.5 mm

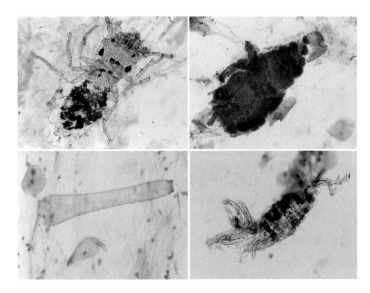

Fig. 15.19. Insects (intermediate magnification images). (*Upper left*) In this image from a voided urine specimen, we can observe the ventral aspect of an entire arthropod. It is possible to identify two antennae and three pairs of segmented legs. The insect is partially covered by a coat of bacteria (Pap stain). (*Bottom left*) In this sputum smear, there is a fragment of an arthropod leg mimicking a Taenia-like organism (Pap stain). (*Upper right*) Sputum smear showing a structure formed by a mixture of mucus and bacteria that may be misinterpreted as a mite (Pap stain). (*Bottom right*) Wood fragment (cellulose fibers) contained within a cervicovaginal smear with an arthropod-like appearance (Pap stain).

long, contain three body sections (head, thorax, foot), have a well-developed cuticle that may bear spines or ridges, exhibit a variety of different shapes (typically somewhat cylindrical), and bear a characteristic ciliated structure (called the corona) on their head. *Vorticella* are ciliated protozoa that mainly live in fresh-water ponds and streams. Each of these cells contains a nucleus (with or without vacuoles) and a characteristic long stalk.

Ancillary Studies

• Expert consultation (e.g., microbiologist, zoologist)

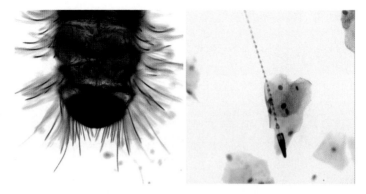

FIG. 15.20. Carpet beetle. (*Left*) Bottom portion of a carpet beetle larva covered with many hairy bristles (low magnification). (*Right*) A carpet beetle hair contaminant present on a cervicovaginal Pap test (Pap stain, high magnification).

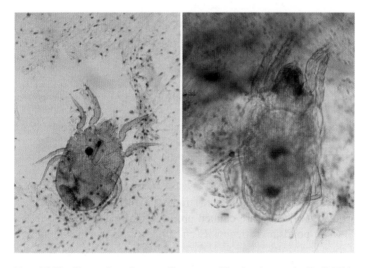

FIG. 15.21. Dust mites (intermediate magnification images). (*Left*) This dust mite specimen was observed as a contaminant within a breast FNA cell block specimen. Note the four pairs of legs (H&E stain). (*Right*) Dust mite found on a sputum smear (Pap stain).

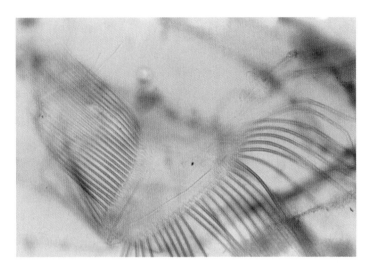

FIG. 15.22.   Water contaminant on a sputum smear. This image shows part of an aquatic insect (*Daphnia* spp.) with numerous filtering filaments (Pap stain, high magnification).

Suggested Reading

Avrin E, Marquet E, Schwarz R, Sobel H. Plant cells resembling tumor cells in routine cytology. Am J Clin Pathol. 1972;57:303–5.

Hadziyannis E, Yen-Lieberman B, Hall G, Procop GW. Ciliocytophthoria in clinical virology. Arch Pathol Lab Med. 2000;124:1220–3.

Martínez-Girón R. Sporangia, sporangium-like spherules and mimicking structures in respiratory cytology. Diagn Cytopathol. 2010;38:897–9.

Martínez-Girón R, González-López JR, Escobar-Stein J, Jou-Muñoz C, García-Miralles M, Ribas-Barceló A. Freshwater microorganisms and other arthropods in Papanicolaou smears. Diagn Cytopathol. 2005;32:222–5.

Martínez-Girón R, González-López JR, Esteban JG, García-Miralles MT, Alvarez-de-los-Heros C, Ribas-Barceló A. Worm-like artifacts in exfoliative cytology. Diagn Cytopathol. 2006;34:636–9.

Martínez-Girón R, Jodra-Fernández O, Tormo-Molina R, Esteban JG, Ribas-Barceló A. Uncommon structures simulating helminth eggs in sputum. Acta Cytol. 2005;49:578–80.

Martínez-Girón R, Ribas-Barceló A. Algae in cytologic smears. Acta Cytol. 2001;45:936–40.

Martínez-Girón R, Ribas-Barceló A, García-Miralles MT, López-Cabanilles D, Tamargo-Peláez ML, Torre-Bayón C, et al. Airborne fungal spores, pollen grains, and vegetable cells in routine Papanicolaou smears. Diagn Cytopathol. 2004;30:381–5.

Martínez-Girón R, Ribas-Barceló A, García-Miralles MT, López-Cabanilles D, Tamargo-Peláez L, Torre-Bayón C, et al. Diatoms and rotifers in cytological smears. Cytopathology. 2003;14:70–2.

Rivasi F, Tosi G, Ruozi B, Curatola C. Vegetable cells in Papanicolaou-stained cervical smears. Diagn Cytopathol. 2006;34:45–9.

Index

L. Pantanowitz et al., *Cytopathology of Infectious Diseases*,
Essentials in Cytopathology 17, DOI 10.1007/978-1-4614-0242-8,
© Springer Science+Business Media, LLC 2011